PAIN MANAGEMENT HANDBOOK

An Interdisciplinary Approach

PAIN MANAGEMENT HANDBOOK

An Interdisciplinary Approach

Evelyn Salerno, BS, PharmD, FASCP
Courtesy Professor,
School of Nursing, Florida International University;
Clinical Assistant Professor,
Nova-Southeastern College of Pharmacy,
Hialeah, Florida

Joyce S. Willens, PhD, RN
Assistant Professor,
College of Nursing, Villanova University,
Villanova, Pennsylvania

with a Foreword by

Ada K. Jacox, RN, PhD, FAAN
Associate Dean for Research,
College of Nursing, Wayne State University,
Detroit, Michigan
and
Panel Co-Chair,
Clinical Practice Guidelines for Acute Pain Management
and Management of Cancer Pain,
Agency for Health Care Policy and Research (AHCPR)

with 40 *illustrations*

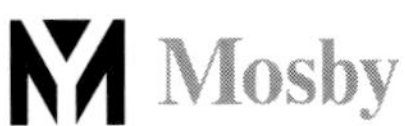

Mosby

St. Louis Baltimore Boston
Carlsbad Chicago Naples New York Philadelphia Portland
London Madrid Mexico City Singapore Sydney Tokyo Toronto Wiesbaden

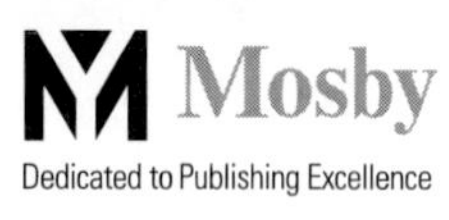

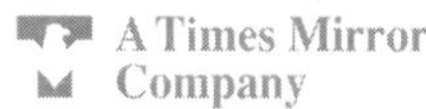

Vice President and Publisher: **Nancy Coon**
Editor: **Robin Carter**
Developmental Editor: **Gina Gay Wright**
Project Manager: **Dana Peick**
Production Editor: **Dottie Martin**
Manuscript Editor: **Dave Mason**
Designer: **Publication Services, Inc.**
Manufacturing Manager: **J. A. McAllister**
Cover designer: **Amy Buxton**
Cover art: **Michael Davidson, Research Scientist, Institute of Molecular Biophysics, The Florida State University, Tallahassee, FL**

Cover depicts micrograph of ibuprofen.

Printed in the United States of America
Editing, production, and composition by Publication Services, Inc.
Printing/binding by R. R. Donnelley and Sons Company

Mosby–Year Book, Inc.
11830 Westline Industrial Drive
St. Louis, Missouri 63146

Library of Congress Cataloging-in-Publication Data

Salerno, Evelyn.
Pain management handbook / Evelyn Salerno, Joyce S. Willens.
p. cm.
ISBN 0-8151-7924-3
1. Pain. 2. Pain—Treatment. 3. Analgesia. I. Willens, Joyce S. II. Title.
[DNLM: WL 39 S163p 1996]
RB127.S25 1996
616′.0472—dc20
DNLM/DLC
for Library of Congress 95-43752
CIP

96 97 98 99 00 / 9 8 7 6 5 4 3 2 1

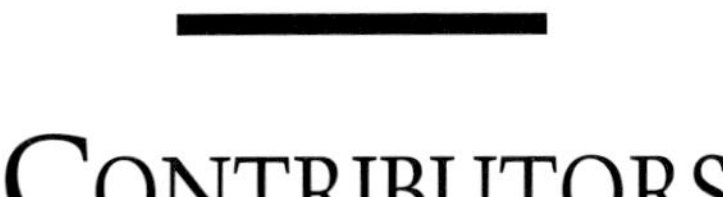

CONTRIBUTORS

Sharon E. Anderson, MS, MA, PhD, RN, ANP
Associate Professor, Graduate Program,
School of Nursing,
Florida International University,
North Miami, Florida
Chapter 12: Geriatric Pain Management

Michael Bozeman, BS, MDiv
Bereavement and Pastoral Care Services Specialist,
Vitas Healthcare Corporation,
Miami, Florida
Chapter 3: Cultural Aspects of Pain Management

Susan M. Bruno, MSW, ACSW, LCSW
Director of Psychosocial Services,
Vitas Healthcare Corporation,
Miami, Florida
Chapter 6: Team Approach to Pain Management

Patricia M. Collins, RN, MSN, OCN
Oncology Nurse Specialist,
South Miami Hospital,
Miami, Florida
Chapter 16: Symptom Management

Nancy Fleming Courts, PhD, RN, NCC
Assistant Professor,
School of Nursing,
University of North Carolina at Greensboro,
Greensboro, North Carolina
Chapter 5: Nonpharmacologic Approaches

Maria L. Cubina, DO
Assistant Professor,
Department of Anesthesia and Critical Care Medicine,
The Children's Hospital of Philadelphia,
Philadelphia, Pennsylvania
Chapter 11: Pediatric Pain Management

Hector Davila, MD
Associate Attending in Anesthesiology and Pain Center,
Mount Sinai Hospital,
Miami Beach, Florida;
Clinical Instructor in Anesthesiology,
University of Miami,
School of Medicine;
Associate Professor of Clinical Anesthesiology,
Barry University,
Miami, Florida
Chapter 12: Geriatric Pain Management

Mary L. Eiman, MSN
Family Nurse Practitioner,
Miami Jewish Home and Hospital for the Aged;
Adjunct Professor,
Barry University,
Miami, Florida
Chapter 12: Geriatric Pain Management

Marianne B. Huml, RN, MS
Head Nurse,
University of Illinois Medical Center;
Adjunct Clinical Faculty,
University of Illinois College of Nursing;
Chicago, Illinois
Chapter 16: Symptom Management

Donna M. Jasinski, CRNA, MS
Nurse Anesthesia Program Director,
School of Nursing,
Georgetown University,
Washington, D.C.
Chapter 14: Invasive Interventions

Barry Kinzbrunner, MD, FACP
Vice President/National Medical Director,
Vitas Healthcare Corporation,
Miami, Florida
Chapter 6: Team Approach to Pain Management
Chapter 10: Cancer Pain Management

Janet Pate McGough, RN, BA, OCN
Clinical Research Nursing Coordinator,
Texas Oncology PA,
Dallas, Texas
Chapter 10: Cancer Pain Management

Barbara Miller, RN, BS, MHA
Nursing Healthcare Consultant,
Pembroke Pines, Florida
Chapter 6: Team Approach to Pain Management

Gayle Newshan, PhD, RN, CS
Adult Nurse Practitioner,
Clinical Nurse Specialist, Pain Management,
AIDS Center Program,
St. Vincent's Hospital,
New York, New York
Chapter 13: Pain in Patients with HIV/AIDS

Mary E. Nossel, MS, CRNP
Nurse Practitioner,
Johns Hopkins Hospital,
Department of Psychiatry,
Chronic Pain Treatment Center;
Instructor,
School of Nursing,
Johns Hopkins University,
Baltimore, Maryland
Chapter 9: Chronic Nonmalignant Pain Management

Jackie Ochsenreither, MSN, CRNP, CCRN
Clinical Nurse Specialist, Pain Management,
Department of Anesthesia and Critical Care Medicine,
The Children's Hospital of Philadephia,
Philadelphia, Pennsylvania
Chapter 11: Pediatric Pain Management

Lynda Peeler, RN, BS Ed, MS in Counseling
Medical Marketing Director/Columnist,
Healthcare People Magazine,
North Bay Village, Florida
Chapter 7: Alternative Approaches to Pain Management

Evelyn Salerno, BS, PharmD, FASCP
Courtesy Professor,
School of Nursing,
Florida International University;
Clinical Assistant Professor,
Nova-Southeastern College of Pharmacy,
Hialeah, Florida
Chapter 4: Pharmacologic Approaches

Michael A. Silverman, MD
Associate Medical Director,
Miami Jewish Home and Hospital for the Aged;
Associate Professor of Clinical Medicine,
School of Medicine,
University of Miami;
Investigator,
Miami VA Hospital,
Geriatric Research, Education, and Clinical Center,
Miami, Florida
Chapter 12: Geriatric Pain Management

Cassandra J. Snyder, RN, MS
Coordinator, Pain Management,
Lehigh Valley Hospital,
Allentown, Pennsylvania
Chapter 14: Invasive Interventions

Avery Spunt, RPh, MEd
Clinical Associate Professor,
Department of Pharmacy Practice,
Assistant Head of Academic Programs,
University of Illinois College of Pharmacy,
Chicago, Illinois
Chapter 16: Symptom Management

Julie A. Stanik-Hutt, PhD, RN, CCRN
Assistant Professor,
School of Nursing,
University of Maryland,
Baltimore, Maryland
Chapter 8: Acute Pain

Janice Fitzgerald Ulmer, RN, PhD
Assistant Professor,
Advanced Practice Nursing Program,
School of Nursing,
Johns Hopkins University,
Baltimore, Maryland
Chapter 2: Identifying and Preventing Pain Mismanagement

Neal Weinreb, MD, FACP
Regional Medical Director for South Florida,
Vitas Healthcare Corporation;
Clinical Assistant Professor of Medicine,
School of Medicine,
University of Miami,
Miami, Florida
Chapter 15: Pain Management in Special Situations

Joyce S. Willens, PhD, RN
Assistant Professor,
College of Nursing,
Villanova University,
Villanova, Pennsylvania
Chapter 1: Introduction to Pain Management

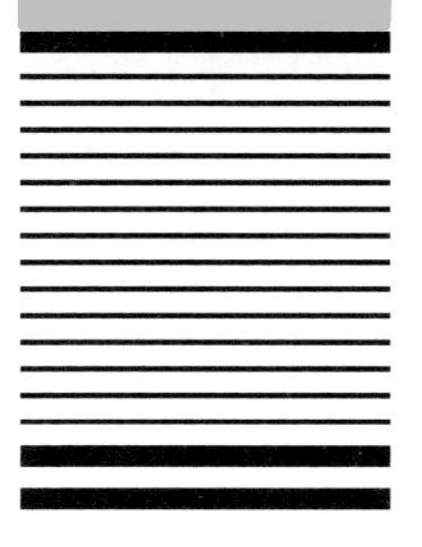

Reviewers

We would like to thank the following reviewers, who provided us with suggestions and constructive comments that were most helpful in guiding us.

Sharon E. Anderson, MS, MA, PhD, RN, ANP
Associate Professor, Graduate Program,
School of Nursing,
Florida International University,
North Miami, Florida

Ellen Barker, RN, MSN, CNRN
President,
Neuroscience Nursing Consultants,
Newark, Delaware

Claudia Borden, RN (AA)
Vitas Regional Education Coordinator,
Miami, Florida

Patricia M. Collins, RN, MSN, OCN
Oncology Nurse Specialist,
South Miami Hospital,
Miami, Florida

Betty Ferrell, RN, PhD, FAAN
Associate Research Scientist,
City of Hope National Medical Center,
Duarte, California

Arthur G. Lipman, PharmD
Professor of Clinical Pharmacy,
College of Pharmacy,
University of Utah,
Salt Lake City, Utah

Irma Rey, MD
Team Physician,
Outreach Inc.,
Vitas Healthcare Corporation,
Miami, Florida

Barbara S. Shapiro, MD
Associate Professor,
Pain Management Service,
Division of General Pediatrics,
Assistant Professor of Pediatrics,
School of Medicine,
University of Pennsylvania,
The Children's Hospital of Philadelphia,
Philadelphia, Pennsylvania

Denice Sheehan, RN, MSN, OCN
Nursing Supervisor,
Hospice of the Western Reserve,
Mentor, Ohio

Yvonne N. Stock, RN, BSN, MS
School of Nursing,
Iowa Western Community College,
Council Bluffs, Iowa

Myron Yaster, MD
Associate Professor,
Anesthesiology and Critical Care Medicine,
Johns Hopkins Medical Institution,
Baltimore, Maryland

E. Ruth Yurchuck, EdD, RN
Senior Test Consultant,
Division of Assessment and Evaluation,
National League for Nursing,
New York, New York

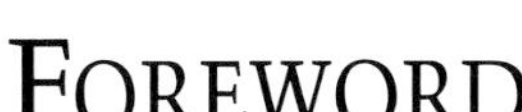

FOREWORD

The field of pain management presently is characterized by the following:

- Increased interest in pain management, with acknowledgment that pain from multiple sources can be prevented or reduced to levels acceptable to patients
- A focus on careful assessment, with an emphasis on believing the patient's report of pain
- Increased awareness of the need to involve the patient and family as part of the pain management team
- Availability of a multitude of interventions for managing pain
- Increased acknowledgment of the value of an interdisciplinary approach to pain management

For far too long, the problem of pain was not addressed seriously by most health professionals. Patients were expected to tolerate pain as well as they could and not to complain too much. A common practice for dealing with postoperative pain was to give intramuscular injections of opioids every 3 to 4 hours prn, a practice that is now recognized as both ineffective and at times harmful. Indeed, basic and clinical research documents the deleterious physiologic and psychologic effects of unrelieved pain.

Fortunately, in the past decade or so, clinicians and researchers alike have placed increasing importance on understanding pain and its management. Professional associations such as the American Pain Society, the American Academy of Pain Medicine, the Oncology Nursing Society, and the American Society of Clinical Oncologists have emphasized the need for patients to receive better pain management. During the past few years, the U.S. Agency for Health Care Policy and Research (AHCPR) has supported the development and dissemination of guidelines for the management of acute pain (1992), cancer pain (1994), and acute low back problems (1994) to enable both clinicians and patients to make better decisions about pain management.

This increased attention is producing better awareness by patients and clinicians that pain is a pervasive problem that can and should be prevented and controlled. Professional, institutional, and societal barriers to effective pain management are being identified and addressed by professional groups, who recognize that improvement of patient care in this area extends beyond learning and using pain management techniques. While effective pain management for individual patients is, without question, important, improving pain management generally will require the implementation of institutionwide quality management programs, changing laws and regulatory practices that unnecessarily restrict the use of drugs for legitimate purposes, and convincing payors and administrators that pain management is important and merits support.

The increased focus on pain management includes the full spectrum of age from neonates to the elderly; recognizes the importance of a multimodal approach; and addresses pain in patients with special problems, such as substance abuse or concurrent health problems. Clinicians in all settings and dealing with all kinds of patients must have access to the most current information on how to manage pain effectively.

This handbook will contribute substantially to helping clinicians become knowledgeable regarding the many recent advances in pain management. The authors make excellent use of the AHCPR guidelines, research, and their own clinical experience to produce a book that should be useful to clinicians as they deal with pain from various causes. They also identify barriers to effective pain management generally and in relation to specific clinical groups.

A second feature characterizing the current focus on pain and its management is the increased awareness of the importance of assessing pain, taking action, and then reassessing the pain. Although there are still gaps in our knowledge of how to assess pain in some patients, such as neonates and cognitively impaired persons, there is a multiplicity of well-developed instruments for measuring the intensity and other characteristics of pain. These are being used in many settings as part of the regular, ongoing clinical data collection and documentation process. Whereas at an earlier time there was a search for "objective" indicators of pain, it is increasingly accepted that the patient is the single most reliable source of information about the pain. Most guidelines today emphasize the need to ask the patient about the pain and to believe what the patient reports. This is a welcome change from the earlier practice in which the subjective expression of pain was seen as less valuable than the objective indicators, which can reflect anxiety, fever, and other symptoms as well as pain.

A related characteristic of current pain management is recognition of the need to include the patient and family in planning and implementing effective pain management strategies. Clinicians are increasingly attuned to the need for patients to have information about their pain and how to alleviate it. The guidelines produced by the AHCPR are mandated by Congress to address patient as well as clinician needs for guidance in managing various clinical conditions. Each guideline produced by the AHCPR has a consumer version, published in both English and Spanish. With so much care being given in clinics, clinicians' offices, and patients' homes, rather than in hospitals, the need for well-informed patients and families will become even more important.

A fourth characteristic of the current pain field is the multiplicity of modalities available. With regard to drugs, researchers and clinicians have given much attention to the development of new drugs, new routes of administration, new delivery technologies that allow patients to control their own drug administration, increased use of various combinations of drugs, and increased awareness of the need to actively prevent and manage undesirable side effects of drugs. Unfortunately, there is still little research that systematically tests the effects of drugs and nondrug interventions used concurrently. In spite of this, clinicians are trying combinations of drug therapies with cognitively based interventions such as patient teaching and relaxation. Many of these interventions, which can be easily learned and used by clinicians in their everyday practice, are described in this handbook.

Finally, pain management currently is characterized by more interdisciplinary research and management. Pain is a complex phenomenon, and a diversity of clinicians are involved in its assessment and management. If pain is to be prevented or managed well, it is imperative that physicians, nurses, and others caring for the patient understand the pain management plan. Many of the chapters in this handbook have been coauthored by nurses, physicians, and others. The result of this collaborative authorship is chapters that include more comprehensive discussions of pain management in particular populations than are usually seen. Descriptions of the mechanisms of pain are accompanied by clinically informed suggestions for managing it, and most chapters have some emphasis on combining phychosocial and drug approaches and on teaching patients and their families about pain.

There is still a multitude of problems to solve in pain management. Although much progress has been made in the past few decades in better understanding pain and how to prevent and manage it, for example, there is still a great need for understanding the circumstances under which these various interventions should be used serially and in combination. Another problem is in disseminating the wealth of new knowledge becoming available on pain management. This handbook should make a substantial contribution in bringing much new information to clinicians in a succinct yet comprehensive book on pain.

Ada K. Jacox, RN, PhD, FAAN

PREFACE

The mismanagement of pain for postoperative, cancer, and chronic pain populations has been a known problem for decades. Health care professionals have recently realized that the denial of the existence of pain in neonates and children has caused pediatric pain management methods to lag behind current standards for adults. The recent publication of clinical practice pain guidelines by many professional organizations and the Agency for Health Care Policy and Research has acknowledged the problem and served to promote methods of change.

The intent of this handbook is to facilitate this process by providing a comprehensive and practical guide to pain management using an interdisciplinary approach. Exemplary pain management should be a major concern for all health care professionals; thus a unified approach is necessary to implement the interventions that work best to relieve a particular individual's pain. The recognition and implementation of assessment instruments and of pharmacologic and nonpharmacologic interventions along with cognizance of cultural influences and the problems of specific age groups and disease states are crucial to achieving effective pain control.

Evelyn Salerno

Joyce S. Willens

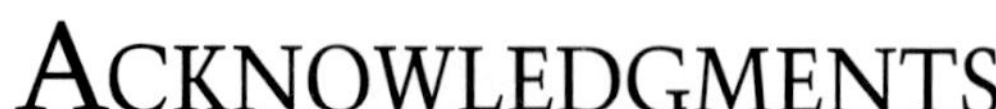

ACKNOWLEDGMENTS

We would like to thank our many contributors to this book. The sharing of their knowledge and expertise is very much appreciated. We also thank our Mosby editors, Robin Carter and Gina Wright, whose help and support was invaluable in seeing the idea through from dream to reality. In addition, we would like to thank Dana Peick, Dottie Martin, Amy Buxton, Connie Salzman, Kris Engberg, Mary Warren, Dave Mason, and Joe Jahde for their hard work and dedication during the production phase of this book. If, as the proverb states, "An hour of pain is as long as a day of pleasure,"* then the anonymous statement applied to pain management is very meaningful: "Don't be afraid to use what talent you possess; the woods indeed would be very silent if no birds sang except those who sang best."

---

*Strauss, M. B. (1968). *Familiar medical quotations.* Boston: Little, Brown, p. 431.

CONTENTS

A NOTE TO THE READER:
The author and publisher have made every attempt to check dosages and nursing content for accuracy. Because the science of pharmacology is continually advancing, our knowledge base continues to expand. Therefore we recommend that the reader always check product information for changes in dosage or administration before administering any medication. This is particularly important with new or rarely used drugs.

SECTION ONE

Pain Management

1

Introduction to Pain Management

Joyce S. Willens

Key Points

- Pain is a subjective experience and must be viewed in those terms to be managed effectively.
- A thorough and comprehensive assessment is key to effective pain management.
- The use of a consistent measurement instrument facilitates communication of pain.
- Behavioral indices are not reliable indicators of pain.
- Published pain guidelines provide a foundation for the development of standard approaches to pain management.

Knowledge of the pain management problem has existed for decades. The publication of the Acute Pain Management Guidelines by the Agency for Health Care Policy and Research (Carr et al., 1992) showed that long-standing awareness of the problem did not readily change clinical practice. Knowledge that postoperative pain is not inevitable and that unrelieved pain, from any type of injury or disease, leads to negative consequences should stimulate the practitioner to make pain relief a priority. This chapter will briefly define and discuss the pathophysiology of pain. Two theories will be reviewed to provide a basis for understanding various pain management methods. Adequate assessment, the cornerstone of effective management, will be stressed. The use of standards, guidelines, and documentation of care will be discussed. Finally, the legal and ethical concerns surrounding adequate pain management will be reviewed.

PAIN DEFINITION

Pain is defined by the International Association for the Study of Pain (IASP) as "an unpleasant sensory and emotional experience associated with actual or potential damage or described in terms of such damage" (IASP, 1979). This well-recognized definition encompasses the multidimensional nature of pain. In addition to having a physiologic dimension, pain is often classified as comprising four components: motivational, cognitive, affective and discriminative (Curro, 1987). The motivational dimension manifests in the form of action or escape, which is often reflexive. The cognitive aspect involves the person's previous experience and memory of the experience. Examples of the affective component are fear, anxiety, and stress. The discriminative component is derived from the peripheral nervous system response to the noxious stimulus. This component includes the onset, duration, intensity, quality, and location of pain.

A broad definition first proposed by McCaffery in 1968 describes the subjective nature of pain. This definition states that "pain is whatever the experiencing person says it is, existing whenever the experiencing person says it does" (McCaffery & Beebe, 1989, p. 7).

These multiple dimensions combined with the highly subjective nature of pain contribute to the problem of adequate assessment and management of pain. Differences in the cognitive and affective dimensions between patients and health care workers contribute to the difficulty in pain management.

TYPES OF PAIN

Pain is categorized according to duration, location, and etiology. *Acute* and *chronic* are commonly used terms to describe pain. Pain has classically been differentiated by time, with acute pain lasting for less than 6 months and chronic pain lasting longer (Fordyce, 1976; Sternbach, 1974). Bonica (1990, p. 19) advocated a different approach, stating that chronic pain is "pain that persists a month beyond the usual course of an acute disease or a reasonable time for an injury to heal or that is associated with a chronic pathologic process that causes continuous pain or the pain recurs at intervals for months or years." Bonica made the point that many acute diseases or injuries heal in 2 or 3 weeks and in some cases up to 6 weeks. Any pain that persists beyond the expected recovery time should, in his opinion, be considered chronic and treated with approaches used for chronic pain. Merskey (1986) defines chronic pain as that which persists "past the time of healing" or more than approximately 3 months.

It would seem prudent to use the patient presentation to classify the pain and plan treatment. Patients suffering from chronic pain present a picture quite different from those in acute pain. Chronic pain eventually depletes the sympathoadrenal responses, and patients begin to experience difficulty with sleep, loss of appetite, irritability, decreased motor function, loss of desire for sex, and become depressed. Their facial expression may be subdued, sad, or perhaps sleepy; all these signs are related to problems with sleep and possibly medications. They may not appear to be suffering from pain but may look exhausted. Most authors in this book use the classic time frame of 6 months to distinguish between acute and chronic pain. In addition to the use of time as a distinguishing feature, chronic pain is further categorized into pain from malignancy (cancer) and nonmalignant chronic pain.

Using location as a classification method assists in the communication of pain and guides treatment. The IASP has named numerous regions, such as head, cervical, thoracic, abdominal, lower limbs, and pelvic.

When pain is classified according to etiology, clinicians can predict the course of pain and plan effective treatment. Examples of pain etiologies are genetic or congenital disorders, trauma, burns, neoplasms, inflammation, and psychologic. The IASP recommends adoption of their classification system in order to facilitate communication, diagnosis, treatment, and reimbursement, but practitioners argue that it is cumbersome. Therefore universal adoption of a classification system has not occurred (Raj, 1994).

INCIDENCE OF INADEQUATE TREATMENT OF PAIN

Research studies and anecdotal experiences of patients and health care providers point to the extent of the pain management problem. Researchers have demonstrated that postoperative analgesia is not sufficient. Inadequate amounts of opioids ordered by physicians, health care professionals' and patients' fear of addiction, waiting too long to request or receive analgesics, and inadequate pain assessment are factors that contribute to the problem. The research studies summarized in Table 1-1 review the extensive nature of the problem. Note that in the span of two decades, the extent of the problem has changed little. Also note that the recommendations are strikingly similar among studies.

The literature about the pathophysiology of pain is extensive. A brief, simplistic review of the pathophysiology of pain and relevant theories of pain provides a basis for adequate pain assessment and management. The cursory review here is intended to provide background information. The reader is referred to pain textbooks for a more in-depth review.

PATHOPHYSIOLOGY OF NOCICEPTION AND PAIN

The perception of pain involves the body's peripheral and central nervous system. There are receptors that detect the noxious (harmful) event and pathways that relay the information to a central processing system to trigger a response.

Peripheral Nervous System

The term *nociception* refers to the body's reaction to a noxious stimulus, and the term *pain* describes the person's perception of the event. Pain receptors are widespread in the skin, periosteum, joint surfaces, arterial walls, subcutaneous tissue, muscle, fascia, and viscera. Most other deep tissues have fewer pain receptors (Bonica, 1990). Located on nerve endings, these receptors, called nociceptors, respond to high-intensity mechanical, thermal, and chemical stimuli. The cutaneous fibers are either myelinated, type Aδ* fibers or unmyelinated, type C fibers. The Aδ fibers conduct acute prickling type pain whereas the C fibers transmit the slower

*δ = Delta.

Table 1-1 Summary of Research Concerning Inadequate Treatment of Pain

Study Authors	Method	Incidence of Pain	Contributing Factors	Recommendations
Marks and Sachar (1973)	Structured interviews (pts and MDs)	32% pts suffered severe and 41% suffered moderate distress Pain interfered with sleep in 78% of pts with marked to moderate pain	MDs had an exaggerated concern about addiction, which contributed to ordering subtherapeutic doses	Need to obtain correct pharmacologic knowledge about adequate dosing and rates of addiction
Kerri-Szanto and Heaman (1972)	Pt interviews ($N = 106$)	40% pts reported some degree of pain 21% reported suffering significant amount of pain despite treatment	By allowing pts to self-administer IV opiates, pain relief was more successful compared with use of doses constrained by prescribed times and amounts	Stressed the need to assess adequacy of analgesic dosing the night of surgery, rather than waiting until morning; need for adequate premedication
Cohen (1980)	Postoperative pts interviewed Nurses given a questionnaire and vignettes	79.8% pts reported adequate pain relief 66.9% stated pain interfered with sleep	Nurses' goals of pain relief differed from pt goals: 25.7% pts felt pain should be relieved completely while 3% of nurses had the same goal Nurses were more likely to give less drug or a placebo to a female pt compared with a similar male pt	Pts should be told preoperatively that they should feel free to request medication when needed Nurses need education about pharmacology of analgesics Need to study process by which nurses choose the amount of opiate to administer

Kuhn, Cooke, Collins, Jones, and Mucklow (1990)	Pt interview (n=133) after IM dose Survey MD and nurses	40% stated postoperative period was painful Pts reported average pain intensity was 60% of maximum	Pt expected less pain than they actually experienced Staff underestimated amount of pain 20% of nurses and 5% of MDs feared addiction	Need to educate pts and nurses to assess pain Use of IV-PCA to manage pain Need to decrease fear of addiction
Owen, McMillan, and Rogowski (1990)	Pt interview	66% said they would wait until they were in severe pain before requesting analgesia 75% expected IM injection immediately after requesting it 50% of pts had pain most or all of the time	Nurses underestimate the lag time between pt request and response Many nurses wait until pt complains of severe pain before giving analgesics Everyone expects some amount of unrelieved pain	Enhanced education on appropriate use of traditional analgesic methods Suggest need for increased attention to pain assessment and management up to 72 hours after surgery Improved pt education about postoperative pain management
Brown (1992)	Experimental—use of pain flow sheet	Pain rating scores and amount of opiates given improved significantly after the introduction of a bedside pain assessment flow sheet	90% of nurses found flow sheet easy to use	Stressed importance of adequate postoperative pain assessment and documentation

Continued.

Table 1-1 Summary of Research Concerning Inadequate Treatment of Pain—cont'd

Study Authors	Method	Incidence of Pain	Contributing Factors	Recommendations
Fife, Irick, and Painter (1993)	Survey—random selection of nurses and MDs in Indiana	84% of nurses and 73% of MDs viewed cancer pain as a major problem 76% of MDs and 67% of nurses believe that cancer pts are undermedicated 25% of respondents in both groups feared addiction $^1/_4$ of MDs and about $^1/_3$ of nurses believe that the need for more analgesics is related to drug tolerance rather than advancing disease	Pts and family members reluctant to discuss problems	Nurses should encourage communication and educate pts and families about pain management Belief that increasing demands for analgesics is probably related to advancing disease should help in prescribing and administering proper doses of analgesics The use of a common, valid, and reliable assessment measure would promote quality of pain relief

Cleeland et al. (1994)	Questionnaire given to outpts diagnosed with recurrent or metastatic cancer Questionnaire given to pts' MDs	42% of pts had inadequate analgesia, with a significantly greater proportion of pts being treated in community clinical oncology programs Those pts whose MDs rated with greater discrepancy the amount of interference with activity related to pain were more likely to report severe pain	The most powerful predictor of successful pain management was the discrepancy between the MD and pt estimates of the severity of pain and its degree of interference with daily activities Older pts (> 70) and minority pts are at greatest risk for poor pain management	Use of standardized assessment forms may eliminate bias

pt, Patient; *MD*, physician; *IV*, intravenous; *IM*, intramuscular; *IV-PCA*, intravenous patient-controlled analgesia.

burning sensations. This explains the double pain sensation felt when a noxious heat stimulus is applied to the skin. The first perception is a stinging sensation, which is followed by a burning pain (Perl, 1976).

Nociception results from tissue damage that stimulates the release of pain-producing substances such as serotonin, H^+, K^+, histamine, bradykinin, and cholecystokinin, which are released from the plasma, and substance P, which is released from nerve terminals. These pain-producing substances are released into the extracellular fluid that surrounds pain fibers. Pain is produced directly by excitation of the pain fiber membranes. Depending on the substance, vasodilation, vasoconstriction, or an increase in capillary permeability results. The increase in capillary permeability disturbs the microenvironment of the pain fibers and contributes to an increase in the excitability, which results in sensitization of the fibers (Bonica, 1990).

Nociceptors rarely adapt to a painful stimulus. However, repeated exposure to noxious stimuli enhances their sensitivity, lowers the threshold to stimulation, and enhances the response to stimulation. Threshold is defined as the intensity and quality of a stimulus that is adequate to produce a response. Thus, when pain receptors are sensitized, smaller-than-usual amounts of a harmful substance may stimulate nociception, which may result in the perception of pain.

Central Nervous System

After tissue injury causes the release of pain-producing substances and the stimulation of nociceptors, nociception is conducted on the Aδ or C fibers to the spinal cord via both the dorsal and ventral roots. The fibers enter the dorsal horn (see Figure 1-1), which is divided into laminae based on cell type. The laminae II cell type is frequently referred to as the substantia gelatinosa (Bonica, 1990). In the substantia gelatinosa are projections that play a role in the transmission of nociception to other parts of the spinal cord. Nociception continues from the periphery through the spinal cord to the reticular formation, the thalamus, the limbic system, and the cortex. The cortex is necessary for a person to determine the location

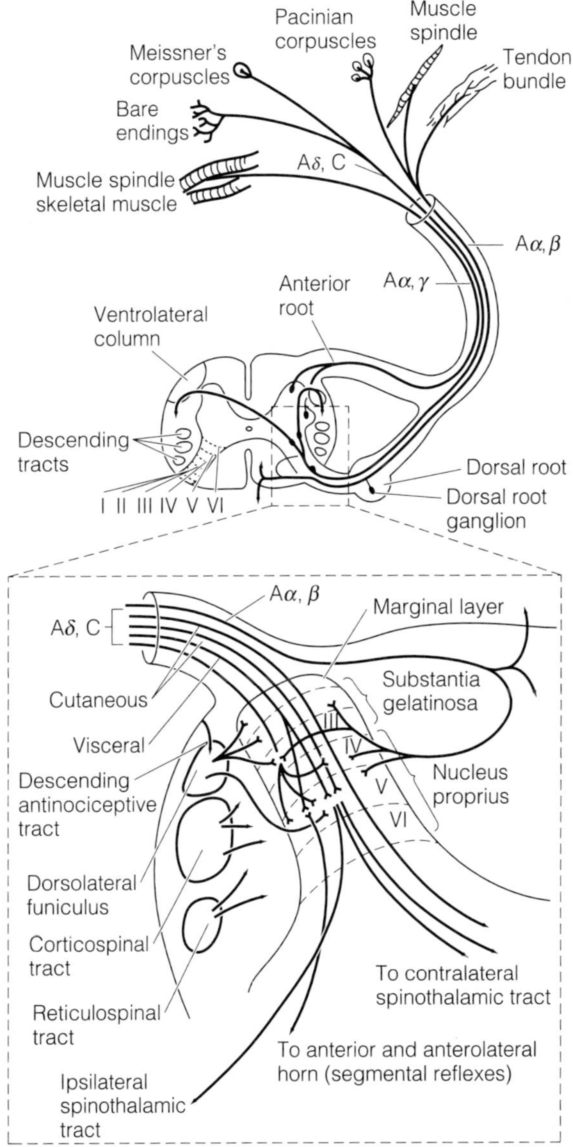

Figure 1-1 Transmission of nociceptive information from the periphery on the Aδ and C fibers with projection into laminae of the spinal cord.

of the pain, its nature, and its intensity. The perception of pain is modulated by a descending mechanism.

Descending Modulation System

Melzack and Wall (1965) first postulated the existence of a descending modulation system. The ability of the brain to control pain sensation, first reported by Reynolds in 1969, is now called stimulation-produced analgesia (SPA). Electrical stimulation of certain areas of the cortex in rats increased the threshold for nociceptive stimuli. Electrical stimulation of the periaqueductal gray areas of the brain also produces analgesia. Impulses are transmitted on descending nerve fibers from the brain to the spinal cord. The impulses are inhibited at the first synapse in the dorsal horn (Raj, 1994).

THEORIES OF PAIN

Theories assist in the description, explanation, and prediction of phenomena for which little is known. The gate control theory stimulated much research into the mechanism of pain (Raj, 1994). The opioid receptor theory serves to emphasize and help explain the role of the descending modulation system. These theories will be reviewed to provide a basis for understanding various pain management methods discussed throughout the book.

Gate Control Theory

The gate control theory (GCT), proposed by Melzack and Wall (1965) and later modified, addresses both the physiologic and psychologic aspects of nociception. The theory proposes that stimulation of the skin evokes nervous impulses that are transmitted by three systems located in the spinal cord. The substantia gelatinosa in the dorsal horn of the spinal cord, the dorsal column fibers, and the central transmission cells act to stimulate or inhibit nociceptive impulses. The transmission of noxious impulses from the afferent fibers to the spinal cord transmission cells is modulated by a spinal gating mechanism in the dorsal horn. This gating mechanism is influenced by the amount of activity in the large-diameter fibers. It is thought that stimulation of the large-diameter fibers inhibits the transmission of pain, thus "closing the gate." The opposite occurs when the smaller fibers are stimulated: pain is transmitted, and "the gate opens." The gating mechanism is influenced by nerve impulses that descend from the brain. The theory proposes a specialized system of large-diameter fibers that activate selective cognitive processes, which then influence, by way of descending fibers, the modulating properties of the spinal gate. Figure 1-2 shows a schematic representation of the GCT.

This theory is useful in explaining how pain interventions such as cutaneous stimulation, heat, massage, and hypnosis work to modulate pain. It is thought that these interventions stimulate the large-diameter fibers and inhibit the transmission of pain by closing the gate. The emotional influences in the perception of pain are depicted by the cognitive control box. This explains how a person's experience and current emotions can influence the gate control system. This theory prophetically hinted at the importance of the spinal cord in the biochemical modulation of pain.

Opioid Receptor Theory

The opioid receptor theory, solely biochemical in focus, emphasizes the role of the descending system that acts to inhibit nociception. The first evidence of an endogenous analgesic system stemmed from reports that electrical stimulation of the periaqueductal gray areas of the brain produced potent analgesia, now called SPA (Mayer, Wolfle, Akil, Carder, & Liebeskind, 1971; Reynolds, 1969). Soon thereafter the discovery of endogenous opiates was reported (Pert & Snyder, 1973), followed by the discovery of endogenous opiate substances in the brains of animals (Hughes, 1975). These substances are now known as enkephalins, meaning "in the head," and endorphins, meaning "endogenous morphine." Much research into the role these substances play in nociception followed.

There are three distinct classes of endogenous opioids: enkephalins, dynorphins, and β-endorphins, which represent three chemically distinct families of opioid peptides and different precursors (Akil et al., 1984; Goldstein, 1976).

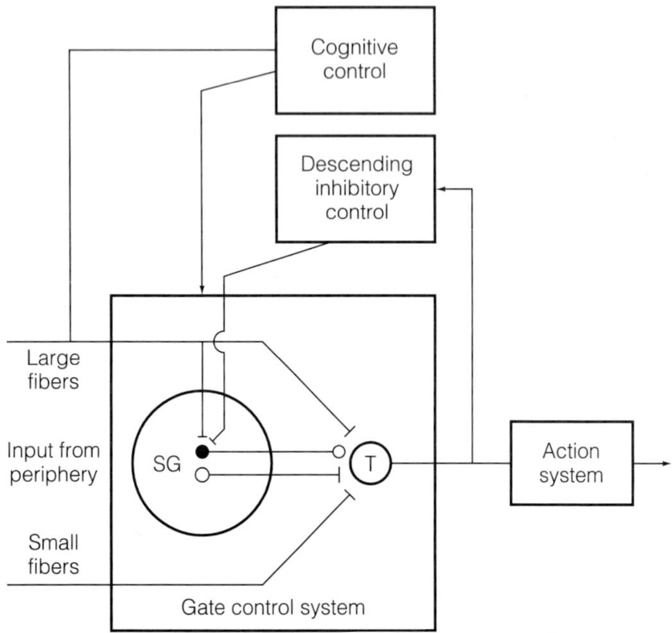

Figure 1-2 The gate control theory (Mark II). The new model includes excitatory (*white circle*) and inhibitory (*black circle*) links from the substantia gelatinosa (*SG*) to the transmission (*T*) cells as well as descending inhibitory control from brainstem systems. The round knob at the end of the inhibitory link implies that its actions may be presynaptic, postsynaptic, or both. All connections are excitatory, except for the inhibitory link from SG to T cell. (Modified from Melzack, R., & Wall, P. D. (1983). *The challenge of pain.* New York: Basic Books; permission granted by Lea & Febiger.)

The opiate binding sites, also referred to as receptors, are classified as mu (μ), kappa (κ), and delta (δ). Each receptor responds in a different manner when activated. Table 1-2 summarizes the effects of each receptor upon stimulation. The function of the δ-receptor in humans is unclear; however, it is thought that this receptor may modulate μ-receptor activity.

Table 1-2 Opiate Receptor Classification and Action

Organ Effect	μ	κ	δ
Pupil	Miosis	Miosis	Mydriasis
Respiratory rate	Stimulation, then depression	No change	Stimulation
Heart rate	Bradycardia	No change	Tachycardia
Body temperature	Hypothermia	No change	Unknown
Affect	Indifference	Sedation	Dysphoria
Gastro-intestine	Constipation	No effects	Nausea

From Willens, J. S. (1994). Pain management in the trauma patient. In V. D. Cardona, P. D. Hurn, P. J. B. Mason, A. M. Scanlon, & S. W. Veise-Berry (Eds.), *Trauma nursing from resuscitation through rehabilitation* (2nd ed., pp. 325-362). Philadelphia: W. B. Saunders. With permission of W. B. Saunders. Copyright 1994 by W. B. Saunders.

The opiate receptors are found in high concentrations in the spinal and medullary dorsal horn, the caudate nucleus, the substantia nigra, periaqueductal gray, hypothalamus, and amygdala as well as other parts of the central nervous system. When these areas are stimulated, the perception of pain is inhibited. The enkephalins, dynorphins, and β-endorphins are concentrated in areas involved in the descending inhibitory system. Figure 1-3 shows the role of enkephalins in pain modulation. It is hypothesized that when enkephalins and β-endorphins are released, they modulate nociception presynaptically and postsynaptically possibly by interfering with calcium or potassium channels (Bonica, 1990, p. 112; Millan, 1986; Yaksh, 1981).

It is believed that exogenous opioids bind with the same opiate receptors to modulate nociception. A given opioid may interact to different degrees with one or more opiate receptors. The opioid may act as an agonist, a partial agonist, or an antagonist. (See Chapter 4 for an in-depth discussion.) Knowledge about the transmission of nociception continues to evolve. It is proposed that a neuron may receive information from many neurotransmitters and that each neurotransmitter may have multiple actions.

In summary, the existence and location of endogenous opiates are well documented. Endorphins and enkephalins bind to opiate receptor sites to modulate pain. What eludes

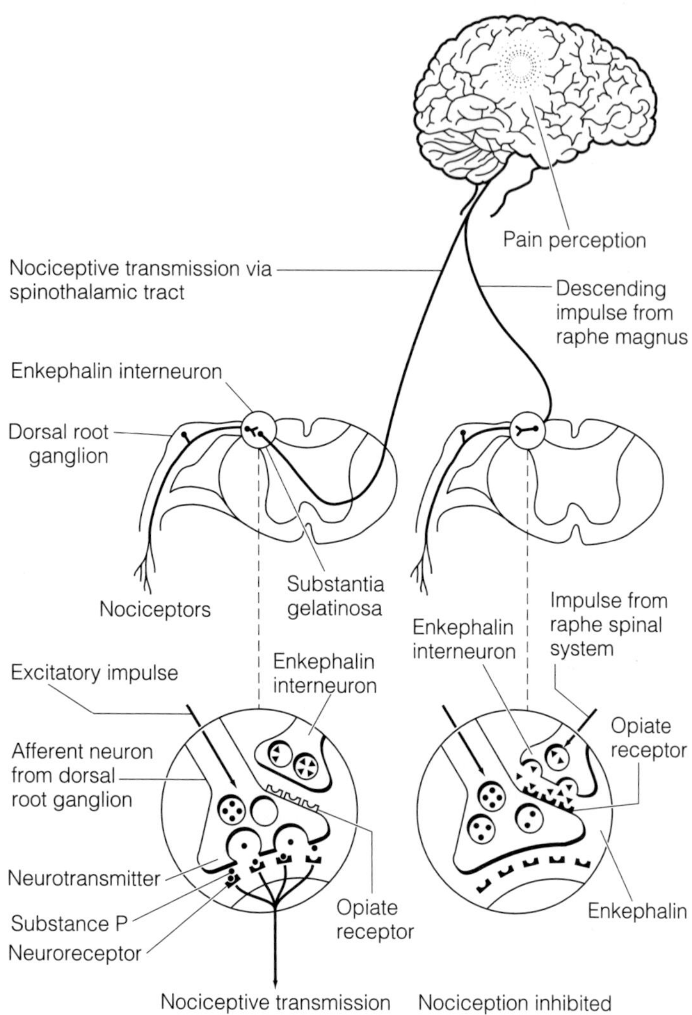

Figure 1-3 The role of enkephalin in pain modulation. (From Chapman, C. R., & Bonica, J. J. (1983). *Acute pain.* Kalamazoo: The Upjohn Company.)

scientists is the exact biochemical mechanism involved in the inhibition of pain when the stimulation of endogenous opioids occurs and when exogenous opioids are administered.

PAIN ASSESSMENT

The following discussion is a general nursing assessment of a patient in pain. The actual questions the nurse uses during a pain assessment will vary with the type and duration of pain. The assessment of acute pain differs in some respects from the assessment of chronic pain. For example, the patient in chronic pain may have tried many different interventions to find relief and suffered greater negative lifestyle effects compared with a patient experiencing acute pain.

The highly subjective nature of pain is what makes assessment and management a challenge for the clinician. The Acute Pain Management Guidelines (Carr et al., 1992) and the Cancer Pain Guidelines (Jacox et al., 1994) contain valuable information regarding pain assessment. The guidelines stress that the reporting of pain is a social transaction between the clinician and the patient. A good rapport with the patient and use of therapeutic communication skills are essential for a thorough pain assessment.

The quantifiable aspects of pain are the intensity, timing, quality, impact, and personal meaning. Other areas to consider include the location, aggravating and alleviating factors, and pain behaviors. The most important and reliable aspect of pain assessment is the report given by the patient. The family may be helpful at times, but the best source is the person who is suffering.

Begin the pain assessment by asking the patient specifically about pain. Try to have the patient use his or her own words to describe the pain. The descriptors used can provide clues about the etiology of the pain. For example, patients who experience chest pain during a myocardial infarction frequently describe the pain as a pressure or as if someone were squeezing the chest. A detailed history should follow the initial query about pain.

Location

To determine the location of the pain, ask the patient to point to the area involved. Along with other aspects of the pain assessment, it is useful for the patient to point to or shade areas in a drawing such as the one in Figure 1-4. This is especially helpful if the pain radiates. The location of the pain can be represented by a circle with shaded areas used to indicate areas of referred pain. The drawing is useful when future assessments are made.

Intensity

The intensity of pain ranges from none, to mild discomfort, to excruciating. The most important thing to remember is that there is no correlation between the stimulus and the patient's perception of pain. The intensity reported is influenced by the person's threshold and tolerance for pain. Threshold refers to the least amount of pain recognized and tolerance to the greatest amount a person can stand. Tolerance varies a great deal from patient to patient. Ask about the present pain intensity as well as the worst and least intensity. Finally, inquire about what level would be acceptable to the patient.

To facilitate accurate reporting of pain intensity, patients should be taught to use some type of scale, and that scale should be used consistently. Figure 1-5 shows several different types of rating scales. A frequently used, easy method is to ask the patient to rate the intensity of the pain on a numerical scale (0 to 10), with zero representing no pain and 10 representing the worst possible pain. To produce a record of pain, the patient can be taught to rate the pain intensity on another type of scale, called a visual analog scale. The patient should be oriented to the anchors at the two ends and requested to mark a perpendicular line straight across the scale. The distance from the *No pain* anchor to the intersecting line is recorded as the pain intensity. Some patients may have difficulty translating their pain intensity into a number. For these patients, the words in the present pain intensity portion of the McGill Pain Questionnaire are useful. The

INITIAL PAIN ASSESSMENT TOOL

Date ________

Patient's Name ______________________________ Age ________ Room ________

Diagnosis ______________________________ Physician ______________________________

Nurse ______________________________

I. LOCATION: Patient or nurse mark drawing.

II. INTENSITY: Patient rates the pain. Scale used ______________________________

Present: ______________________________

Worst pain gets: ______________________________

Best pain gets: ______________________________

Acceptable level of pain: ______________________________

III. QUALITY: (Use patient's own words, e.g., prick, ache, burn, throb, pull, sharp) ______________________________

IV. ONSET, DURATION VARIATIONS, RHYTHMS: ______________________________

V. MANNER OF EXPRESSING PAIN: ______________________________

VI. WHAT RELIEVES THE PAIN? ______________________________

VII. WHAT CAUSES OR INCREASES THE PAIN? ______________________________

VIII. EFFECTS OF PAIN: (Note decreased function, decreased quality of life.)

Accompanying symptoms (e.g., nausea) ______________________________

Sleep ______________________________

Appetite ______________________________

Physical activity ______________________________

Relationship with others (e.g., irritability) ______________________________

Emotions (e.g., anger, suicidal, crying) ______________________________

Concentration ______________________________

Other ______________________________

IX. OTHER COMMENTS: ______________________________

X. PLAN: ______________________________

Figure 1-4 Pain assessment instrument. (From McCaffery, M., & Beebe, A. (1989). *Pain: Clinical manual for nursing practice.* St. Louis: Mosby.)

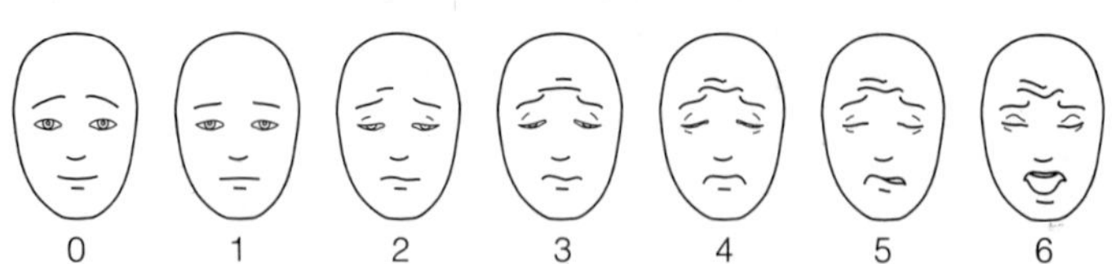

Faces Pain Scale (Bieri, Reeve, Champion, Addicoat, & Aigler, 1990; with permission)

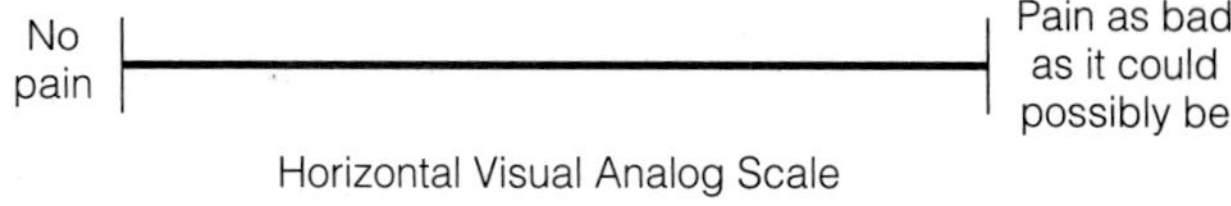

Horizontal Visual Analog Scale

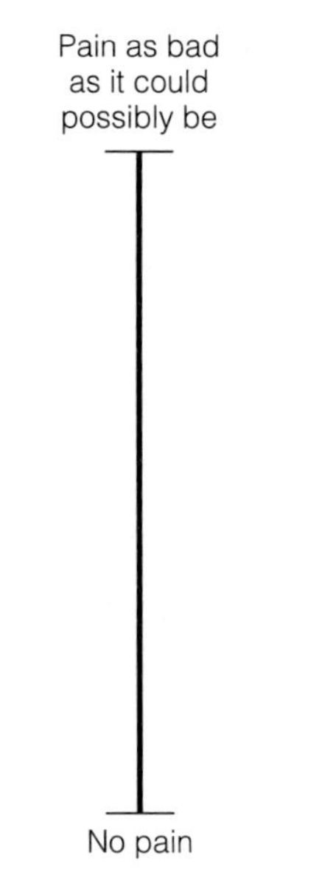

Vertical Visual Analog Scale

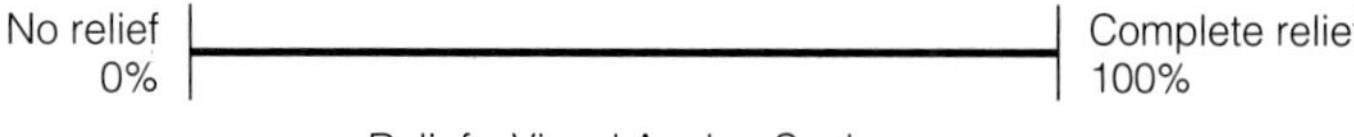

Relief—Visual Analog Scale

Figure 1-5 Pain intensity rating scales. To guarantee reliability, lines should be 10 cm in length when used.

words *mild, discomforting, distressing, horrible,* and *excruciating* are quantified from 1 (mild) to 5 (excruciating). The clinician can use either the word or the number to make judgments about the treatment indicated or the effectiveness of treatment. A detailed explanation and an illustration of this questionnaire appear in Chapter 8.

Quality

Ask the patient to describe the quality of the pain without offering cues. For example, asking the patient to describe what the pain feels like should elicit a descriptive answer. Allow adequate time for the patient to describe the pain and record as many adjectives as offered. The exact words should be documented for future reference. If the patient is unable to state words that describe the quality of the pain, words can be offered, and the fact that the words were suggested by the clinician should be included in the documentation.

Timing

The etiology of pain can sometimes be determined when time aspects are known. The patient should be asked about the onset, duration, time-intensity relationship, and changes in the rhythmic patterns. It is important to determine whether the pain occurred suddenly or increased gradually. Pain of a sudden nature that rapidly reaches maximum intensity is often indicative of tissue rupture. On the other hand, ischemic pain gradually increases and becomes more intense with time. The time-intensity relationship is useful in detecting diurnal relationships that may occur with chronic pain. For example, arthritic pain is most intense in the morning or after periods of inactivity.

Aggravating and Alleviating Factors

Questions about aggravating and alleviating factors tell the clinician what activity worsens pain or what a patient may have tried to lessen it. Ask the patient what makes the pain worse, and ask specifically about the relationship between pain and activity. This can lead to detection of factors associated with the pain. For example, pain with coughing or defecation may signal spinal cord compression in a patient with cancer. It is important to inquire about how environmental factors such as temperature and noise affect pain. These may be easily controlled to lessen pain. Finally, determine whether the pain affects or is affected by sleep deprivation and anxiety. Both can significantly affect pain intensity and the quality of life.

Knowledge of the alleviating factors will help treatment of the pain. Ask the patient what medications, both prescription and over-the-counter, have helped. Ask specifically about the amount of medication taken and the frequency. This assists in determining teaching needs in addition to providing information for pain assessment. Inquire whether nonpharmacologic interventions such as massage, warm baths, position changes, or hypnosis have decreased the pain.

Daily Activities

To learn how the pain affects activities of daily living, ask what the pain means to the patient. Pain can mean many different things, such as impending death, the need for escalating doses of an opiate, or that an injury has just occurred. This helps in understanding what the patient thinks may happen because of the pain. Knowledge of how pain is viewed will help the practitioner plan for educational or psychologic interventions to help the patient cope with the pain. If the pain is chronic, ask whether and how it interferes with basic needs such as sleep, nutrition, relationships, and finances for treatment.

Other Aspects

Other assessment areas include nonverbal, behavioral expressions of pain. Patients may grimace, cry, rock, rub the affected area, moan, or withdraw. These expressions of pain are not exhibited by all patients and are not easily quantifiable. Thus they should not be used as indicators of the pres-

Table 1-3 Behaviors Associated with Pain

Type of Behavior	Examples
Facial expression	Grimacing, clenching teeth, tightly shutting lips, gazing/staring, wrinkling forehead, tearing
Vocalization	Moaning, groaning, grunting, sighing, gasping, crying, screaming
Verbalization	Praying, counting, swearing or cursing, repeating nonsensical phrases
Body action	Thrashing, pounding, biting, rocking, rubbing
Behaviors	Massaging, immobilizing, guarding, bracing, eating/drinking, applying pressure/heat/cold, assuming special position/posture, reading, watching television, listening to music

From Puntillo, K., & Wilkie, D. (1991). Assessment of pain in the critically ill. In K. Puntillo (Ed.), *Pain in the critically ill: Assessment and management.* Gaithersburg, MD: Aspen. Reprinted by permission.

ence or absence of any degree of pain. Table 1-3 lists many behaviors typically associated with pain.

Physiologic responses such as tachycardia, hypertension, tachypnea, pallor, diaphoresis, mydriasis, hypervigilance, and increased muscle tone are related to stimulation of the autonomic nervous system (Wells, 1984). These responses are short lived because the body adapts to the stress response over time. These physiologic responses could be the result of other physical events such as the onset of hypovolemic shock. It is imperative to look for and note any observations of pain; however, it is equally important not to assume that the absence of clinical signs indicates there is no pain. Resist the temptation to rely on physiologic observations as indicators of pain in any patient, and especially in nonresponsive patients.

Accurate pain assessment is vital to effective pain management. The patient must be assessed thoroughly to determine proper treatment as well as to evaluate the effectiveness of intervention. Accurate assessment allows the clinician to assist the patient in making judgments about what is and what is not working. Figure 1-6 shows an algorithm that summarizes the assessment process.

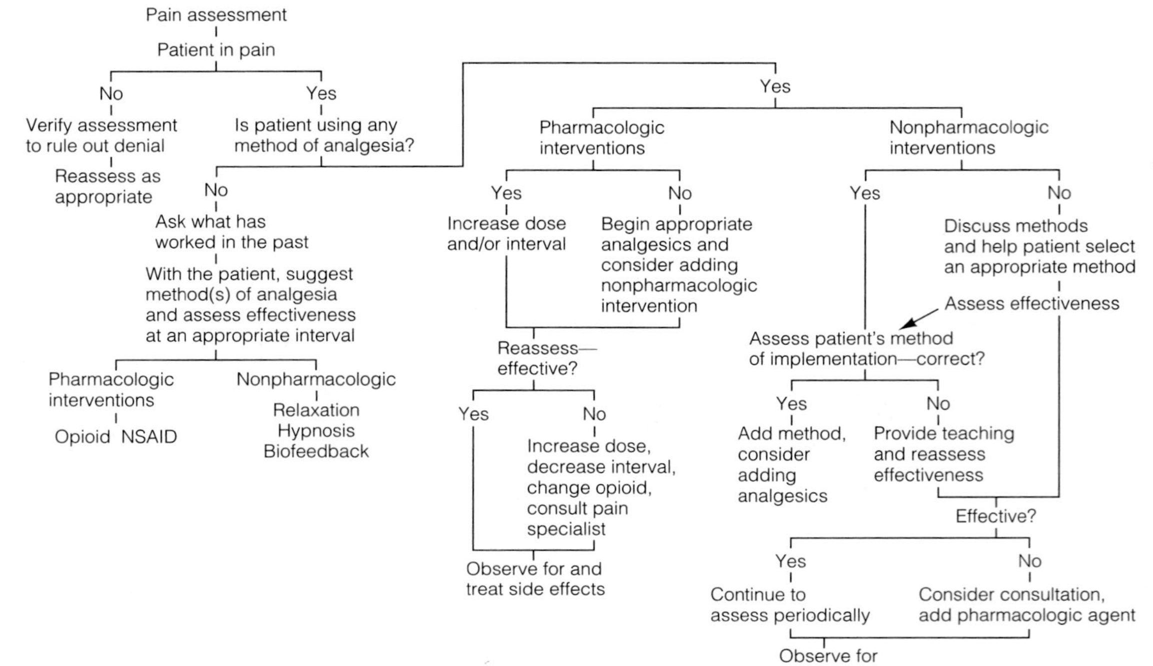

Figure 1-6 Pain assessment algorithm.

DEVELOPMENTAL ASPECTS OF PAIN

To adequately assess pain, the clinician must consider the patient's developmental level. It was previously assumed that neonates and infants do not experience pain. This myth existed in part because neonates and infants are unable to express pain. The clinician must develop a good rapport with the child and family to ensure adequate assessment and successful management.

Observation of behavior is the primary approach for assessing neonates, infants, and children unable to verbalize pain. Vocalizations such as crying or whining, facial expressions, muscle tension and rigidity, guarding of body parts, temperament, activity, and general appearance may indicate the presence of pain. The CRIES scale (see Table 1-4), developed for use with neonates up to 6 months of age in the postoperative period, considers behaviors as indicating the severity of pain. Preliminary evidence for reliability or validity was published by the creators (Krechel & Bildner, 1995) of the instrument; however, more studies need to be conducted. These behaviors are an educated guess at best and should be used as such. Behavioral changes over time can serve as indicators for the onset of pain or a change in intensity.

Table 1-4 CRIES Score

	0	1	2
Crying	No	High-pitched	Inconsolable
Requires O_2 for $SaO_2 > 95\%$	No	$< 30\%$ of time	$> 30\%$ of time
Increased vital signs from preoperative values	$\leq$	$< 20\%$ increase	$> 20\%$ increase
Expression	None	Grimace	Grimace and grunt
Sleepless	No	Wakes at frequent intervals	Constantly awake

Reprinted with permission of S. W. Krechel and J. Bildner, University of Missouri-Columbia, Department of Anesthesiology.

Generally, children more than 4 years of age can verbalize pain (McGrath, 1990). Children should be asked what pain is. Ask the parents what words the child uses to express pain. It is important to ask about previous experiences with pain. This will give some information about how the child deals with pain. Ask what the child does when in pain, what is not done, and what the child's preferences are for treatment. Question the child and parent about the effectiveness of previous interventions.

Assessment instruments frequently used for children more than 4 years of age include the Oucher (Beyer, Villarruel, & Denyes, 1993) and the Poker Chip scale (Hester, Foster, & Kristensen, 1990). Figure 1-5 includes commonly used assessment scales for children. The Faces Pain Scale (Bieri, Reeve, Champion, Addicoat, & Aiegler, 1990) has demonstrated reliability with children in grades 1 and 3 (mean ages 6.7 and 8.7). Children more than 7 years of age may begin to effectively understand the concepts of order and numbers. These children may prefer to use a numerical scale or a visual analog scale (VAS). Researchers (Tesler et al., 1991) have reported that the VAS was the least preferred of five horizontal pain scales. Refer to Chapter 11 for a more thorough discussion of pediatric assessment.

Flexibility in pain assessment in the elderly is necessary for those who have problems with memory or cognition. The older adult without those deficits does not require any changes in the assessment approach. Hopefully, the myth that older adults have an increased tolerance for pain is decreasing. Those with memory problems often can report present pain (Carr et al., 1992), but their integration of past pain with present pain and its relationship to current treatment is less reliable. This suggests that pain assessments should be more frequent than for other age groups. Cognitive impairment and delirium present special problems for which there are no solutions. Observation of the person's functional abilities for changes that may be related to pain may be the only method available, and not necessarily a reliable one. See Chapter 12 for a more thorough discussion of assessment in the geriatric patient.

STANDARDS AND GUIDELINES FOR PAIN MANAGEMENT

Guidelines are systematically developed statements designed to assist clinicians and patients in attaining appropriate health care for certain clinical conditions. Standards, developed from guidelines, are established methods for the assessment, treatment, and evaluation of care. The American Pain Society and many specialty organizations have studied pain and made recommendations for future research. The guidelines developed by the Agency for Health Care Policy and Research (Carr et al., 1992; Jacox et al., 1994) resulted from an enormous interdisciplinary study that reviewed drug and nondrug literature. These guidelines are broader and serve to eliminate overlap from single specialty efforts.

The Acute Pain Management guidelines (Carr et al., 1992) had four main goals:

1. Reduce the incidence and severity of patients' acute postoperative or posttraumatic pain.
2. Educate patients about the need to communicate unrelieved pain so they can receive prompt evaluation and effective treatment.
3. Enhance patient comfort and satisfaction.
4. Contribute to fewer postoperative complications and in some cases shorter stays after surgical procedures.

Similar goals were developed in the Cancer Pain Management guidelines (Jacox et al., 1994):

1. Inform clinicians and patients and their families that most cancer pain can be relieved by available methods.
2. Dispel unfounded fears that addiction results from the appropriate use of medications to control cancer pain.
3. Inform clinicians that cancer pain accompanies both disease and treatment; changes over time; may have multiple, simultaneous causes; and if unrelieved

can affect the physical, psychologic, social, and spiritual well-being of the patient.

4. Promote prompt and effective assessment, diagnosis, and treatment of pain in patients with cancer.
5. Strengthen the ability of patients with cancer and their families to communicate new or unrelieved pain to secure prompt evaluation and effective treatment.
6. Provide clinicians with a synthesis of the literature and expert opinion for application to the management of cancer pain.
7. Familiarize patients and their families with options available for pain relief and promote their active participation in selecting among these.
8. Provide a model for cancer pain management to guide therapy in selected painful, life-threatening conditions such as acquired immunodeficiency syndrome (AIDS).
9. Provide information and guidelines on the use of controlled substances for the treatment of cancer pain that distinguish the use of these drugs for legitimate medical purposes from their abuse as illegitimate drugs.
10. Identify health policy and research issues that affect cancer pain management.

Both sets of guidelines (Carr et al., 1992; Jacox et al., 1994) emphasize a collaborative, interdisciplinary approach to pain management; an individualized approach; the need for adequate and frequent assessment; the use of pharmacologic and nonpharmacologic interventions; and a formalized institutional approach to the management of pain.

Using these guidelines, each institution should develop standard approaches to patients in pain. Any health care professional responsible for some aspect of care should be taught how to assist the patient in pain. Ferrell and Leek (1991) have suggested many ways to improve pain management using the AHCPR guidelines. See the box on pp. 32 and 33 for a list of ways to improve pain management. Finally, all health care professionals should document the methods used to treat pain as well as the effectiveness of the treatment.

Abram and Gillespie (1992) argue that standards and guidelines are necessary to develop and oversee certification processes and to provide a basis for care and fair reimbursement. They propose separate standards for chronic pain clinics, cancer pain services, and acute pain services. They suggest the type of health care professionals that should be involved in patient care, the amount of time they should be available, their educational preparation, physical environment, and other services for each type of care.

LEGAL ISSUES IN THE MANAGEMENT OF PAIN

Liability concerns surrounding pain management involve four main areas: health care professional liability to patients, liability to the professional discipline for inappropriate pain management, liability to third parties for injury caused by patients treated for pain, and liability for side effects of treatment. All these issues should be considered by health care professionals who are involved in pain management.

It is the responsibility of health care providers to ensure the proper administration of pain medications. Proper administration includes the right drug, amount, and route. Courts are willing to recognize improper pain management as a breach of good and acceptable practice (Shapiro, 1994). Failure to provide adequate pain management to a patient in a nursing home resulted in a $15 million verdict, which was settled out of court. Citing the "patient's bill of rights" and standards of proper care, the nursing home and a nurse were found to be negligent by undermedicating a dying patient. This should be disconcerting to all health care professionals in light of the vast recent documentation of the undermedication of many hospitalized patients.

It is possible for physicians who fail to meet professional standards to face discipline from a medical board for negligent medical treatment and unprofessional conduct (Shapiro, 1994). This is especially important following the

TWENTY-SEVEN WAYS TO IMPROVE PAIN MANAGEMENT IN YOUR SETTING

1. Obtain copies of the APCPR guidelines and distribute them widely to your staff.
2. Perform a pain audit including review of charts and patient interviews. The first step toward change is demonstrating that a problem exists.
3. Create an awareness of the status of pain management in your institution. Inform physicians, nursing staff, and administrators of the status of pain control and areas in need of improvement.
4. Designate an "expert nurse" on each shift as the consultant to colleagues on pain. Support that nurse in getting additional pain education and in becoming the unit "watchdog" for untreated pain.
5. Educate the physicians. Circulate articles, monographs, or audiotapes of interest. Work to sponsor a continuing medical education offering on pain management.
6. Adopt a uniform pain assessment tool for use during admission to the unit of any patient whose pain is a significant problem.
7. Adopt a uniform system for pain assessment (e.g., a 0-10 pain rating scale).
8. Establish standards of care. (Nurses do not accept uncontrolled infection rates, extravasations, and falls, so why accept uncontrolled pain?)
9. Involve others in pain management. Develop an army of supporters such as volunteers and personnel from physical therapy, occupational therapy, social services, and the pharmacy.
10. Educate the patients. Patients must know that pain is preventable and treatable. Pain management should become a consumer issue, and patients should not settle for unrelieved pain.
11. Involve families in every aspect of pain management. Family members can be the greatest asset to pain relief or the greatest barrier.

TWENTY-SEVEN WAYS TO IMPROVE PAIN MANAGEMENT IN YOUR SETTING—cont'd

12. Develop a "bag of tricks" of nondrug interventions for pain management such as heat and cold therapy, instructions for breathing exercises, music and videotapes used for relaxation, and audiotapes used for imagery or relaxation.
13. Educate the nursing staff about basic principles of pain management.
14. Post equianalgesic charts on the unit. They are required nursing knowledge.
15. Develop a working relationship with someone in the pharmacy who can advocate for pain management.
16. Include pain management philosophy and strategies in new employee orientation.
17. Develop a pocket card for every nurse that includes the pain assessment scale and equianalgesia guides.
18. Make pain management accessible. Ensure that the pharmacy stocks appropriate medications and doses of drugs.
19. Develop an expectation in the unit that *pain can be relieved.* Nurses and patients often beleieve that cancer pain is inevitable and uncontrollable.
20. Plan for continuity in pain management. Coordinate pain efforts between inpatient units, the outpatient area, physician offices, and home or hospice sevices.
21. Document pain assessment. The patient's pain experience must be effectively communicated among all disciplines involved.
22. Evaluate your efforts.
23. Ask the patient. The patient is the best authority on his or her pain and our treatment of it.
24. Educate yourself, your professional organizations, and your institution regarding regulatory barriers to pain relief, and work to overcome these barriers.
25. Sponsor a public education forum on pain.
26. Incorporate pain content into patient support groups.
27. Provide the kind of pain management that you would seek for your own family members.

Modified from Ferrell, B. R., & Leek, C. J. (1991). Pain. In J. L. Creasia & B. Barker (Eds.), *Conceptual foundations of professional nursing practice.* Philadelphia: Mosby.

wide dissemination of the pain guidelines (Carr et al., 1992; Jacox et al., 1994) aimed at health care professionals and patients. With growing acceptance of these guidelines and suggestions for institutional standards, the possibility for professional discipline has increased.

The recent passage of the Patient Self-Determination Act (1991), requiring all health care institutions to provide written information about advanced directives, has implications in the realm of pain management. It is possible for patients to specify pain management preferences to be followed by their health care proxy. The physician is compelled (in some states) to comply with such wishes, and failure to do so may cause legal difficulties.

Caution must be exercised in medicating patients for pain. If the patient causes injury to a third party because of side effects from a medication, the physician may be held liable to the third party for causing harm. Careful patient teaching (and documentation about the teaching) concerning medications and side effects that could impair the operation of dangerous machinery should help the practitioner avoid legal action.

Manufacturers of drugs and pain management devices are required to provide instructions about product use and potential side effects. The prescribing physician or health care provider acts as an intermediary when prescribing, providing, or administering medications and pain management devices. As an intermediary, the health care professional should exercise independent and informed judgment about use of the product and warn the patient about harmful effects. Lawsuits could result if the manufacturer does not provide adequate information or if adequate information is not passed on to the patient, and this results in injury. Protection against such liability centers around gaining as much information as possible about a medication or pain management device and making certain that patients are well educated in using such products. Thorough documentation of such teaching to verify the patient's understanding is another form of protection against liability.

In conclusion, the inadequate treatment of pain is now considered to be more than a problem for the patient. The move toward implementation of pain guidelines and standards will result in greater accountability for pain management. As a result, pain management is a liability issue for health care professionals.

SUMMARY

The incidence of inadequate pain management has been well documented. Classification of pain is helpful in determining the method of treatment. Knowledge of the pathophysiology of pain is essential in the understanding of pain assessment, management, and evaluation. The person experiencing the pain plays a key role in the successful management of pain. The patient's developmental level must be considered for adequate assessment of pain. Even though physiologic and nonverbal behaviors are not reliable indicators, for some patient populations they may be all the clinician has to work with, but they should be used with caution. The recent publication of pain guidelines (Carr et al., 1992; Jacox et al., 1994) serves as a vehicle for institutions to develop and formalize standards of care.

References

Abram, S. E., & Gillespie, B. M. (1992). Standards of care and reimbursement issues in pain management. In P. P. Raj (Ed.), *Practical management of pain* (2nd ed., pp. 40-55). St. Louis: Mosby.

Akil, H., Watson, S. J., Young, E., Lewis, M. E., Khachaturian, H., & Walker, J. M. (1984). Endogenous opioids: Biology and function. *Annual Review of Neuroscience, 7*, 223-255.

Beyer, J. E., Villarruel, A. M., & Denyes, M. (1993). The Ouchers: The new user's manual and technical report. Denver: University of Colorado Health Sciences Center.

Bieri, D., Reeve, R. A., Champion, G. D., Addicoat, L., & Aiegler, J. B. (1990). The Faces Pain Scale for the self-assessment of the severity of pain experienced by children: Initial validation, and preliminary investigation for ratio scale properties. *Pain, 41*,139-150.

Bonica, J. J. (1990). *The management of pain* (2nd ed.). Philadelphia: Lea & Febiger.

Brown, J. (1992). Nurses' analgesic choices and postoperative patients' perceived pain: The effect of a pain flow sheet. *American Journal of Pain Management, 2*(4), 192-197.

Carr, D. B., Jacox, A. K., Chapman, C. R., Ferrell, B., Fields, H. L., Heidrich, G., Hester, N. K., Hill, C. S., Lipman, A. G., McGarvey, C. L., Miaskowski, C., Mulder, D. S., Payne, R., Schecter, N., Shapiro, B. S., Smith, R. S., Tsou, C. V., & Vecchiarelli, L. (1992). *Acute pain management: Operative or medical procedures and trauma. Clinical practice guideline.* AHCPR Pub. No. 92-0032. Rockville, MD: Agency for Health Care Policy and Research, PHS, USDHHS.

Cleeland, C. S., Gonin, R., Hatfield, A. K., Edmonson, J. H., Blum, R. H., Stewart, J. A., & Pandya, K. J. (1994). Pain and its treatment in outpatients with metastatic cancer. *New England Journal of Medicine, 330*(9), 592-596.

Cohen, F. L. (1980). Postsurgical pain relief: Patients' status and nurses' medication choices. *Pain, 9,* 265-274.

Curro, F. (1987). Assessing the physiologic and clinical characteristics of acute versus chronic pain. *Dental Clinics of North America, 31*(4), xiii-xxiii.

Ferrell, B. R., & Leek, C. J. (1991). Pain. In J. L. Creasia & B. Barker (Eds.), *Conceptual foundations of professional nursing practice* (pp. 345-362). Philadelphia: Mosby.

Fife, B. L., Irick, N., & Painter, J. D. (1993). A comparative study of the attitudes of physicians and nurses toward cancer pain. *Journal of Pain and Symptom Management, 8*(3), 132-139.

Fordyce, W. E. (1976). *Behavioral methods for chronic pain and illness.* St. Louis: Mosby.

Goldstein, A. (1976). Opioid peptides (endorphins) in pituitary and brain. *Science, 193*(4258), 1081-1086.

Hester, N. O., Foster, R., & Kristensen, K. (1990). Measurement of pain in children: Generalizability and validity of the Pain Ladder and the Poker Chip Tool. In D. C. Tyler & E. J. Drane (Eds.), *Pediatric pain: Vol. 15. Advances in pain research and therapy* (pp. 79-84). New York: Raven Press.

Hughes, J. (1975). Isolation of an endogenous compound from the brain with pharmacological properties similar to morphine. *Brain Research, 88,* 295-308.

International Association for the Study of Pain (IASP) Subcommittee on Taxonomy. (1979). Pain terms: A list with definitions and notes on useage. *Pain, 6*(2), 249.

Jacox, A., Carr, D. B., Payne, R., Berde, C. B., Breitbart, W., Cain, J. M., Chapman, C. R., Cleeland, C. S., Ferrell, B. R., Finley, R. S., Hester, N. O., Hill, C. S., Leak, W. D., Lipman, A. G., Logan, C. L., McGarvey, C. L., Miaskowski, C. A., Mulder, D. S., Paice, J. A., Shapiro, B. S., Silberstein, E. B., Smith, R. S., Stover, J., Tsou, C. V., Vecchiarelli, L., & Weissman, D. E. (1994). *Management of cancer pain: Clinical practice guideline.* AHCPR Pub. No. 94-0592. Rockville, MD: Agency for Health Care Policy and Research, PHS, USDHHS.

Keeri-Szanto, M., & Heaman, S. (1972). Postoperative demand analgesia. *Surgery, Gynecology and Obstetrics, 134,* 647-651.

Krechel, S. W., & Bildner, J. (1995). CRIES: A new neonatal postoperative pain measurement score. Initial testing of validity and reliability. *Pediatric Anesthesia, 5,* 53-61.

Kuhn, S., Cooke, K., Collins, M., Jones, M. J., & Mucklow, J. C. (1990). Perceptions of pain relief after surgery. *British Medical Journal, 300,* 1687-1690.

Marks, R. M., & Sachar, E. J. (1973). Undertreatment of medical inpatients with narcotic analgesics. *Annals of Internal Medicine, 78*(2), 173-181.

Mayer, D. J., Wolfle, T. L., Akil, H., Carder, B., & Liebeskind, J. C. (1971). Analgesia from electrical stimulation in the brainstem of the rat. *Science, 174,* 1351-1354.

McCaffery, M., & Beebe, A. (1989). *Pain: Clinical manual for nursing practice.* St. Louis: Mosby.

McGrath, P. A. (1990). *Pain in children: Nature, assessment, and treatment.* New York: Guilford Press, pp. 88-110.

Melzack, R., & Wall, P. D. (1965). Pain mechanisms: A new theory. *Science, 150*(3699), 971-979.

Merskey, H. (1986). Classification of chronic pain: Description of chronic pain syndromes and definitions of pain terms. *Pain, 3*(suppl.), 1-226.

Millan, M. J. (1986). Multiple opioid systems and pain. *Pain, 27,* 303-347.

Owen, H., McMillan, V., & Rogowski, D. (1990). Postoperative pain therapy: A survey of patients' expectations and their experiences. *Pain, 41,* 303-307.

Patient Self-Determination Act. (1991). 42 U. S. Congress Sect. 1395 et seq.

Perl, E. R. (1976). Sensitization of nociceptors and its relation to sensation. *Advances in Pain Research and Therapy, 1,* 17-28.

Pert, C. B., & Snyder, S. H. (1973). Opiate receptor: Demonstration in nervous tissue. *Science, 179,* 1011-1014.

Raj, P. P. (1994). *Practical management of pain* (2nd ed.). St. Louis: Mosby.

Reynolds, D. V. (1969). Surgery in the rat during electrical analgesia induced by focal brain stimulation. *Science, 164,* 444-445.

Shapiro, R. S. (1994). Liability issues in the management of pain. *Journal of Pain and Symptom Management, 9*(3), 146-152.

Sternbach, R. A. (1974). *Pain patients' traits and treatment.* New York: Academic Press.

Tesler, M. D., Savedra, M. C., Holzemer, W. L., Wilkie, D. J., Ward, J. A., & Paul, S. M. (1991). The word-graphic rating scale as a measure of children's and adolescent's pain intensity. *Research in Nursing and Health, 14*(5), 361-371.

Wells, N. (1984). Responses to acute pain and the nursing implications. *Journal of Advanced Nursing, 9,* 51-58.

Yaksh, T. (1981). Spinal opiate analgesia: Characteristics and principles of action. *Pain, 11,* 293-346.

2

Identifying and Preventing Pain Mismanagement

Janice Fitzgerald Ulmer

Key Points

- Professional organizations and government agencies have acknowledged pain as a public health problem.
- Societal lack of expectation for pain relief is the major contributing factor to pain mismanagement.
- Health care professionals lack adequate basic education in pain assessment and pain management.
- Recent trends and societal attitudes toward drug abuse discourage the legitimate use of analgesics.
- Clinicians should take a proactive approach to pain management by acquiring education and implementing the recommendations of research-based clinical practice guidelines.

The science and technology of pain management has advanced over the last 2 decades, stimulated by an increase in our understanding of the mechanisms of pain and analgesia. The new technologies should assure patients today that most acute and chronic pain can be relieved. Clinical guidelines that recommend approaches to pain management have been available since 1986 (American Pain Society, 1986; World Health Organization, 1990). These guidelines and the acute and cancer pain guidelines recently released by the Agency for Health Care Policy and Research (Carr et al., 1992a; Jacox et al., 1994a) suggest that most pain can be relieved by relatively simple means. Research studies (Anonymous, 1994; Teoh & Stjernsward, 1992) are accumulating that evaluate the implementation of the World Health Organization (WHO) Guidelines for Cancer Pain Relief and Palliative Care. These studies clearly demonstrate that most cancer pain can be relieved using oral analgesics, routine or scheduled analgesic administration, and the WHO ladder to guide analgesic decisions.

Two decades after publication of Marks and Sachar's classic report (1973), researchers continue to discover significant levels of unrelieved pain in medical, surgical, and cancer pain patients (Cleeland et al., 1994; Kuhn, Cooke, Collins, Jones, & Mucklow, 1990; Owen, McMillan, & Rogowski, 1990). (See Table 1-1 in Chapter 1.) This chapter will discuss patient, clinician, and health care system barriers to effective pain relief. The importance of pain management standards and quality monitoring will be emphasized, and recommendations will be made for ensuring the effectiveness of pain management approaches.

UNDERTREATMENT OF PAIN

Pain often is the primary symptom for which a patient seeks medical care. Patients with complaints of pain are generally evaluated, and diagnostic, medical, or in some instances surgical treatment is initiated. Often, however, once the initial evaluation is completed and treatment is initiated, little attention is given to ongoing management of the pain complaint. Even professionals who consider themselves pain specialists sometimes do not look beyond their own area of expertise to ensure adequate treatment of pain.

Professional organizations and governmental agencies have acknowledged pain as a public health problem and responded by developing guidelines for pain management and providing clinicians with information and opportunities for professional education. Yet pain mismanagement continues. Max (1990) advises that education alone may not be enough to improve the outcomes of analgesic treatment. Pain management must be recognized as a national priority and as every patient's right.

In 1992 the U.S. government raised public awareness of acute pain problems and recognized pain management as a national priority through its release of *Acute Pain Management: Operative or Medical Procedures and Trauma Clinical Practice Guideline* (Carr et al., 1992a). More recently, a second guideline was released to address the special needs of patients with cancer (Jacox et al., 1994a). Within the

Table 2-1 Barriers to Cancer Pain Management

- Problems related to health care professionals
  - Inadequate knowledge of pain management
  - Poor assessment of pain
  - Concern about regulation of controlled substances
  - Fear of patient addiction
  - Concern about side effects of analgesics
  - Concern about patients becoming tolerant to analgesics
- Problems related to patients
  - Reluctance to report pain
    - Concern about distracting physicians from treatment of underlying disease
    - Fear that pain means disease is worse
    - Concern about not being a "good" patient
  - Reluctance to take pain medications
    - Fear of addiction or of being thought of as an addict
    - Worries about unmanageable side effects
    - Concern about becoming tolerant to pain medications
- Problems related to the health care system
  - Low priority given to cancer pain treatment
  - Inadequate reimbursement
    - The most appropriate treatment may not be reimbursed or may be too costly for patients and families
  - Restrictive regulation of controlled substances
  - Problems of availability of treatment or access to it

Reprinted from Jacox, A., Carr, D. B., Payne, R., Berde, C. B., Breitbart, W., Cain, J. M., Chapman, C. R., Cleeland, C. S., Ferrel, B. R., Finley, R. S., Hester, N. O., Hill, C. S., Leak, W. D., Lipmann, A. G., Logan, C. L., McGarvey, C. L., Miaskowski, C. A., Mulder, D. S., Paice, J. A., Shapiro, B. S., Silberstein, E. B., Smith, R. S., Stover, J., Tsou, C. V., Vecchiarelli, L., & Weissman, D. E. (1994). *Management of cancer pain. Clinical practice guideline.* AHCPR Pub. No. 94-0592. Rockville, MD: Agency for Health Care Policy and Research, PHS, USDHHS.

latter guideline, factors were identified that act as major barriers to effective pain relief (Table 2-1). These factors can be categorized as problems that relate to health care professionals, to patients, and to the health care system. Although most of the work concerning barriers to effective pain relief was initiated to improve cancer pain relief, this information has relevance for patients with other acute and chronic pain conditions.

PROFESSIONAL AND PATIENT-RELATED BARRIERS

Professional and patient-related barriers to effective pain management will be discussed from six perspectives: societal expectations; knowledge deficits; inadequate assessment techniques; ineffective communication; attitudes and beliefs; and fear of tolerance, addiction, and analgesic side effects. First, however, studies that report barriers described by care providers and patients will be reviewed.

Researchers (Ryan, Vortherms, & Ward, 1994; Von Roenn, Cleeland, Gonin, Hatfield, & Pandya, 1993; Vortherms, Ryan, & Ward, 1992) recently reported care provider barriers to pain relief for cancer patients. The five most prevalent barriers reported by physicians and nurses were inadequate pain assessment, patient reluctance to report pain, patient reluctance to take opioids, physician reluctance to prescribe opioids, and inadequate staff knowledge about pain management (Ryan et al., 1994; Von Roenn et al., 1993). Other barriers included nurse reluctance to administer opioids, restrictive state regulation of analgesics, and issues related to lack of access to, or skill in the use of, advanced pain technologies (see Table 2-2).

Patients and families were most concerned about opioid addiction and tolerance, analgesic side effects, disease progression, and the desire to be perceived as a "good" patient (Ward & Gatwood, 1994; Ward et al., 1993). Patients who were categorized as undermedicated based on analgesics they reported using had a significantly higher level of concern than those who were categorized as adequately medicated. Patients who were older, were less educated, or had less income also tended to have more concerns about analgesic use.

Societal Expectations

The factor that perhaps contributes most to pain mismanagement is the lack of societal expectation of pain relief. Unrelieved pain is expected and accepted during medical

Table 2-2 Barriers to Cancer Pain Management in Care Providers' Own Practice Setting

	PERCENTAGE	
Barriers to Pain Relief	MDs[1] (*n* = 897)	RNs[2] (*n* = 327)
Inadequate assessment of pain	76	77
Patient reluctance to report pain	62	80
Patient reluctance to take opioids	62	57
Physician reluctance to prescribe opioids	61	59
Inadequate staff knowledge about pain management	52	72
Nursing staff reluctance to give opioids	38	50
Excessive state regulation of analgesics	18	
Lack of access to professional methods	12	
Lack of access to specialized methods or professionals who practice specialized methods		53
Lack of psychologic support services	11	62
Lack of equipment or skills in using equipment	6	35

Modified from [1]Von Roenn, J. H., Cleeland, C. S., Gonin, R., Hatfield, A. K., & Pandya, K. J. (1993). Physician attitudes and practice in cancer pain management: a survey from the Eastern Cooperative Oncology Group. *Annals of Internal Medicine, 119* (2), 121-126; and [2]Vortherms, R., Ryan, P., Ward, S. (1992). Knowledge of, attitudes toward, and barriers to pharmacologic management of cancer pain in a statewide random sample of nurses. *Research in Nursing & Health, 15*, 459-466.

procedures, following surgery, and during treatment for chronic benign and malignant conditions. Pain also is sometimes considered a normal part of the aging process, and older adults with pain may be encouraged to endure their pain. Untreated pain places the older adult at risk for depression and functional limitation (Harkins & Price, 1993). Such attitudes have a restrictive influence and can lead to treatment delay and unnecessary suffering.

In addition to relieving pain, early intervention with over-the-counter nonsteroidal antiinflammatory drugs (NSAIDs) will enhance the resolution of traumatic or inflammatory conditions. Yet the tendency for many professionals is to prescribe these drugs on an "as needed" basis for pain relief. Such a practice encourages patients to delay the use of NSAID analgesics until a sanctioned level of pain is attained. Such advice is counter to pharmacologic knowledge and clinical practice guidelines that recommend NSAID analgesics be administered on an around-the-clock basis for the period of expected inflammatory pain.

Of greater concern is the more recent trend for patients, families, teachers, and others to avoid or discourage the legitimate use of analgesics, particularly opioid analgesics, due to societal attitudes toward drug abuse (Angarola, 1990; Benton, 1993; Hill, Fields, & Thorpe, 1989; Joranson, 1990). Programs such as the "Just Say No to Drugs" campaign interfere with effective pain relief, particularly for children with cancer or other chronic pain conditions.

Knowledge Deficits

Professional Knowledge

Numerous studies have documented the tendency for physicians to underprescribe analgesics and for nurses to not administer the full amount of a prescribed analgesic (see Table 1-1 for a review of such studies). These studies show that physicians and nurses are unable to differentiate among physical dependence, tolerance, and addiction; they lack pharmacokinetic knowledge and skill in performing equianalgesic conversions; and they find decisions about analgesics difficult because of their limited knowledge of these drugs (Grossman & Sheidler, 1985; Sheidler, McGuire, Grossman, & Gilbert, 1992; Ferrell, Eberts, McCaffery, & Grant, 1991; see National Institute for Nursing Research, 1994, for an extensive review).

One reason that pain is managed poorly is that physicians and nurses receive little information about pain management in their basic educational programs. Watt-Watson and Watson (1989) surveyed medical and nursing school facilities and found that 78% of the medical schools and 48% of the nursing schools reported minimal (<3.5 hours) or no pain-related content. Bonica (1984) reviewed 22,000 pages in 17 medical-surgical and oncology medicine textbooks and found only 58 pages containing information about pain. Oden (1989) found no mention of pain in three of the five most popular surgery textbooks and only 7 pages of pain-related text in the 10,000 pages he reviewed. Pharmacologic information provided in text and reference books do not accurately represent the analgesic needs of patients with ongoing pain because it is often based on single-dose studies (Hill, 1990).

Medical and nursing textbooks lack adequate information on the mechanisms of pain and analgesia, pain assessment, and pain management. Lacking is information that would provide physicians and nurses with the knowledge needed for making clinical decisions related to pain management, including (a) sequelae of unrelieved pain; (b) comprehensive pain assessment techniques; (c) selecting the appropriate analgesic class and discriminating among drugs within a given class; (d) calculating equivalent dosages to use when converting from one drug to another or from one route of administration to another; (e) accurate information about opioid tolerance, physical dependence, and addiction; (f) indications for prescribing adjuvant analgesics; and (g) information about and practice in using nonpharmacologic interventions.

Both physicians and nurses gain most of their information about pain and pain management through clinical practice by assimilation of customary knowledge and practices (Edwards, 1990; Foster, 1990; Morgan, 1989). Both groups come to accept informal standards that assign pain management a low priority and practices that are not recommended by current standards, such as "as needed" administration, intramuscular injections, and preferential use of meperidine.

Inadequate Consumer Knowledge

Consumer lack of knowledge also contributes to pain mismanagement. Consumers commonly are not aware that most pain can be relieved or that unrelieved pain negatively affects physical, psychologic, and social functioning and quality of life. Patients lack knowledge regarding pain assessment, the use of analgesic medications, side effects of medications, and how to manage side effects when they occur. Through modeling, patients develop negative views regarding the use of analgesics; such attitudes discourage patients from advocating for pain relief and leave them unprepared to manage their own pain. These negative views are reinforced by public awareness initiatives like the "Just Say No to Drugs" campaign.

Inadequate Assessment Techniques

Another reason for pain mismanagement is a lack of knowledge about and skill in assessing pain. Although relatively simple, valid, and reliable instruments are available to measure pain in adult and pediatric patients, they are seldom used in clinical practice. Researchers (Donovan & Dillon, 1987; Donovan, Dillon, & McGuire, 1987; Marks & Sachar, 1973) have found that in many instances medical-surgical or cancer patients are not asked about their pain or, when they are, cursory or nonspecific questions are used. Seldom is an initial pain history and assessment obtained. Follow-up assessments are generally performed in a haphazard manner even when moderate to severe levels of pain are expected, such as following surgery or trauma, or for patients with progressive malignant conditions (Choiniere, Melzack, Girard, Rondeau, & Paquin, 1990; Foster, 1990; Watt-Watson, 1987). For example, Morgan, Lindley, and Berry (1994) recently reported that pain assessments for hospice patients were obtained at entry and at 1-month intervals rather than as a routine part of nursing care.

A second problem related to pain assessment is that when nurses ask about pain they often are hesitant to believe patient self-reports and choose instead to rely on vital signs (McCaffery & Ferrell, 1992) or behavioral cues (Ferrell, Wisdom, Rhiner, & Alletto, 1991; Ferrell, McCaffery, & Grant, 1991; Hester, 1989). Because of this reliance on nonspecific indicators, nurses have difficulty differentiating pain from other conditions such as anxiety. Nurses also lack knowledge of cultural differences in the expression of pain or cultural influences on their interpretation of pain behaviors (Martin & Belcher, 1986).

Pain assessment is particularly troublesome in patients who are not able to communicate pain, such as infants and young children, some older adults, and the cognitively impaired. Pain assessment is difficult in critically ill patients because these patients often have cognitive impairments and because survival and treatment needs are given greater priority than pain management. Further work is needed in developing appropriate assessment instruments and techniques for critically ill and injured patients. Later chapters will discuss how pain should be assessed and how culture influences pain and pain management (see Chapter 3).

Ineffective Communication Skills

Professional Communications

Poor communication skills on the part of patients and health care providers contribute to pain mismanagement. Communication about pain is difficult for professionals because pain has not been made a priority socially or professionally and because they lack the knowledge and skill to adequately assess pain and negotiate for effective relief. The failure to use standard valid and reliable instruments to measure pain makes it difficult to monitor progress toward pain relief. Although this is changing, clinical documentation forms typically do not highlight pain assessment information as they do other symptoms, such as fever, nausea, diarrhea, or vomiting.

Consumer Communications

Patients may not report pain because they are unaware that pain can be managed; they think it is not severe enough (Taylor & Curran, 1985), or they do not want to distract care providers from treatment of the primary disease (Cleeland, 1984). Patients also may conceal pain because they fear that pain signals disease progression (Ahles, Blanchard, & Ruckdeschel, 1983) or they fear diagnostic tests (Watt-Watson, Evernden, & Lawson, 1990). Patients sometimes fail to report pain because of the desire to be viewed as a "good" patient (Ward et al., 1993). Fagerhaugh (1977) found that patients in a variety of settings and situations, including burn wound debridement, were socialized not to report pain. Studies with burn-injured patients show that even when pain is severe to excruciating and they believe a pain medication would be helpful, the patients themselves or the parents of children may not ask for pain medication (Atchison, Guercio, & Monaco, 1986; Perry, Heidrich, & Ramos, 1981). Other patients delay requesting pain medication because they believe they will receive medication immediately when they do request it (Owen et al., 1990).

Patients have particular difficulty advocating for themselves when the interventions they would like to use are not sanctioned by the professionals responsible for their care (i.e., nonpharmacologic or nontraditional interventions, parental presence). Other patients have special needs and are unable to report pain. These include children, older adults, critically ill or injured patients, and patients who are cognitively impaired.

Attitudes and Beliefs

Inappropriate Professional Attitudes and Beliefs

In some instances, pain is not managed because of inappropriate beliefs or misconceptions held by health professionals. For example, neonates, infants, and children often are not medicated for pain because of a belief that they do not feel pain. Although most pediatric anesthesiologists, pediatricians, family practitioners, and surgeons now believe that young children experience pain, most are hesitant to prescribe opioids after surgery (Purcell-Jones, Dormon, & Sumner, 1988; Schechter, Allen, & Hanson, 1986). For example, Johnston, Jeans, Abbott, Grey-Donald, and Edgar (1988) found that 60% of children for whom pain was estimated as moderate to severe received no analgesic in the previous 24 hours.

In other instances pain is mismanaged because health care professionals have been socialized not to view pain relief as a priority. Complete pain relief is not a goal for most nurses, and for many nurses the goal is to relieve pain "just enough to function" (Burokos, 1985; Cohen, 1980; Gadish, Gonzalez, & Hayes, 1988). Regardless of stated goals, studies have shown that physicians prescribe subtherapeutic analgesic dosages and nurses are hesitant to administer prescribed analgesics, or they administer less than the maximum dose for patients who report moderate to severe pain (Chapman, Ganendran, Scott, & Basford, 1987; Donovan & Dillon, 1987; Donovan et al., 1987; Foster & Hester, 1989; Marks & Sachar, 1973; Mather & Mackie, 1983; Weis, Sriwantanakul, Alloza, Weintraub, & Lasagna, 1983).

Many examples of such practices have been reported. In their classic study of pain in medical inpatients, Marks and Sachar (1973) found that although 73% of patients were experiencing moderate to severe distress, the average amount of medication received by these patients in the previous 24 hours was 9 mg of a morphine sulfate equivalent. Von Roenn and others (1993) found that although 86% of oncologists and other cancer specialists believed that the majority of cancer patients are undermedicated, 31% reported that they would wait until the patient's life expectancy was less than 6 months to begin maximum-tolerated opioid analgesia. Examples such as these highlight the ways in which professional attitudes contribute to pain mismanagement.

Inappropriate Consumer Attitudes and Beliefs

Patient attitudes, beliefs, and behaviors also contribute to pain mismanagement. Many patients believe that pain builds character, that medication should be used only when the pain becomes unbearable, or that bearing pain is a quality of a "good" patient (Cleeland, 1984; Weis et al., 1983). Watt-Watson and colleagues (1990) cite situations in which even young children were expected to bear their pain. Patients do not like to be bothersome, and they find it particularly difficult to tell health care providers when treatments are ineffective or troublesome (Cleeland).

Fear of Tolerance, Addiction, and Analgesic Side Effects

Professionals and patients alike fear addiction, and studies (Atchison et al., 1986; Lander, 1990; McCaffery, Ferrell, O'Neil-Page, Lester, & Ferrel, 1990; Morgan, 1989) have shown that physicians and nurses have difficulty differentiating among physical dependence, tolerance, and addiction. Addiction often is defined inappropriately as the need for increased analgesic medication or more frequent analgesic dosing than is prescribed (i.e., tolerance). Patients who require opioid analgesics for legitimate medical purposes will develop tolerance and physical dependence (i.e., adaptation of the body to opioid dose).

Addiction or psychologic dependence is a pattern of compulsive drug use characterized by a continued craving for an opioid and the need to use the opioid for effects other than pain relief (Jacox et al., 1994a). In reality, addiction in patients treated with opioids is rare (Porter & Jick, 1980). Patients who require opioids for medical reasons do not develop the drug-seeking behavior of the addict. Rather, opioids taken for pain relief often enable patients to resume normal functional lifestyles or improve the quality of their remaining life.

The fear of addiction is so strong that professionals may hesitate to follow analgesic guidelines that recommend use of opioids for treatment of moderate to severe pain. Care providers who withhold or delay use of opioids when they are medically indicated are legally accountable for the pain and suffering their patients endure. In the 1991 case of *Estate of Henry James v. Hillhaven Corporation* (cited in Shapiro, 1994b), the Hillhaven Corporation was held liable for pain and suffering made intolerable by a nurse, their employee, who "with the advice, consent, or orders of a physician" withheld opioids because she believed Mr. James to be addicted.

Hill (1990) has identified four types of cancer patients who are particularly vulnerable to undertreatment of pain. These are cancer patients who (a) require "unusual" doses over an extended time, (b) have predominantly neuropathic pain or pain that only partially responds to opioids, (c) have pain for which no organic cause can be demonstrated, and (d) have a history of drug abuse or fit the profile of someone who abuses drugs. Cleeland and others (1994) were able to demonstrate that discrepancies between physician and patient estimates of pain, pain that physicians did not attribute to cancer, and absence of performance impairment predicted pain mismanagement.

Physicians and nurses also tend to overestimate the incidence of respiratory depression and withhold opioid doses because of fear of respiratory depression or early death. This is because they do not know or do not believe that opioid tolerance includes tolerance to the respiratory depressant effect of the drug. They also mistakenly believe that patients may become immune to the drug when, in fact, there is no ceiling effect for opioids (see Chapter 4).

Patients' fears mirror those of health care providers. Cancer patients fear that if they use opioid analgesics too early, the opioids will not work later when they may really need them, or they fear becoming addicts. They also fear the side effects of opioid analgesics (e.g., altered mental state, constipation) and are not aware that side effects can be managed. (See Chapter 16 for an in-depth discussion of symptom management.) Also, patients' families, like nurses, fear that high doses of opioids may lead to respiratory depression and early death. Such fears would be less likely if patients and professionals had an adequate understanding of tolerance, physical dependency, and addiction.

HEALTH CARE SYSTEM BARRIERS

Health care system issues that contribute to pain mismanagement include the low priority given to pain management, restrictive regulation of controlled substances, access to care, and inadequate reimbursement policies. Health care system barriers, as well as many of the professional and patient-related barriers, stem from a lack of societal concern for pain and pain management (Dahl, Joranson, Engberg, & Dosch, 1988; Hill et al., 1989; Max, 1990).

These issues and others (costs associated with analgesic therapies, professional liability, and the ethics of pain management) were identified by the Cancer Pain Guideline Panel (Jacox et al., 1994a) as factors that contribute to pain mismanagement. Readers are referred to a series of seven papers published in the April and May 1994 issues of the *Journal of Pain and Symptom Management* for in-depth discussion and analyses of these topics (see Cain & Hammes, 1994; Ferrell & Griffith, 1994; Hammes & Cain, 1994; Joranson, 1994; Kolassa, 1994; Shapiro, 1994a, b).

Low Priority for Pain Management

Societal attitudes toward pain management, as discussed earlier, have greatly influenced the quality of pain management services. For many reasons, society does not expect pain relief, and professionals have attitudes, misconceptions, and training that do little to promote effective pain management. Max (1990) describes the phenomenon of failure in pain management in terms of its lack of visibility. Health care provider and patient communications about pain typically are ineffective. Professionals ask vague questions, and patients underreport their pain. When pain is reported, often it is treated as a low-priority issue, leaving treatment delayed. Documentation about pain historically has been absent or incomplete (Camp & O'Sullivan, 1987; Donovan et al., 1987; Fox, 1982; Paice, Mahon, & Faut-Callahan, 1991). Unlike the recording of vital signs, until recently there was no routine place where health professionals documented patients' pain. Quality review programs seldom monitored pain management (National Institute for Nursing Research, 1992), and in cases where pain mismanagement occurred, professionals seldom were held accountable.

Restrictive Regulation

Legislative regulation that contributes to pain mismanagement includes (a) use of terminology in state legislature that does not clearly distinguish legal and illegal usage of opioids,

(b) restriction of the number of pain prescription dosage units that can be prescribed in a given time, and (c) use of multi-copy prescription programs (Shapiro, 1994a). Each of these policies contributes to pain mismanagement by placing restrictions on what practitioners can legally prescribe or by instilling fear of recrimination for the prescription of medically indicated opioids to patients whose pain management requires large doses (Hill, 1993; Shapiro).

Access to Care

Researchers are beginning to identify inequities in the delivery of health care services, including pain management. Cleeland and others (1994) found that patients treated at oncology centers that treat predominantly minority patients were three times more likely than patients treated elsewhere to experience pain mismanagement. They also found that elderly and female patients were more likely than younger or male patients to have pain mismanagement. These findings are similar to those of earlier researchers who reported that black cancer patients were more likely to suffer pain mismanagement (Blendon, Aiken, Freeman, & Corey, 1989; Freeman & Wasfie, 1989) and that Hispanic patients were less likely to receive analgesics for emergency room treatment of long bone fracture (Todd, Samaroo, & Hoffman, 1993) than nonminority patients treated in the same setting.

Other factors also limit access to prescribed therapies. For example, Kanner and Cooper (1989) found that, for a variety of reasons (fear of robbery, inadequate demand, etc.), retail pharmacies often do not stock potent opioids. Also, skilled professionals (pain specialists) and advanced technologies are not equally distributed across health care settings. Patients who receive care in rural settings, smaller hospitals, institutions that are not affiliated with educational institutions, publicly funded institutions, or ambulatory care and home settings often have less access to advanced technologies and skilled professionals.

Cost and Reimbursement

Long-term pain frequently requires costly professional services, prescription drugs, medical equipment, and supportive care that may or may not be reimbursable. The various third-party payors have different reimbursement policies for pain management, many of which leave a substantial number of people underinsured (Earnest, 1990; Joranson, 1994). Those with low income and the elderly are particularly vulnerable and, as a result, often are not offered the same pain management as someone who is well insured.

A second problem is that some policies, including Medicare, favor more expensive technologies over less expensive ones. For example, patients may be treated with intravenous opioids when they could be managed as effectively and at less expense on oral analgesics, because the more complex and costly therapy is reimbursed and the oral opioid is not. Such complex care not only is costly but also decreases quality of life by limiting function, increasing anxiety, or producing side effects or caregiver burden (Ferrell & Griffith, 1994).

A third problem is variance in the cost of analgesic drugs and other therapies. Analgesic drugs with similar efficacy can vary markedly in cost. Kolassa (1994) reported that the cost of NSAID analgesic drugs in 1992 ranged from $10.50 to $127.80 for a 30-day supply. Ferrell and Griffith (1994) examined cost issues related to pain management and provided a 13-point framework for analyzing the cost of pain management (see Table 2-3). In using this framework, clinicians are urged to consider costs and risks/benefits when choosing among analgesic therapies. Ferrell and Griffith's framework is particularly useful for clinicians because it considers costs to the consumer as well as costs to the health care system, and it encourages use of the most effective yet least expensive and least invasive treatment possible.

Often health care providers have the option of selecting from a variety of equally efficacious therapies. In doing so, providers should be aware of the cost of analgesics and other

Table 2-3 Framework for Cost Analysis Related to Pain

1. Costs associated with oral medications
2. Costs associated with parenteral and spinal medications
3. Personnel costs
4. Costs of surgical and anesthetic procedures
5. Costs of radiation therapy
6. Costs of unrelieved pain at home
7. Costs of nondrug interventions
8. Cost savings by various care settings
9. Costs associated with morbidity
10. Costs to justify services
11. Reimbursement biases
12. Conflict of interest
13. Indirect costs to patients and families

Reprinted by permission of Elsevier Science Inc. from "Cost issues related to pain management: report from the Cancer Pain Panel of the Agency for Health Care Policy and Research," by B.R. Ferrell and H. Griffith, *Journal of Pain and Symptom Management,* Vol. 9(4), pp. 221–234. Copyright 1994 by the U.S. Cancer Pain Relief Committee.

therapies and whether the therapies they prescribe place a financial burden on the patients they treat. In addition, care providers should educate politicians and health insurers about how reimbursement policies influence pain management practices, patient quality of life, and the cost of health care.

ACTIONS FOR IMPROVED PAIN MANAGEMENT

The U.S. government, with the release of the acute and cancer pain guidelines (Carr et al., 1992a; Jacox et al., 1994a), took the first step toward making pain management a treatment priority. These and other guidelines (American Pain Society, 1986) recommend the following: (a) an institutional policy designate who is responsible for pain management and for determining how and when pain should be assessed; (b) that patients be told that pain relief is an important part of their care, that pain will be routinely assessed, and that actions will be taken to relieve pain; (c) policies that define acceptable levels of pain and actions to take when pain is not relieved; (d) that institutions review available technologies in light of their resources and design treatment approaches that will optimize pain relief for the populations they serve; and (e) that institutions monitor the quality of the care they provide on an ongoing basis, implementing changes based on quality review findings and advances in institutional technology and skill.

Clinicians and researchers have responded by developing institutional quality assurance programs for improving pain management (see Table 2-4). Clinical documentation and patient management forms are being revised to include pain assessment and pain management documentation. Clinicians are beginning to incorporate standard valid and reliable instruments into their documentation forms to measure pain and related symptoms or side effects (see Chapter 16).

Critical pathways or care maps that are used to manage patients with complex conditions often include goals and objectives for effective pain relief. Programs have been designed to provide clinicians access to expert knowledge and clinical role models. Many institutions have added pain services to provide consultation to clinicians who manage patients with acute and chronic pain problems. Others (Ferrell, Grant, Ritchey, Ropchan, & Rivera, 1993) have developed and evaluated programs that educate nurses to act as pain resource nurses within their own clinical units. For these programs to be successful, clinicians must be provided with tools for change (i.e., concise guides to analgesic use, concise information about drug dosages and timing on order sheets, and computerized programs for prescribing drugs and making equianalgesic conversions) that they can use to make decisions about analgesic therapies (Max, 1990).

Programs have also been developed to teach patients and their families about pain. For example, many institutions are now teaching patients and their families about pain using the acute and cancer pain guideline consumer brochures

Table 2-4 Recommended Actions for Nursing Administration in Achieving Improved Pain Outcomes

1. Implement an interdisciplinary chart audit to determine the status of pain assessment and treatment in your facility.
2. Conduct an ongoing assessment of care provider attitudes regarding pain and pain treatment.
3. Establish a uniform method of assessing pain for all patients, such as a numerical rating scale or faces scale for children.
4. Implement a method for uniform interdisciplinary documentation of pain assessment in the patient record.
5. Establish standards of care for patients in pain. How much pain is acceptable in your setting? Develop the expectation that pain can be relieved.
6. Work collaboratively with other care providers to sponsor a continuing education program on pain management.
7. Incorporate pain education into new staff orientation, including basic principles of pain, assessment of pain, and nonpharmacologic and pharmacologic pain-relief methods.
8. Provide ongoing interdisciplinary education for staff to maintain knowledge and skill in pain assessment.
9. Involve other departments in pain management such as physical therapy, occupational therapy, social service, and pharmacy.
10. Design education for the patients and families about pain and its management.
11. Post essential references such as pain guidelines or handbooks and equianalgesic charts in areas where clinicians provide patient care.
12. Provide pocket cards for clinicians who manage pain that include a pain-assessment scale and equianalgesic guides.
13. Promote interdisciplinary pain rounds for discussion of patients with complex pain problems.
14. Coordinate continuity of care in pain management efforts between inpatient units, the outpatient areas, physician offices, and home care or hospice.
15. Provide opportunities for maintaining and updating clinical knowledge about pain management such as interdisciplinary journal clubs and educational seminars.

Modified from Ferrell, B. R., McCaffery, M., & Ropchan, R. (1992). Pain management as a clinical challenge for nursing administration. *Nursing Outlook, 40*(6), 263-268.

(Carr et al., 1992b, c; Jacox et al., 1994b, c). Pain management is being addressed as a quality of care outcome (Dietrick-Gallagher, Polomano, & Carrick, 1994; Ferrell et al., 1991), and patient satisfaction is being monitored and evaluated within such programs (Miaskowski, Nichols, Brody, & Synold, 1994).

For these initiatives to be successful in alleviating unnecessary pain and suffering, individual clinicians will need to assess their own attitudes and beliefs and educate themselves about pain and pain management. Clinicians are encouraged to use the information provided in this book and elsewhere (American Pain Society, 1986; Carr et al., 1992a, d, e; Jacox et al., 1994a, d) to learn more about pain assessment and pharmacologic and nonpharmacologic management approaches. Clinicians are also encouraged to assess pain management within their own clinical or institutional setting and to intervene to develop appropriate programs for ensuring cost-effective, quality pain management for the patients they treat.

References

Ahles T. A., Blanchard E. B., & Ruckdeschel J. C. (1983). The multidimensional nature of cancer-related pain. *Pain, 17,* 277-288.

American Pain Society. (1986). *Principles of analgesic use in the treatment of acute pain and chronic cancer pain: A concise guide to medical practice.* Skokie, IL: American Pain Society [updated 1989, 1992].

Angarola, R. T. (1990). National and international regulation of opioid drugs: Purpose, structures, benefits and risks. *Journal of Pain and Symptom Management, 5*(2) (suppl), S6-S11.

Anonymous. (1994). WHO guidelines for cancer pain relief: Validation studies. *Cancer Pain Release, 7*(1), 5-7.

Atchison, N., Guercio, P., & Monaco, C. (1986). Pain in the pediatric burn patient: Nursing assessment and perception. *Issues in Comprehensive Pediatric Nursing, 9,* 399-409.

Benton, O. (1993). Innocent victims of the drug war? *APS Bulletin, 3*(1), 17-19.

Beyer, J. E., DeGood, D. E., Ashley, L. C., & Russell, G. A. (1983). Patterns of postoperative analgesic use with adults and children following cardiac surgery. *Pain, 17,* 71-81.

Blendon, R. J., Aiken, L. H., Freeman, H. E., & Corey, C. R. (1989). Access to medical care for black and white Americans: A matter of continuing concern. *JAMA, 261,* 278-281.

Bonica, J. J. (1984). Pain research and therapy: Recent advances and future needs. In L. Kruger & J. C. Liebeskind (Eds.), *Advances in pain research and therapy* (pp. 1-22). New York: Raven Press.

Burokas, L. (1985). Factors affecting nurses' decisions to medicate pediatric patients after surgery. *Heart & Lung, 14*(4), 373-379.

Cain, J. M., & Hammes, B. (1994). Ethics and pain management: Respecting patient wishes. *Journal of Pain and Symptom Management, 9*(3), 160-165.

Camp, D. L., & O'Sullivan, P. S. (1987). Comparison of medical, surgical and oncology patients' descriptions of pain and nurses' documentation of pain assessments. *Journal of Advanced Nursing, 12,* 593-598.

Carr, D. B., Jacox, A., Chapman, C. R., Ferrell, B., Fields, H. L., Heidrich, G., Hester, N. K., Hill, C. S., Lipman, A. G., McGarvey, C. L., Miaskowski, C., Mulder, D., Payne, R., Schechter, N., Shapiro, B. S., Smith, R. S., Tsou, C. V., Vecchiarelli, L. (1992a). *Acute pain management: Operative or medical procedures and trauma. Clinical practice guideline.* AHCPR Pub. No. 92-0032. Rockville, MD: Agency for Health Care Policy and Research, PHS, USDHHS.

Carr, D. B., et al. (1992b). *Pain control after surgery. A patient's guide.* AHCPR Pub. No. 92-0021. Rockville, MD: Agency for Health Care Policy and Research, PHS, USDHHS.

Carr, D. B., et al. (1992c). *Pain control after surgery. Guia para el paciente* (Spanish version). AHCPR Pub. No. 92-0068. Rockville, MD: Agency for Health Care Policy and Research, PHS, USDHHS.

Carr, D. B., et al. (1992d). *Acute pain management in adults: Operative procedures. Quick reference for clinicians.* AHCPR Pub. No. 92-0019. Rockville, MD: Agency for Health Care Policy and Research, PHS, USDHHS.

Carr, D. B., et al. (1992e). *Acute pain management in infants, children and adolescents: Operative procedures. Quick reference for clinicians.* AHCPR Pub. No. 92-0020. Rockville, MD: Agency for Health Care Policy and Research, PHS, USDHHS.

Chapman, P. J., Ganendran, A., Scott, R. J., & Basford, K. E. (1987). Attitudes and knowledge of nursing staff in relation to management of postoperative pain. *Australian and New Zealand Journal of Surgery, 57,* 447-450.

Choiniere, M., Melzack, R., Girard, N., Rondeau, J., & Paquin, M.J. (1990). Comparisons between patients' and nurses' assessment of pain and medication efficacy in severe burn injuries. *Pain, 40,* 143-152.

Cleeland, C. S. (1984). The impact of pain on the patient with cancer. *Cancer, 54,* 2635-2641.

Cleeland, C. S., Gonin, R., Hatfield, A. K., Edmonson, J. H., Blum, R. H., Stewart, J. A., & Pandya, K. J. (1994). Pain and its treatment in outpatients with metastatic cancer. *New England Journal of Medicine, 330*(9), 592-596.

Cohen, F. L. (1980). Postsurgical pain relief: Patients' status and nurses' medication choices. *Pain, 9,* 265-274.

Dahl, J. L., Joranson, D. E., Engberg, D., Dosch, J. (1988). The cancer pain problem: Wisconsin's response. A report on the Wisconsin Cancer Pain Initiative. *Journal of Pain and Symptom Management, 3*(1), S1-S20.

Dietrick-Gallagher, M., Polomano, R., & Carrick, L. (1994). Pain as a quality management initiative. *Journal of Nursing Care Quality, 9*(1), 30-42.

Donovan, M. I., & Dillon, P. (1987). Incidence and characteristics of pain in a sample of hospitalized cancer patients. *Cancer Nursing, 10*(2), 85-92.

Donovan, M. I., Dillon, P., & McGuire, L. (1987). Incidence and characteristics of pain in a sample of medical-surgical inpatients. *Pain, 30,* 69-78.

Earnest, M. (1990). Access to health care in the United States: Barriers for neurologic patients, challenges for neurologic physicians. *Neurology, 14,* 1815-1819.

Edwards, W. T. (1990). Optimizing opioid treatment of postoperative pain. *Journal of Pain and Symptom Management, 5*(1), S24-S36.

Fagerhaugh, S. Y. (1977). *Politics of Pain Management.* Reading, MA: Addison-Wesley.

Ferrell, B. R., Eberts, M. T., McCaffery, M., & Grant, M. (1991). Clinical decision making and pain. *Cancer Nursing, 14*(6), 289-297.

Ferrell, B. R., Grant, M., Ritchey, K. J., Ropchan, R., & Rivera, L. M. (1993). The pain resource nurse training program: A unique approach to pain management. *Journal of Pain and Symptom Management, 8*(8), 549-556.

Ferrell, B. R., Griffith, H. (1994). Cost issues related to pain management: Report from the Cancer Pain Panel of the Agency for Health Care Policy and Research. *Journal of Pain and Symptom Management, 9*(4) 221-234.

Ferrell, B. R., McCaffery, M., & Ropchan, R. (1992). Pain management as a clinical challenge for nursing administration. *Nursing Outlook, 40*(6), 263-268.

Ferrell, B. R., Wisdom, C., Rhiner, M., & Alletto, J. (1991). Pain management as a quality of care outcome. *Journal of Nursing Quality Assurance, 5*(2), 50-58.

Foster, R. L. (1990). A multi-method approach to the description of factors influencing nurses' pharmacologic management of children's pain. Unpublished doctoral dissertation, University of Colorado Health Sciences Center, Denver.

Foster, R., & Hester, N. (1989). The relationship between assessment and pharmacologic intervention for pain in children. In S. G. Funk, E. M. Tornquist, M. T. Champagne, L. A. Copp, & R. A. Wiese (Eds.), *Key aspects of comfort: Management of pain, fatigue, and nausea* (pp. 72-79). New York: Springer.

Fox, L. S. (1982). Pain management in the terminally ill cancer patients: An investigation of nurses' attitudes, knowledge, and clinical practice. *Military Medicine, 147*, 455-460.

Freeman, H. P., & Wasfie, T. J. (1989). Cancer of the breast in poor black women. *Cancer, 63*, 2562-2569.

Gadish, H. S., Gonzalez, J. L., & Hayes, J. S. (1988). Factors affecting nurses' decisions to administer pediatric pain medication postoperatively. *Journal of Pediatric Nursing, 3*(6), 383-389.

Grossman, S. A., & Sheidler, V. R. (1985). Skills of medical students and house officers in prescribing narcotic medications. *Journal of Medical Education, 60*, 552-557.

Hammes, B. J., Cain, J. M. (1994). The ethics of pain management for cancer patients: Case studies and analysis. *Journal of Pain and Symptom Management, 9*(3), 166-170.

Harkins, S. W., & Price, D. D. (1993). Are there special needs for pain assessment in the elderly? *APS Bulletin, 3*(1), 1, 5-6.

Hester, N. O. (1989). Comforting the child in pain. In S. G. Funk, E. M. Tornquist, M. T. Champagne, L. A. Copp, & R. A. Weise (Eds.), *Key aspects of comfort: Management of pain, fatigue, and nausea* (pp. 290-298). New York: Springer.

Hill, C. S., Jr. (1990). Relationship among cultural, educational, and regulatory agency influences on optimum cancer pain treatment. *Journal of Pain and Symptom Management, 5*(1) (suppl.), S37-S45.

Hill, C. S., Jr. (1993). The barriers to adequate pain with opioid analgesics. *Seminars in Oncology, 20*(2) (suppl. 1), 1-5.

Hill, S. C., Fields, W. S., & Thorpe, D. M. (1989). A call to action to improve relief of cancer pain. *Advances in Pain Research and Therapy, 11,* 353-361.

Jacox, A., Carr, D. B., Payne, R., Berde, C. B., Breitbart, W., Cain, J. M., Chapman, C. R., Cleeland, C. S., Ferrell, B. R., Finley, R. S., Hester, N. O., Hill, C. S., Leak, W. D., Lipman, A. G., Logan, C. L., McGarvey, C. L., Miaskowski, C. A., Mulder, D. S., Paice, J. A., Shapiro, B. S., Silberstein, E. B., Smith, R. S., Stover, J., Tsou, C. V., Vecchiarelli, L., Weissman, D. E. (1994a). *Management of cancer pain. Clinical practice guideline.* AHCPR Pub. No. 94-0592, Rockville, MD: Agency for Health Care Policy and Research, PHS, USDHHS.

Jacox, A., et al. (1994b). *Managing cancer pain. Patient guide.* AHCPR Pub No 94-0595. Rockville, MD: Agency for Health Care Policy and Research, PHS, USDHHS.

Jacox, A., et al. (1994c). *El control del dolor causado por el cancer. Guia para el paciente.* AHCPR Pub. No. 94-0596, Rockville, MD: Agency for Health Care Policy and Research, PHS, USDHHS.

Jacox, A., et al. (1994d). *Management of cancer pain: Adults. Clinical practice guideline.* AHCPR Pub. No. 94-0593. Rockville, MD: Agency for Health Care Policy and Research, PHS, USDHHS.

Johnston, C. C., Jeans, M. E., Abbott, F. V., Grey-Donald, K., & Edgar, L. (1988). A survey of pain in hospitalized children: Preliminary results. In *Proceedings of the 1st International Symposium on Pediatric Pain.* p. 80, Seattle.

Joranson, D. E. (1990). Federal and state regulation of opioids. *Journal of Pain and Symptom Management, 5*(1), S12-S23.

Joranson, D. E. (1994). Are health-care reimbursement policies a barrier to acute and cancer pain management? *Journal of Pain and Symptom Management, 9*(4), 244-253.

Kanner, R., & Cooper, E. S. (1989). Availability of narcotic analgesics for ambulatory patients with pain. *Advances in Pain Research and Therapy, 11,* 191-195.

Kolassa, M. (1994). Guidance for clinicians in discerning and comparing the price of pharmaceutical agents. *Journal of Pain and Symptom Management, 9*(4), 235-243.

Kuhn, S., Cooke, K., Collins, M., Jones, M. J., & Mucklow, J. C. (1990). Perceptions of pain relief after surgery. *British Medical Journal, 300,* 1687-1690.

Lander, J. (1990). Clinical judgments in pain management. *Pain, 42,* 15-22.

Marks, R. M., & Sachar, E. J. (1973). Undertreatment of medical inpatients with narcotic analgesics. *Annals of Internal Medicine, 78*(2), 173-181.

Martin, B. A., & Belcher, J. V. (1986). Influence of cultural background on nurses' attitudes and care of the oncology patient. *Cancer Nursing, 9*(5), 230-237.

Mather, L., & Mackie, J. (1983). The incidence of postoperative pain in children. *Pain, 15*(3), 271-282.

Max, M. B. (1990). Improving outcomes of analgesic treatment: Is education enough? *Annals of Internal Medicine, 113*(11), 885-889.

McCaffery, M., & Ferrell, B. R. (1992). Opioid analgesics: Nurses' knowledge of doses and psychological dependence. *Journal of Nursing Staff Development, 8*(2), 77-84.

McCaffery, M., Ferrell, B. R., O'Neil-Page, E., Lester, M., & Ferrell, B. (1990). Nurses' knowledge of opioid analgesic drugs and psychological dependence. *Cancer Nursing, 13*(1), 21-27.

Miaskowski, C., Nichols, R., Brody, R., & Synold, T. (1994). Assessment of patient satisfaction utilizing the American Pain Society's quality assurance standards on acute and cancer-related pain. *Journal of Pain and Symptom Management, 9*(1), 5-11.

Morgan, A. E., Lindley, C. M., & Berry, J. I. (1994). Assessment of pain and patterns of analgesic use in hospice patients. *American Journal of Hospice and Palliative Care, 11*(1), 13-19, 22-25.

Morgan, J. P. (1989). American opiophobia: Customary underutilization of opioid analgesics. *Advances in Pain Research Therapy, 11,* 181-189.

National Institute for Nursing Research. (1994). *Symptom management: Acute pain. National nursing research agenda.* NIH Pub. No. 94-2421, Bethesda, MD: NINR, NIH, PHS, USDHHS.

Oden, R. (1989). Management of postoperative pain. *Anesthesiology Clinics of North America, 7*(1), xi-xiii.

Owen, H., McMillan, V., & Rogowski, D. (1990). Postoperative pain therapy: A survey of patients' expectations and their experiences. *Pain, 41*(3), 303-307.

Paice, J. A., Mahon, S. M., & Faut-Callahan, M. (1991). Factors associated with adequate pain control in hospitalized postsurgical patients diagnosed with cancer. *Cancer Nursing, 14*(6), 298-305.

Perry, S., Heidrich, G., & Ramos, E. (1981). Assessment of pain by burn patients. *Journal of Burn Care and Rehabilitation, 2*(6), 322-326.

Porter, J., & Jick, H. (1980). Addiction rare in patients treated with narcotics [letter]. *New England Journal of Medicine, 302,* 123.

Purcell-Jones, G., Dormon, F., & Sumner, E. (1988). Paediatric anaesthetists' perceptions of neonatal and infant pain. *Pain, 33,* 181-187.

Ryan, P., Vortherms, R., & Ward, S. (1994). Cancer pain: Knowledge, attitudes of pharmacologic management. *Journal of Gerontological Nursing, 20*(1), 7-16.

Schechter, N. L., Allen, D. A., & Hanson, K. (1986). Status of pediatric pain control: A comparison of hospital analgesic usage in children and adults. *Pediatrics, 77*(1), 11-15.

Shapiro, R. S. (1994a). Legal bases for the control of analgesic drugs. *Journal of Pain and Symptom Management, 9*(3), 153-159.

Shapiro, R. S. (1994b). Liability issues in the management of pain. *Journal of Pain and Symptom Management, 9*(3), 146-152.

Sheidler, V. R., McGuire, D. B., Grossman, S. A., & Gilbert, M. R. (1992). Analgesic decision-making skills of nurses. *Oncology Nursing Forum, 19,* 1531-1534.

Taylor, H., & Curran, N. M. (1985). *The Nuprin pain report (No. 851017).* New York: Louis Harris and Associates.

Teoh, N., & Stjernsward, J. (1992). WHO cancer pain relief program—Ten years on. *IASP Newsletter,* 5-6.

Todd, K. H., Samaroo, N., & Hoffman, J. R. (1993). Ethnicity as a risk factor for inadequate emergency department analgesia. *JAMA, 269,* 1537-1539.

Von Roenn, J. H., Cleeland, C. S., Gonin, R., Hatfield, A. K., & Pandya, K. J. (1993). Physician attitudes and practice in cancer pain management: A survey from the Eastern Cooperative Oncology Group. *Annals of Internal Medicine, 119*(2), 121-126.

Vortherms, R., Ryan, P., & Ward, S. (1992). Knowledge of, attitudes toward, and barriers to pharmacologic management of cancer pain in a statewide random sample of nurses. *Research in Nursing and Health, 15,* 459-466.

Ward, S., & Gatwood, J. (1994). Concerns about reporting pain and using analgesics: A comparison of persons with and without cancer. *Cancer Nursing, 17,* 200-206.

Ward, S. E., Goldberg, N., Miller-McCauley, V., Mueller, C., Nolan, A., Pawlik-Plank, D., Robbins, A., Stormoen, D., & Weissman, D. E. (1993). Patient-related barriers to management of cancer pain. *Pain, 52*(3), 319-324.

Watt-Watson, J. H. (1987). Nurses' knowledge of pain issues: A survey. *Journal of Pain and Symptom Management, 2*(4), 207-211.

Watt-Watson, J. H., Evernden, C., & Lawson, C. (1990). Parents' perceptions of their child's acute pain experience. *Journal of Pediatric Nursing, 5*(5), 344-349.

Watt-Watson, J. H., & Watson, C. P. N. (1989). Pain curriculum. *Canadian Nurse, 85*(9), 44-45.

Weis, O. F., Sriwantanakul, K., Alloza, J. L., Weintraub, M., & Lasagna, L. (1983). Attitudes of patients, housestaff, and nurses toward postoperative analgesic care. *Anesthesia and Analgesia, 62,* 70-74.

World Health Organization. (1990). *Cancer pain relief and palliative care. Report of a WHO expert committee.* World Health Organization Technical Report Series, No. 804. Geneva: World Health Organization, pp. 1-75.

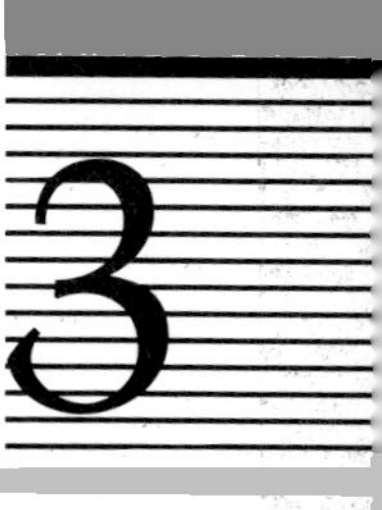

Cultural Aspects of Pain Management

Michael Bozeman

Key Points

- Cultural diversity is a rich resource and invaluable nursing aid rather than a handicap in managing pain and providing optimal patient outcomes.
- One's culture influences perceived causal factors of pain, emotional responses to pain, meaning attached to pain, reported pain intensity, how pain should be treated, and who should treat the pain.
- The foundational element in transcultural nursing is sensitivity to the unique cultural and ethnic differences of each patient. Stereotyping severely limits the ability to adequately assess and treat pain.
- Transcultural assessment requires a thorough cultural history assessment.
- The primary strategy for working with a patient in pain of a different culture is to establish a relationship with the patient by listening, showing respect, and

allowing the patient to help formulate and choose treatment options.

- Pharmacologic effects of medications differ among cultural groups.

Dealing with cultural differences is often viewed as a handicap to health care practitioners, a view that hinders and slows effective patient care and pain management. This chapter presents cultural diversity as a rich resource and an invaluable nursing aid in both managing pain and providing optimal patient outcomes. Transcultural nursing, which is grounded in cultural awareness and sensitivity, leads to cultural synergy that integrates and builds on cultural differences to produce creative and effective pain and symptom management. The clinician must be willing to identify and shed any ethnocentric tendencies (feelings that one's ethnic group and, for the purposes of this chapter, accepted Western medical practices are superior), which prevent cultural appreciation and ultimately hinder the clinician-patient relationship. Effective pain management in a multicultural environment requires fidelity to and respect for the patient's cultural needs and preferences. It also requires an ability to adapt accepted Western health care practices to the particular cultural needs of the patient. This chapter, divided into five sections, discusses the meaning of culture and its relevance to health care, avoidance of ethnocentrism and cultural stereotypes, cultural meanings of pain, cultural assessment and pain management, and transcultural interventions. Also addressed are pharmacologic, nonpharmacologic, and nontraditional interventions.

MEANING AND RELEVANCE OF CULTURE

Culture is a way of life, extending much further than one's country of origin, language, or body features. Social scientists, although differing as to a precise definition of culture, agree that it is a rich tapestry into which are woven language, ritual, values, beliefs, and differing views of illness, pain, suffering, and death. A working definition of culture offered by Bates and Edwards (1992, p. 64) is "the patterned ways in which humans have learned to think about and act in their world." As Harris and Moran (1991) have pointed out, culture can be thought of as primarily a tool for problem solving that helps people cope in their environments and create a distinctive world around them. Cultural orientation is further conditioned by one's ethnic group and the quality of ties to this group. Ethnicity refers to one's social group within the larger culture, which further provides identity and a sense of belonging and gives particular shape to one's values and attitudes. In opposition to the transcultural theory that individuals vary widely within a given culture, stereotyping often overlooks the importance of ethnicity within the larger culture and of cultural differences in one's ethnic group. Researchers have long pointed out the pervasive influence of culture on one's understanding of and attitudes toward pain; individuals respond to pain according to attitudes and behaviors learned within their respective cultures (Zborowski, 1969; Wolff, 1985).

Perhaps because of the increased mobility of families and loss of the extended family, the last two decades have witnessed something of a resurgence of cultural identity and the desire to be grounded beyond one's situation. The "melting pot" theory of cultural blending and assimilation has been a significant social phenomenon during this century, as evidenced by increasing numbers of Americans claiming a multiple ancestry rather than a single country of origin. It is, however, less than an accurate representation of cultural patterns within the United States. Many Americans associate their identities with cultural or ethnic groups. The rich pluralism and multicultural diversity that exemplifies the desire to preserve culture perhaps could be crudely but more accurately described as a "salad bowl" where people desire to retain or reclaim their cultural heritage. Examples of this phenomenon include the strong ethnic communities of "Chinatown" in San Francisco, "Little Haiti" in Miami, and the predominantly African-American "South Side" in Chicago.

Clinicians face enormous challenges as they seek to provide health care to people pouring into the United States from all over the world. Although the percentage of European immigration is decreasing, large numbers of Asians—especially Chinese, Indians, Filipinos, and Vietnamese—as well as Pacific Islanders and Hispanics, are arriving on U.S. shores in increasing numbers. Other cultural groups on the move to the United States include Mexicans, Russians, Indians, Poles, Israelis, Dominicans, Irish, and Germans (Bureau of the Census, 1994). If trends continue, it is estimated that more than 10 million immigrants will settle in the United States this decade alone (Miller, 1994). As Table 3-1 illustrates, this will lead to dramatic shifts in the ethnic makeup of the U.S. population, with the Asian, Pacific Islander, and Hispanic populations growing significantly by the year 2025.

Clinicians will increasingly come into intimate contact with people of cultures other than their own, whose attitudes toward illness, pain, and health care will likely be different from their own. Therefore nursing must be transcultural both in assessing patient needs and in providing appropriate in-

Table 3-1 Census Bureau Projections of U.S. Resident Population

Race	1995	2000	2010	2025
White	218,334,000	226,267,000	240,297,000	261,531,000
Black	33,117,000	35,469,000	40,224,000	48,005,000
Hispanic	26,798,000	31,166,000	40,525,000	56,927,000
Asian and Pacific Islander	9,756,000	12,125,000	17,191,000	25,524,000

Modified from Bureau of the Census. (1994, September). *Statistical abstract of the United States.* (114th ed.). U.S. Dept. of Commerce, Economics and Statistics Division, pp. 24, 25. Figures are approximate projections based on trends. "White" and "black" are Census Bureau terms. Persons listed as "Hispanic" may be of any race.

terventions. This begins with cultural awareness and sensitivity, which requires that the clinician spend time learning from the patient during the assessment process. This learning will allow the clinician to see how strongly the patient identifies with his or her group within the larger culture, which will help to indicate the meaning of pain for the individual and their expectations from the health care provider. It also requires objectivity in terms of allowing the patient to share cultural norms and attitudes rather than engaging in cultural stereotyping, which diminishes the possibility of effective pain management as well as the clinician's appreciation for the richness of the patient and his or her culture. As the cultural face of America changes, the clinician needs to be a cosmopolitan who can function effectively in a variety of cultural settings free from prejudice and provincialism—as the colloquial expression goes, someone who can "think globally and act locally."

When visiting another country, tourists tread lightly at first, curious to learn the customs of the country, often reading brochures and learning at least a few important native expressions both to cope in an alien environment and to show respect for the residents of the particular country. Walking into a patient's room is very similar to stepping into the patient's country of origin. The clinician must first be a "tourist" who, rather than "passing through," tries to learn all that can be learned about the culture of the patient in order to best meet the patient's needs and expectations. Learning, relating, respecting, and providing helpful interventions depends, to a large degree, on the clinician's openness to studying the patient's particular culture.

AVOIDING ETHNOCENTRISM AND CULTURAL STEREOTYPES

A person's culture has been called his or her "assumptive world" (Cantril, 1950, p. 87; Frank & Frank, 1991, pp. 24-34). That is, what is assumed to be the norm in a culture shapes the individual's assumptions and expectations of others and their cultures. For example, if we have been brought up to greet someone by shaking hands, we will naturally assume that this is the "acceptable" way for all persons to show respect until we witness other ways of greeting, such as bowing the head or kissing the cheek. Although to some degree this is unavoidable, mistaken assumptions and ethnocentrism can be decreased by valuing and learning from differences and by appreciating diversity. Ethnocentrism invariably leads to stereotyping, or viewing all persons of a certain culture or ethnic group as alike and not being cognizant of significant differences. In terms of managing pain, cultural stereotyping not only decreases the likelihood of effective pain and symptom management, but it prevents any opportunity for professional growth or broadening of the clinician's world.

"Generalizing," however, can be a positive activity so long as it incorporates the consideration that the patient may not fit the generalizations assumed about the larger culture (Geissler, 1994). Generalizing begins with some assumptions based on the patient's culture, which are constantly revised as the clinician has more contact with the patient and hence develops increased understanding of the patient's cultural characteristics (Geissler, 1994). Although it is helpful to have an internal as well as a written cultural "data bank" on the various constituencies served by the particular health care provider, any such data bank needs to consider the wide variety of differences within a given culture. For example, to assume that a patient from India is Hindu when in fact she is Muslim or Buddhist may have profound negative implications for the clinician-patient relationship. The same is true for the assumption that all Hindus are alike in customs and beliefs. The challenge in using generalizations is to use them as a starting place for understanding and to avoid drawing stereotypic conclusions (Geissler, 1994).

It is difficult to make conclusions about ethnic and cultural differences in pain severity because age, gender, education, religion, socioeconomic class, and acculturation are additional, confounding factors (Faucett, Gordon, & Levine, 1994). Bates and Edwards (1992, p. 79) reported that "within several ethnic groups, those who are immigrants or first-generation U.S.-born, who have high degrees of heritage consistency, and who believe they have strong support of family and friends report less severe (although not necessarily less expressive) responses to the pain in several areas." Thus patients who maintain strong ethnic ties will be less likely to assimilate or respond to pain than the typical middle-class American (Bates, Edwards, & Anderson, 1993).

Although some clinicians will quickly deny any ethnocentrism or prejudice in their associations with others, and especially in their work with patients, in reality very few individuals are free of negative feelings about some cultural or ethnic group. One cannot easily shed childhood or ethnic influences that portray other groups negatively, especially when these have been strongly ingrained over a number of years. Overcoming these influences is not usually accomplished through attending a course in ethnic appreciation or reading an article on how to avoid prejudice. Although gaining secondhand "classroom" knowledge of ethnic appreciation is helpful, because ethnocentrism and prejudice are born primarily of fear and insecurity, individuals who become more culturally accepting and appreciative usually do so through positive personal associations with those of other cultures and ethnic groups. These personal associations and friendships challenge one's assumptions and fears, increase one's sense of security and self-esteem, and gradually lead to a positive revision in how one perceives others. An ancient Native American proverb is a helpful reminder: "Don't try to understand me unless you've walked a mile in my shoes." For the clinician, understanding the patient of another culture or ethnic group may involve the courage to leave one's cultural comfort zone and step *into* the patient's world rather than "reading up" on the patient's ways or customs.

CULTURAL VARIATIONS IN THE EXPERIENCE OF PAIN

Culture greatly influences one's response to pain. Culture influences (a) perceived causal factors of pain (e.g., fate, lifestyle, punishment, witchcraft); (b) emotional responses to pain, including appropriate and inappropriate expressions of pain; (c) meaning attached to pain; (d) reported pain intensity; (e) feelings of how pain should be treated; and (f) beliefs on who should treat the pain. As stated in Chapter 1, a helpful definition for understanding the subjective nature of pain is that "pain is whatever the experiencing person says it is, existing whenever the experiencing person says it does" (McCaffery & Beebe, 1989, p. 7). Pain is not only physiologic but is a multidimensional phenomenon experienced on many different levels, including affective and cognitive. The cognitive dimension of pain is especially influenced by culture in that one's total upbringing, experiences, and memory determines the experience of pain.

Although it is not the purpose of this section to provide an exhaustive comparative examination of cultural variations in the experience of pain, some variations will be mentioned to demonstrate that cultural differences must be considered in achieving effective pain management. Although most of what is known about pain has been observed through the "lens" of the medical profession, which has focused on the physiologic and neurologic experience of pain, a growing body of research suggests that pain is as much a cultural and social experience as it is a biologic and psychologic one. In his classic work on cultural and social aspects of the pain experience, Zborowski (1969) studied the pain responses of four European ethnic groups in a Veterans' Administration hospital, all of which consisted of men suffering from chronic back pain. These ethnic groups were first-generation or second-generation Jewish, Italian, and Irish and a fourth group of third-generation "Old American" or predominantly Anglo-Saxon Protestant. Whereas both the "Old American" and Irish men were typically unexpressive and unemotional, avoiding crying or complaining, the Italian and Jewish men were emotional and expressive in their responses to pain.

Zatzick and Dimsdale (1990, p. 553) have stated that "first and second generation immigrants are more likely to retain idiosyncratic beliefs and behaviors that may influence the response to painful stimuli." Later generations are believed to be less apt or more limited in their expression of ethnic behaviors. Thus pain tolerance, which is considered a reflection of the behavioral response to pain, is more influenced culturally than pain threshold. Intergroup and intragroup variations abound (Zatzick & Dimsdale, 1990), so more research is needed to identify the variables that most influence an individual patient's response to pain.

Whereas the "Old American" and Irish men viewed their pain as a private occurrence that made them tend to withdraw from others, the Jewish and Italian men desired the presence of family and friends. The psychologic state of the men also differed among groups in terms of the effect of the pain on one's general outlook on life. Zborowski (1969) concluded that the response to pain is affected by beliefs, attitudes, and behaviors learned by the individual within his or her particular culture and serves different functions in different cultures. Since Zborowski's study, interethnic differences have been studied among chronic pain patients of Japanese, Italian, Polish, African-American, Puerto Rican, French Canadian, New Zealander, Mexican, Columbian, and other European groups. Comparative studies in pain have also been made between Americans and cultural groups living outside of the United States. Although some may view their pain as a medical problem, studies have indicated that chronic pain may be experienced as a personal, social (Kotarba, 1977, 1983), or spiritual (Ohnuki-Tierney, 1984) issue, which suggests the importance of psychospiritual interventions. Weisenberg and Caspi (1989) found that Western women rated their delivery pain as less intense than Middle Eastern women.

Pain studies have also indicated that the experience of pain is affected by influencces other than culture and ethnicity. Lawlis, Achterberg, Kenner, and Kopetz (1984) and Kleinman (1988) examined the role of gender in the experience of pain and noted that women tend to express their pain more frequently and openly than men. Bendelow (1993) reported similar findings using a phenomenologic approach with 53 men and 54 women. Two statistically significant gender differences in the perception of pain were noted: the role of emotions in the process and social expectations of the ability to cope with the pain. Most of the subjects felt that women coped better with pain than men. The experience of pain also differs by socioeconomic class (Haywood et al., 1993), religion (Lambert, Libman, & Poser, 1960; Poser, 1963), and education (Weisenberg & Caspi, 1989).

Bates and colleagues (1993) studied pain intensity of 372 chronic pain patients from six ethnic groups at a multidisciplinary pain treatment center. The researchers found that "ethnocultural affiliation is important to chronic pain perception and response variation" (p. 101) and that "it appears that pain intensity variation may be affected by differences in attitudes, beliefs and emotional and psychological states associated with the different ethnic groups" (p. 101).

Meanings and perceptions of pain vary significantly from culture to culture. In the West, body locations where pain is experienced are not usually viewed as symbolic of emotional or spiritual imbalance. Eastern cultures, on the other hand, attach much symbolism to the location of pain. For example, to many Japanese abdominal pain is viewed as the result of an emotional or spiritual imbalance since the abdomen represents the seat of the soul (Ohnuki-Tierney, 1984). Eastern cultures often place importance on the "chakras," or perceived energy centers of the body, which must be unblocked and balanced for healing to take place. For example, most Chinese do not view the body as organs and tissues that perform vital functions; rather, "the body consists of energy spheres to which physically demonstrable organs and tissues are attached" (Tu, 1987, p. 147). For pain treatment, medical interventions such as acupuncture must be directed at restoring the vitality of or unblocking each of these energy centers, since pain is caused by a blockage in the flow of energy. (See Chapter 7 for further information.)

In Hindu philosophy, physical pain and the body are inconsequential compared with the immortality of the soul. It is believed that the self can transcend and control the experience of pain. Therapy is directed at the spirit, not the body, with the goal of strengthening the patient's spiritual resources and attitude (Pandya, 1987). Prescribing large doses of medication to patients in intractable pain is unacceptable in Hindu philosophy because it reduces the patient's ability to draw upon inner resources to transcend pain (Pandya). Muslims similarly believe that the patient must not be too lethargic from medication to recite scripture from the Qur'an and pray to Allah (The Qur'an, 1990 ed.).

Cultures that have been affected by African influences, such as Haitian and Hispanic, may believe that pain is caused by either voodoo (vodoun) or witchcraft, in which another person is responsible for the patient's illness and pain. Pain and illness therefore may be understood as "cause and effect" and not as natural or accidental processes. Patients may be nonreceptive to Western medication, not because they are opposed to it, but because of the belief that spiritually based illness and pain must be dealt with on spiritual terms through a spiritual person who can break the "spell" cast on the afflicted person (Porter & Porter, 1993). In other words, perceived causal factors for illness vary from culture to culture. To the patient, the cause of the illness may be as significant as the illness itself. Moreover, the patient may perceive the problem as being much deeper than the illness itself.

In contrast with the notion that illness is primarily caused by malicious human intervention, some Christians believe that illness can be a form of punishment from God for wrongdoing. Many Christians believe that confession or faith healing may be necessary to remove or manage illness. Other cultures attach less significance to causal factors. For example, many Jews, downplaying causal factors of pain, turn their attention to finding meaning and hope in the midst of suffering. For many Holocaust survivors, the experience of pain brings memories of coping and surviving in concentration camps, and these memories often serve as tools to deal with present pain. In the Catholic tradition, pain and suffering are to be accepted rather than questioned and are an opportunity for spiritual growth as well as an opportunity to share in the crucifixion and resurrection of Christ (O'Rourke, 1992).

Although there are many other cultural groups and aspects of pain and culture that could be mentioned, the lesson is that the experience of pain is culturally determined and that the clinician must carefully listen for these differences. The clinician should be mindful that each individual's expression of pain is different; people associate different meanings with pain and have different goals for treatment. Therefore it is necessary to consider using teaching methods and instruments appropriate for the individual's culture.

CULTURAL ASSESSMENT AND PAIN MANAGEMENT

An openness to revise one's "assumptive world" leads to cultural sensitivity, which, for the clinician, leads to more effective assessment of the patient's needs and expectations. This requires an understanding that although Western medicine is "advanced," certain standard clinical interventions for pain treatment were developed out of Western values. An example is the treatment of arthritic pain with a mild analgesic whereas the standard intervention in another culture may be acupuncture. For interventions to be appropriate and effective, they may need to be very different for two patients of different cultures as well as for patients within the same culture with the same condition.

Most research reports describing the measurement of pain do not mention the ethnicity of the subjects involved (Wilkie, Savedra, Holzemer, Tesler, & Paul, 1990). For this reason, Turk (1989) calls pain an elusive construct that is difficult to measure. For many pain measurement instruments, the assumption must be made that all individuals respond to pain descriptors in the same manner. However, pain is a multidimensional and highly individual phenomenon.

Because some persons are threatened by questionnaires or an interrogative type of communication, cultural and pain assessment may be best accomplished using conversation rather than a question-and-answer format, with clues taken from the patient's comfort level and body language. Patients should be questioned and prompted using language such as: "Tell me about your family." "Tell me about your pain."

"What do people believe about illness in your culture?" "What are some of the causes?" "How do people deal with it?" These are preferable to questions that make the patient feel evaluated or uncomfortable in responding.

Assessment must go beyond fitting the patient within one's routine assessment parameters. Many if not most Western pain assessment instruments focus heavily on the physical aspects of pain assessment. Assessment instruments are often inadequate means for performing effective transcultural or pain assessment since such instruments are culturally influenced. This is especially true for patients who (a) view illness and pain as being nonphysically or spiritually based, (b) feel it is unacceptable to express pain or significantly limit expressions of pain, or (c) are reluctant to discuss pain because of the age, culture, gender, or discipline of the clinician (e.g., nurse as opposed to spiritual healer).

In general, most people of other cultures like to discuss aspects of their culture and feel respected when clinicians invite them to share their preferences and customs before initiating treatment. The initial goal, therefore, is to make the patient feel comfortable and as nonthreatened as possible so that he or she is willing to share useful information with the clinician (Pachter, 1994). It is also important to recognize that transcultural assessment is a continual process as the clinician learns more from the patient, the patient's family, and other clinicians in contact with the patient and family. Whereas initial assessments in Western medical environments are sometimes completed during an initial visit with the patient, this may not be the case for a transcultural assessment. Knowledge of the patient's culture evolves over time as rapport is established and more personal information is shared with the clinician.

INTERVENTIONS

As stated previously, cultural differences are often seen as a handicap to effective nursing. Dealing with language difficulties, relating to people who think and behave differently, and taking the time to understand the customs and preferences of the patient can be a laborious task. There may also be an uneasiness that the clinician, no matter how sensitive, does not understand the needs of the patient sufficiently to provide optimal treatment outcomes. Healing involves more than appropriate assessment and interventions. It is aided by the patient's perception that the clinician has sought to provide understanding and concern, even if needs are not completely met. Most people of other cultures have experienced being misunderstood and at times treated with insensitivity, and their expectations may be that health care providers will be no different. Showing sensitivity and working with the patient to address his or her needs may significantly surpass the patient's expectations, even if needs are not completely addressed. When the clinician and patient explore and build on each other's cultural resources to achieve effective pain and symptom management (synergy), patient outcomes may exceed original expectations.

The primary strategy for working with a patient in pain from a different culture is to establish a relationship by listening, showing respect, and allowing the patient to help formulate and choose treatment options. The quality of the relationship is an important component in providing pain relief. Since the clinician may not understand non-Western pain remedies, the patient must be free to ask for what is needed. It is also important to respect the patient's attitudes and beliefs about pain, as well as preferred treatment options, even if these are in conflict with the clinician's beliefs about pain treatment. For example, if a patient prefers folk remedies to an opioid for pain relief, the clinician needs to honor the patient's preferences if approved by the health care provider. During the assessment process the clinician may explore patient beliefs about combining therapies so that the patient is made familiar with a range of pain treatment options.

Research is gradually uncovering much needed information about significant variances in the pharmacologic effects of medications on cultural groups (Levy, 1993). These variances include many types of drugs, as shown in Table 3-2. To individualize the drug regimen for each patient, the nurse

Table 3-2 Ethnic and Racial Differences in Response to CNS Agents

Comparison Groups	Drug Class/Example	Clinical Response
Chinese/whites	Benzodiazepines (diazepam, alprazolam)	Chinese require lower doses; more sensative to sedative effects
Chinese/whites Hispanics/Anglos	Antidepressants (imipramine, desipramine, amitriptyline, cloipramine)	Chinese and Hispanics require lower doses; side effects greater in Hispanics
Asians/whites	Neuroleptics (e.g., haloperidol)	Asians require lower doses
Asian Indians/whites	Analgesics (e.g., acetaminophen, codeine)	Asian Indians have greater clearance rates
Chinese/whites	Analgesics (e.g., morphine)	Chinese less sensitive to cardiovascular and respiratory effects, but more sensitive to GI side effects
Asians/whites	Alcohol	Asians more sensitive to side effects
Native Americans/ whites	Alcohol	Native Americans have faster metabolism and less tolerance

From McKenry, L., & Salerno, E. (1995). *Mosby's pharmacology in nursing,* (19th ed.). St. Louis: Mosby.

needs to note these differences among cultural groups and ask the patient about prior use of the particular drug. Fortunately, the vast majority of pharmaceutical companies now include minorities in their clinical trial groups for testing and evaluating drugs (Levy, 1993).

The clinician also needs to be aware that the patient may never have taken a Western medication or may have a very limited experience with prescription and OTC drugs. It is important to explain the drug's purpose and the side effects the

TRANSCULTURAL ASSESSMENT

It is important to make the assessment a "conversation" rather than a question-and-answer session. Many of the following questions—such as "What is the usual distance when talking?"—are answered from observation. The clinician needs to tailor questions to the specific situation, always noting signs of patient discomfort. The clinician is not expected be able to assess the patient on all of the following questions. The goal is to gain as much information about the patient's cultural preferences and customs as possible.

1. **Social structure and family:**

   What is the patient's country of origin? Parent's origin?

   Who makes the decisions? The patient? The patient and family? The oldest?

   Are families matriarchal or patriarchal? What are the roles and expectations of women and children?

   How do the patient's views and attitudes vary (ethnicity) within his or her cultural group? What is known about the particular culture and ethnic group, and are these generalizations accurate for the patient? How do they need to be revised?

2. **Views on health care:**

   Who should be told of the illness? How should the news be conveyed?

   What are the patient's views on self-determination?

   What are the roles of the physician and nurse?

   What are common treatments and interventions for pain and other symptoms?

3. **Attitudes and beliefs about illness, pain, and suffering:**

   To what does the patient attribute the illness, pain, or suffering?

   What remedies (traditional and nontraditional) are acceptable to the patient?

TRANSCULTURAL ASSESSMENT—cont'd

What is known or believed by the patient about Western medications? What Western medications has the patient received?

Are there other "folk" remedies (such as herbal "teas," rituals, laying on of hands, or acupuncture) believed to be helpful?

Is the person puzzled by, fearful of, or accepting of illness, pain, and suffering?

To what degree is it acceptable to the patient to express and complain about pain, and how is this expressed?

What role does suffering play? For example, is it punishment from God, a "curse" from another person, a form of testing, or a source of meaning?

What role does religion play in the illness and experience of pain?

Where are meaning and hope derived from? The present? The afterlife?

What other rituals or resources can provide pain relief or help the patient feel comfortable?

4. **Communication and building relationships:**

What is the primary means of communication? Verbal or nonverbal?

What languages does the patient speak?

Would the patient prefer someone who speaks his or her primary language?

What is the usual distance when talking? (Two feet? Four feet?)

Are promises viewed as "oaths" that are binding?

Are there taboos such as handshaking, touching, eye contact between males and females, or other customs that may affect the provision of health care?

Continued.

TRANSCULTURAL ASSESSMENT—cont'd

How are "outsiders" viewed? What is the process for building trust?

5. **Diet and food:**

What are customary foods? What foods may not be eaten?

Does the patient need permission from a spiritual leader to eat food (e.g., Muslims)?

What preparation must be made to eat food (e.g., special hand washing rituals)?

Do certain foods have symbolic meaning?

patient may experience. If the patient desires to use an herbal remedy, it is equally important to evaluate the herb's properties and interactions with other medications prescribed. *The Honest Herbal* (Tyler, 1993) lists over 100 herbs and related remedies with helpful, brief descriptions of their uses. This book provides a "quick reference" summary chart (pp. 336-351) in which the uses, "efficacy," and safety of each herb and remedy are easily identified.

The clinician should be open to exploring nontraditional interventions with the patient. These include relaxation and imagery as well as all of the expressive therapies, especially music and art therapy, therapeutic touch involving the balancing of energy centers, acupuncture or acupressure, and spiritual and religious interventions associated with the patient's pain or culture. Such interventions are reviewed in the chapters on nonpharmacologic and alternative pain management in this book.

Whereas in the United States the patient's right to be informed of an illness by the physician as well as to choose treatment options is valued and respected, to many Japanese and Ethiopians, as well as other cultural groups, disclosing "bad news" to the patient is viewed as either inappropriate, harmful, or both (Beyene, 1992; Gordon, 1991; Holland,

1987). As Beyene points out in referring to the inappropriateness of frank disclosure of terminal illness to Ethiopian patients, who to tell and what to tell are deeply embedded in culture (Beyene). (See the previous box on transcultural assessment.)

SUMMARY

Effective transcultural nursing demands sensitivity, patience, and creativity. Treatment plans are not quickly or easily formulated, especially where there are significant language barriers or when the patient views the cause or treatment of the illness as nonmedical. Transcultural nursing is, however, unavoidable as health care organizations seek to meet the health care needs of an increasingly multicultural U.S. population. The clinician may not be from a comparable culture or religion; therefore the key is to assess the patient's needs, ways, and customs as thoroughly and sensitively as possible. This helps to establish a relationship in which the patient feels heard and respected and is more likely to explore treatment options with the clinician. The time spent can often result in cultural synergy in which the clinician and patient build on each other's cultural differences and resources to creatively and effectively address not only the patient's pain but a variety of physical, emotional, and spiritual needs.

References

Bates, M. S., & Edwards, W. T. (1992). Ethnic variations in the chronic pain experience. *Ethnicity and Disease, 2*(1), 63-68.

Bates, M. S., Edwards, W. T., & Anderson, K. O. (1993). Ethnocultural influences on variation in chronic pain perception. *Pain, 52*(1), 79, 101-112.

Bendelow, G. (1993). Pain perceptions, emotions and gender. *Sociology of Health and Illness, 15*(3), 273-294.

Beyene, Y. (1992). Medical disclosure and refugees: Telling bad news to Ethiopian patients. *Western Journal of Medicine,* September, 328-332.

Bureau of the Census, (1994, September). *Statistical abstract of the United States* (114th ed.). U.S. Department of Commerce, Economics and Statistics Division, pp. 11-25.

Cantril, H. (1950). *The "why" of man's experience.* New York: Macmillian, p. 87.

Faucett, J., Gordon, N., & Levine, J. (1994). Differences in postoperative pain severity among four ethnic groups. *Journal of Pain and Symptom Management, 9*(6), 383-389.

Frank, J. D. & Frank, J. B. (1991). *Persuasion and healing* (3rd ed.). Baltimore: Johns Hopkins University Press, pp. 24-34.

Geissler, E. (1994). *Pocket guide to cultural assessment.* St. Louis: Mosby, pp. xiii-xv.

Gordon, D. R. (1991). Culture, cancer, and communication in Italy. *Anthropological Medicine,* July, 137-159.

Harris, P. R., & Moran, R. T. (1991). *Managing cultural differences* (3rd ed.). Houston: Gulf Publishing, p. 23.

Haywood, L., Ell, K., deGuman, M., Norris, S., Blumfield, D., & Sobel, E. (1993). Chest pain admissions: Characteristics of black, Latino, and white patients in low- and mid-socioeconomic strata. *Journal of the National Medical Association, 85*(10), 749-757.

Holland, J. C., (1987). An international survey of physician attitude and practice in regard to revealing the diagnosis of cancer. *Cancer Investigation, 5,* 151-154.

Kleinman, A. (1988). *The illness narratives.* New York: Basic Books.

Kotarba, J. (1977). The chronic pain experience. In J. D. Douglas (Ed.), *Existential sociology.* (pp. 257-272). Cambridge: Cambridge University Press.

Kotarba, J. (1983). *Chronic pain: Its social dimensions.* Beverly Hills: Sage.

Lambert, W. E., Libman, E., & Poser, E. G. (1960). The effects of increased salience of a membership group on pain tolerance. *Journal of Personality, 38,* 350-357.

Lawlis, G., Achterberg, J., Kenner, L., & Kopetz, K. (1984). Ethnic and sex differences in response to clinical and induced pain in chronic spinal pain patients. *Spine, 9,* 751-754.

Levy, R. A. (1993). *Ethnic and racial differences in response to medicines. Preserving individualized therapy in managed pharmaceutical programs.* Reston, VA: National Pharmaceutical Council, p. 3.

McCaffery, M., & Beebe, A. (1989). *Pain: Clinical manual for nursing practice.* St. Louis: Mosby.

Miller, J. (1994). Assimilation enriches America's melting pot. *Insight on the News, 10*(3), 20.

Ohnuki-Tierney, E. (1984). *Illness and culture in contemporary Japan.* Cambridge: Cambridge University Press, pp. 56-60.

O'Rourke, K. (1992). Pain relief: The Catholic perspective. *Journal of Pain and Symptom Management,* 7(8), 485-491.

Pachter, L. M. (1994). Culture and clinical care—Folk illness beliefs and behaviors and their implications for health care delivery. *Journal of the American Medical Association, 271*(9), 690-694.

Pandya, S. K. (1987). Hindu philosophy on pain: An outline. *Acta Neurochirurgica, 38*(suppl.), 136-146.

Porter, E. T., & Porter, L. K. (1993). Haiti: Death and dying issues. Unpublished manuscript.

Poser, E. (1963). Some psychosocial determinants of pain tolerance. Paper presented at the 16th International Congress of Psychology, Washington, D.C.

The Qur'an. (1990). 6th U.S. ed. Elmhurst, NY: Tahrike Tarsile Qur'an.

Tu, W. M. (1987). A Chinese perspective on pain. *Acta Neurochirurgica, 38*(suppl.), 147.

Turk, D. C. (1989). Assessment of pain: The elusiveness of latent constructs. In C. R. Chapman & J. D. Loeser (Eds.), *Issues in pain management.* New York: Raven Press.

Tyler, V. (1993). *The honest herbal* (3rd ed.). Binghamton, NY: Haworth Press.

Weisenberg, M., & Caspi, Z. (1989). Cultural and educational influences on pain of childbirth. *Journal of Pain and Symptom Management, 4,* 13-19.

Wilkie, D. J., Savedra, M. C., Holzemer, W. L., Tesler, M. D., & Paul, S. M. (1990). Use of the McGill Pain Questionnaire to measure pain: A meta-analysis. *Nursing Research, 39*(1), 36-41.

Wolff, B. B. (1985). Ethnocultural factors influencing pain and illness behavior. *Clinical Journal of Pain, 1,* 23-30.

Zatzick, D. F., & Dimsdale, J. E. (1990). Cultural variations in response to painful stimuli. *Psychosomatic Medicine, 52,* 544-557.

Zborowski, M. (1969). *People in pain.* San Francisco: Jossey-Bass.

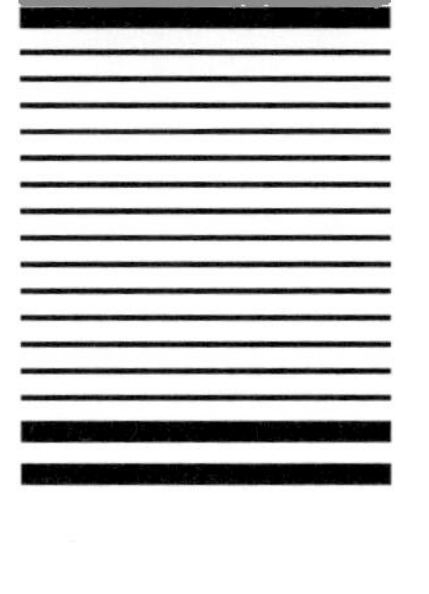

SECTION TWO

Therapeutic Approaches to Pain Management

4

Pharmacologic Approaches

Evelyn Salerno

Key Points

- Pain is a universal health problem; it is more distressing and disabling than nearly any other patient symptom.
- The currently available analgesics are potent and adequate to treat mild to very severe pain, if properly utilized.
- Analgesics are selected according to the patient's diagnosis, concurrent illnesses, and the degree of pain as identified by the patient.
- Application of the opioid agonist, agonist-antagonist, nonopioid, and adjuvant analgesics is based on their pharmacokinetics, clinical indicators, and individual patient presentation.
- Fear of dependence, tolerance, and addiction does not justify withholding opioid analgesics in patients suffering with pain.
- Adhere to established ceiling dose levels for acetaminophen, the NSAIDs, and the nonopioid with opioid drug combinations. Monitor for serious side or adverse drug effects.
- Provide information to the patient, family, and patient caregivers about the safe and effective use of analgesics.

This chapter will review the pharmacokinetics, clinical indicators, major drug interactions, and dosage guidelines for the various pharmacologic agents used to treat pain. The review is divided into four sections: opioid agonist analgesics (morphine, hydromorphone, etc.), opioid agonist-antagonist and partial agonist analgesics (buprenorphine, pentazocine, etc.), nonopioid analgesics (acetaminophen and the NSAIDs), and the adjuvant medications (anticonvulsants, antidepressants, etc.). To properly treat and monitor a patient in pain, the nurse needs to be informed regarding the pharmacologic principles of the various analgesic and adjuvant medications and the step approach to pain management, that is, the appropriate medications to treat mild, moderate, and severe pain. (See Chapter 10 for the World Health Organization's ladder approach to treating cancer pain.)

OPIOID AGONIST ANALGESICS

Opioid Receptor Activity

The term *agonist* means "to do," and the term *antagonist* means "to block." Opioids have been classified as agonist, partial agonist, or mixed agonist-antagonist medications. An agonist drug binds with the receptor(s) to activate and produce the maximum response of the individual receptor, whereas a partial agonist produces a partial response. A mixed agonist-antagonist substance will produce mixed effects; that is, it will activate one type of receptor (agonist) and block a different receptor (antagonist). Selected examples of these classifications are listed in Table 4-1.

The mechanism of action for opioids is related to their binding to specific opioid receptors in and outside of the central nervous system (CNS) (Jacox et al., 1994). Although a number of types and subtypes of receptors have been identified, the primary opioid receptors concentrated in the CNS are the mu (μ), kappa (κ), delta (δ), and sigma (σ) receptors. Analgesia has been associated with μ-, κ-, and δ-receptors, but research with the δ-receptor is limited, primarily due to the lack of a strong δ-agonist; therefore, only μ- and κ-receptors will

Table 4-1 Selected Opioid Receptor Responses

Receptor	Medication Examples	Response
Mu	Strong agonist: morphine, hydromorphone Partial agonist: buprenorphine Weak agonist: meperidine	Supraspinal analgesia, euphoria, respiratory depression, sedation, constipation, urinary retention, drug dependence
	Antagonist: naloxone, nalbuphine	Reverses opioid effects, induces acute withdrawal in opioid dependency
Kappa	Agonist: pentazocine, morphine Little or no activity: levorphanol, methadone, meperidine	Spinal analgesia, sedation
	Antagonist: naloxone, buprenorphine	Reverses opioid effects, induces acute withdrawal in opioid dependency

be discussed in this chapter (Twycross, 1994). σ-Receptors are primarily associated with psychotomimetic or unwanted effects, such as dysphoria, hallucinations, and confusion. The opioid agonist-antagonist drugs, especially pentazocine (Talwin), may induce these undesirable effects as a result of their σ-receptor activity. Agonist-antagonist medications may also cause an acute withdrawal reaction and enhanced pain if administered to opioid-dependent patients or if given concurrently with an opioid in a clinical setting (Carr et al., 1992a). See Table 4-1 for analgesic receptor effects.

Morphine

Morphine is the prototype opioid most commonly prescribed for the treatment of moderate to severe pain. On the World Health Organization (WHO) ladder (1990) for the treatment of cancer and palliative care, morphine and other agonist opioids are used to treat step 3, or severe pain. See Figure 4-1. Morphine is available in various dosage forms and is admin-

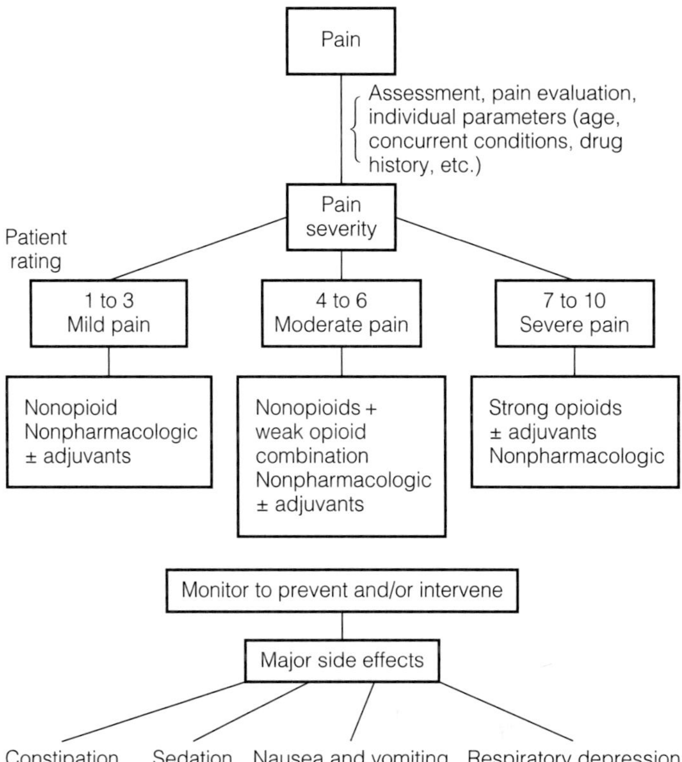

Figure 4-1 Pharmacologic approaches flow chart.

istered through a wide variety of routes, depending on the patient's diagnosis, physical condition, and individual response (Table 4-2). It is considered the drug of choice for cancer pain (Jacox et al., 1994).

Morphine has additional pharmacologic effects that are useful in treating symptoms other than pain. For example, morphine may be used in the treatment of clients with lung cancer, to treat pain aggravated by coughing or an unproductive nagging cough. Small doses of morphine may cause

Table 4-2 Morphine Analgesic Dosage and Administration

Route*	Adult Dosage
IV	4-10 mg diluted in 4-5 ml sterile water administered slowly
IM	5-20 mg every 4 hr
SC	5-20 mg every 4 hr
Epidural	1-5 mg initially; assess in 1 hr; if inadequate for pain relief, 1-2 mg increments may be administered; 10 mg in 24 hr maximum
Intrathecal	0.2-1 mg as single dose only; repeated dosage by this route not recommended
Oral (individualized)	Initially 10-30 mg every 4 hr for morphine sulfate syrup, oral solution, and tablets; may be increased according to pain severity and client's response
Rectal suppositories	20-30 mg rectally every 4-6 hr

From McKenry, L., & Salerno, E. (1995). *Mosby's pharmacology in nursing* (19th ed.). St. Louis: Mosby.
**IV*, Intravenous; *IM*, intramuscular; *SC*, subcutaneous.

depression of the cough center, and this secondary effect is useful in selected situations. For patients with a cough caused by a cold, less potent and potentially safer medications, such as codeine or the nonnarcotic antitussive dextromethorphan, are usually preferred.

Another indication for morphine therapy is the treatment of acute pulmonary edema secondary to congestive heart failure or left ventricular failure. Morphine's peripheral vasodilation effect on veins and arteries can be very useful in decreasing heart workload, resulting in enhanced cardiac function and a reduction of fluid in the lungs. Morphine's effectiveness in treating myocardial infarction is due to (a) its failure to significantly alter heart rate and blood pressure at the usual dosages and (b) its calming effect, which along with the peripheral vasodilation effect may result in a decreased cardiac workload (McKenry & Salerno, 1995).

Morphine may be administered orally, intramuscularly, intravenously, subcutaneously, epidurally, intrathecally, or rectally. For onset, peak, and duration of action, see Table 4-3. Morphine is distributed widely in body tissues, is metabolized in the liver primarily to morphine 3-glucuronide (M3G) and morphine 6-glucuronide (M6G, an active metabolite), and is excreted primarily by the kidneys.

The most frequently reported side effects of morphine and the other opioids are related to their receptor stimulation effects, which include vertigo, constipation, fatigue, sedation, nausea and vomiting, increased sweating, and hypotension. Less frequently reported side effects include dry mouth, headache, anorexia, abdominal cramping, anxiety, mental confusion, urinary retention or painful urination, visual disturbances, and nightmares.

Among the more serious adverse reactions reported are seizures (particularly with meperidine and propoxyphene), tinnitus, jaundice (hepatic toxicity), pruritus, skin rash or facial edema (allergic reaction), breathing difficulties,

Table 4-3 Pharmacokinetics of Morphine Dosage Forms

Dosage Form	Onset of Action (min)	Peak Effect (min)	Duration of Action (hr)
Oral			
Solution,* syrup,† tablets	10-30	60-120	4-5
Extended-release tablets‡	—	—	8-12
IM	10-30	30-60	4-5
IV		20	4-5
SC	10-30	50-90	4-5
Epidural§	15-60	—	Up to 24
Intrathecal§	15-60	—	Up to 24
Rectal‖	20-60	—	4-5

*Roxanol, M.O.S., MSIR.
†Morphite, Morphitex-1, Morphitec-5 (not commercially available in United States).
‡MS Contin, Roxanol SR.
§Duramorph (preservative-free).
‖RMS suppositories.

respiratory depression, excitability (paradoxical reaction seen mainly in children), confusion, and tachycardia.

Analgesic Drug Interactions

Each patient's drug regimen should be assessed for possible drug interactions. Following is a list of significant drug interactions, potential effects, and management.

When morphine or another opioid is given with:

1. Alcohol or other CNS depressant drugs, enhanced CNS depression, respiratory depression, and hypotension may result. The dosage of one or both drugs should be reduced and the patient monitored closely for decreased respiratory rate, blood pressure, slowed reflexes, and drowsiness.
2. Buprenorphine, an additive effect of respiratory depression may result if given concurrently with low doses of a μ-receptor agonist or a κ-receptor agonist. Avoid concurrent usage. Buprenorphine has partial agonist effects on the μ-receptor. If given prior to or after an opioid agonist, it may reduce the analgesic effects of the opioid.
3. Carbamazepine administered concurrently with propoxyphene, the carbamazepine metabolism may be reduced, resulting in an increased carbamazepine serum level, which increases the potential for toxicity. Avoid concurrent drug administration.
4. Monamine oxidase (MAO) inhibitor drugs, such as procarbazine (Matulane), phenelzine (Nardil), and tranylcypromine (Parnate), or in patients who have received an MAO inhibitor within the previous 2 to 3 weeks. Concurrent administration with meperidine has resulted in very severe and even fatal reactions. The effects include sudden excitation, increased sweating, rigidity, severe hypertension (or hypotension), coma, seizures, hyperpyrexia, and collapse. Smaller doses of other opioids may be used cautiously with close monitoring. It is also suggested

that the opioid dose be tested by administering one quarter of the usual prescribed dose to ascertain compatibility of the medications (USP DI, 1994).

5. Phenytoin and rifampin chronically administered, methadone metabolism may be increased, resulting in withdrawal symptoms in persons treated for opioid dependence. They should be monitored closely, as methadone drug dosages may need to be adjusted (USP DI, 1994).
6. Morphine and zidovudine (AZT, Retrovir), hepatic metabolism and zidovudine excretion may be inhibited, resulting in toxicity of either or both drugs. Therefore, concurrent drug use is not recommended (USP DI, 1994).

Other Selected Opioids

Opium Preparations

Opium contains several alkaloids, including morphine and small amounts of codeine and papaverine. The effects of opium result from the presence of morphine in the preparations. The mechanism of action and pharmacokinetics are similar to those of morphine.

Opium tincture contains 10 mg morphine per milliliter and is used as an antidiarrheal agent (an agent inhibiting diarrhea) and, when diluted, for the treatment of neonatal opioid dependence.

Camphorated tincture of opium (paregoric) contains 2 mg morphine per 5 ml. It also is an antidiarrheal agent. In some instances, it has been used to treat neonatal opioid dependence, but this use is controversial. Paregoric contains camphor, which can cause serious toxicity (including seizures and respiratory depression), and benzoic acid, which can displace bilirubin from albumin. Both substances may enhance the problems typically seen in such infants (such as convulsions and hyperbilirubinemia); therefore, many physicians seem to prefer the use of diluted opium tincture to paregoric.

Opium and belladonna suppositories (B & O Supprettes, No. 15A) contain 30 mg powdered opium (10% morphine and other alkaloids) and 16.2 mg powdered belladonna alkaloid (the principal alkaloids of belladonna are atropine and scopolamine). B & O Supprettes No. 16A contains 60 mg powdered opium and 16.2 mg belladonna extract. The preparations are used to relieve moderate to severe pain reported with ureteral spasms and have also been prescribed for breakthrough pain between injections of opioids.

Codeine (Methylmorphine)

Codeine is available in sulfate and phosphate salts and is marketed in oral tablet, oral solution, and injectable dosage forms. Codeine is absorbed well after either oral or parenteral administration and is excreted by the kidneys. Oral administration is used for analgesic, antitussive (cough suppressant), and antidiarrheal effects. Codeine may also be injected for treatment of mild to moderate pain. See Table 4-4 for a pharmacokinetic overview of selected opioid dosage forms and Table 4-5 for dosing data for opioid analgesics.

Hydrocodone Bitartrate (Vicodin, Hycodan)

Hydrocodone is marketed in combination with homatropine in the United States. Hydrocodone bitartrate is used as an analgesic and antitussive. See Tables 4-4 and 4-5 for additional information.

Hydromorphone (Dilaudid, Dilaudid HP)

Hydromorphone, a semisynthetic opioid, has a faster onset of action but a shorter duration of action than morphine. It is prescribed for its analgesic effects but also has antitussive effects. See Tables 4-4 and 4-5 for additional information.

Meperidine (Demerol)

Meperidine is an effective analgesic for short-term use but is considered "the least potent of the common opioid

Table 4-4 Pharmacokinetic Overview of Selected Opioid Dosage Forms

Drug/Dosage Form	Onset of Action (min)	Peak Effect (min)	Duration of Action (hr)
Codeine			
Oral	30-45	60-120	4
IM	10-30	30-60	4
SC	10-30		4
Hydrocodone bitartrate			
Oral	10-30	30-60	4-6
Hydromorphone hydrochloride			
Oral	30	90-120	4
IM	15	30-60	4
IV	10-15	15-30	2-3
SC	15	30-90	4
Rectal	Not available	Not available	6-8
Meperidine			
Oral	15	60-90	2-4 (usually 3)
IM	10-15	30-50	2-4 (usually 3)
IV	1	5-7	2-4 (usually 3)
SC	10-15	30-50	2-4 (usually 3)
Methadone			
Oral	30-60	90-120	4-6*
IM	10-20	60-120	4-5*
IV		15-30	3-4
Levorphanol			
Oral	10-60	90-120	4-5
IM	Not available	60	4-5
IV	Not available	Within 20	4-5
SC	Not available	60-90	4-5
Oxycodone			
Oral	Not available	60	3-4
Oxymorphone			
IM	10-15	30-90	3-6
IV	5-10	15-30	3-4
SC	10-20	Not available	3-6
Rectal	15-30	2	3-6
Propoxyphene			
Oral	15-60	120	4-6

From McKenry, L., & Salerno, E. (1995). *Mosby's pharmacology in nursing* (19th ed.). St. Louis: Mosby.

*With active metabolites and continuous dosing, half-life and duration of action may increase to 22 to 48 hours.

Table 4-5 Dosing Data for Opioid Analgesics

Drug	Approximate Equianalgesic Oral Dose	Approximate Equianalgesic Parenteral Dose	Recommended Starting Dose (Adults More than 50 kg Body Weight)		Recommended Starting Dose (Children and Adults Less than 50 kg Body Weight)*	
			Oral	Parenteral	Oral	Parenteral
			Opioid Agonist			
Morphine†	30 mg q 3-4 hr (around-the-clock dosing) 60 mg q 3-4 hr (single dose or intermittent dosing)	10 mg q 3-4 hr	30 mg q 3-4 hr	10 mg q 3-4 hr	0.3 mg/kg q 3-4 hr	0.1 mg/kg q 3-4 hr
Codeine‡	130 mg q 3-4 hr	75 mg q 3-4 hr	60 mg q 3-4 hr	60 mg q 2 hr (intramuscular/ subcutaneous)	1 mg/kg q 3-4 hr§	Not recom-mended
Hydromorphone† (Dilaudid)	7.5 mg q 3-4 hr	1.5 mg q 3-4 hr	6 mg q 3-4 hr	1.5 mg q 3-4 hr	0.06 mg/kg q 3-4 hr	0.015 mg/kg q 3-4 hr
Hydrocodone (in Lorcet, Lortab, Vicodin, others)	30 mg q 3-4 hr	Not available	10 mg q 3-4 hr	Not available	0.2 mg/kg q 3-4 hr§	Not available

Levorphanol (Levo-Dromoran)	4 mg q 6-8 hr	2 mg q 6-8 hr	4 mg q 6-8 hr	2 mg q 6-8 hr	0.04 mg/kg q 6-8 hr	0.02 mg/kg q 6-8 hr
Meperidine (Demerol)	300 mg q 2-3 hr	100 mg q 3 hr	Not recommended	100 mg q 3 hr	Not recommended	0.75 mg/kg q 2-3 hr
Methadone (Dolophine, others)	20 mg q 6-8 hr	10 mg q 6-8 hr	20 mg q 6-8 hr	10 mg q 6-8 hr	0.2 mg/kg q 6-8 hr	0.1 mg/kg q 6-8 hr
Oxycodone (Roxicodone, also in Percocet, Percodan, Tylox, others)	30 mg q 3-4 hr	Not available	10 mg q 3-4 hr	Not available	0.2 mg/kg q 3-4 hr§	Not available
Oxymorphone† (Numorphan)	Not available	1 mg q 3-4 hr	Not available	1 mg q 3-4 hr	Not recommended	Not recommended
Opioid Agonist-Antagonist and Partial Agonist						
Buprenorphine (Buprenex)	Not available	0.3-0.4 mg q 6-8 hr	Not available	0.4 mg q 6-8 hr	Not available	0.004 mg/kg q 6-8 hr
Butorphanol (Stadol)	Not available	2 mg q 3-4 hr	Not available	2 mg q 3-4 hr	Not available	Not recommended

Continued.

Table 4-5 Dosing Data for Opioid Analgesics—cont'd

Drug	Approximate Equianalgesic Oral Dose	Approximate Equianalgesic Parenteral Dose	Recommended Starting Dose (Adults More than 50 kg Body Weight)		Recommended Starting Dose (Children and Adults Less than 50 kg Body Weight)*	
			Oral	Parenteral	Oral	Parenteral
Nalbuphine (Nubain)	Not available	10 mg q 3-4 hr	Not available	10 mg q 3-4 hr	Not available	0.1 mg/kg q 3-4 hr
Pentazocine (Talwin, others)	150 mg q 3-4 hr	60 mg q 3-4 hr	50 mg q 4-6 hr	Not recommended	Not recommended	Not recommended

From Carr, D. B., Jacox, A., Chapman, C. R., Ferrell, B., Fields, H. L., Heidrich, G., Hester, N. K., Hill, C. S., Lipman, A. G., McGarvey, C. L., Miaskowski, C., Mulder, D., Payne, R., Schechter, N., Shapiro, B. S., Smith, R. S., Tsou, C. V., Vecchiarelli, L. (1992). *Accute pain management: Operative or medical procedures and trauma. Clinical practice guideline.* AHCPR Pub. No. 92-0032. Rockville, MD: Agency for Health Care Policy and Research, PHS, USDHHS.

Note: Published tables vary in the suggested doses that are equianalgesic to morphine. Clinical response is the criterion that must be applied for each patient; titration to clinical response is necessary. Because there is not complete cross tolerance among these drugs, it is usually necessary to use a lower than equianalgesic dose when changing drugs and to retitrate to response.

Caution: Recommended doses do not apply to patients with renal or hepatic insufficiency or other conditions affecting drug metabolism and kinetics.

**Caution:* Doses listed for patients with body weight less than 50 kg cannot be used as initial starting doses in babies less than 6 months of age. Consult the *Acute Pain Management: Operative or Medical Procedures and Trauma Clinical Practice Guideline* section on management of pain in neonates for recommendations.

†For morphine, hydromorphone, and oxymorphone, rectal administration is an alternative route for patients unable to take oral medications, but equianalgesic doses may differ from oral and parenteral doses because of pharmacokinetic differences.

‡*Caution:* Codeine doses above 65 mg often are not appropriate due to diminishing incremental analgesia with increasing doses but continually increasing constipation and other side effects.

§*Caution:* Doses of aspirin and acetaminophen in combination opioid-NSAID preparations must also be adjusted to the patient's body weight.

analgesics and is administered in the largest doses" (Mather & Denson, 1992, p. 81). A commonly prescribed analgesic, it has a pharmacologic profile similar to morphine, with the following noted differences:

1. Meperidine is less apt to release histamine or to increase biliary tract pressure than morphine; thus it is often prescribed for patients with acute asthma, biliary colic, and pancreatitis (Sinatra & Savarese, 1992).
2. Its duration of action is shorter than that of morphine; thus a more frequent dosing schedule is necessary. See Table 4-4.
3. Meperidine has poor oral bioavailability; that is, to achieve an approximate analgesic equivalency to 75 mg IM of meperidine requires an oral dose of 300 mg (USP DI, 1994). Because the largest oral form of meperidine marketed is a 100-mg tablet, this preparation is often prescribed in dosages that are less effective than the injectable form. See Table 4-5 for dosing data.
4. Meperidine is metabolized in the liver to normeperidine, a CNS neurotoxic metabolite. Normeperidine has a half-life between 15 and 20 hours in persons with normal renal function. Prolonged administration or use of high doses of meperidine, or use in older adults or in patients with impaired renal or hepatic function, has resulted in normeperidine-induced CNS toxicity. This neurotoxicity may produce significant mood changes such as sadness, anger, restlessness and apprehension, increased irritability, nervousness, tremors, agitation, quivering, convulsions, and myoclonus (AHFS, 1994; Jacox et al., 1994). Neurotoxicity has also been reported in patients with sickle cell anemia, burn patients, and cancer patients that had normal renal and hepatic function but were receiving repeated, large doses of meperidine (AHFS).

Although the use of meperidine for only a few days in appropriate patients generally results in mild and tolerable side effects, meperidine should be avoided in those who require prolonged usage or high-dose therapy, for continuous infusions, or when renal or liver dysfunction is present. The nurse should be aware that naloxone (opioid antagonist) will antagonize meperidine but not normeperidine-induced seizures (Twycross, 1994).

5. Meperidine may produce a vagolytic effect, resulting in significant tachycardia; therefore, its use should probably be avoided or closely monitored in clients with dysrhythmias or myocardial infarction.
6. Review the drug interaction section, especially for concurrent use of MAO-inhibitors with meperidine. Very severe, unpredictable reactions may result.

Methadone (Dolophine, Methadose)

Methadone is an effective analgesic with properties similar to those of morphine, with the exception of its extended half-life. The duration of analgesic action for methadone is usually listed at 4 to 6 hours, but with repeated oral dosing the plasma half-life may extend from 22 to 48 hours (perhaps even longer in the elderly and patients with renal dysfunction). This extended half-life is *not* related to its analgesic effect. To control pain, methadone is administered every 6 or 8 hours, based on the individual's response. See Table 4-5 for dosing data.

Because of its extended half-life, methadone is approved by the FDA for use in detoxification and maintenance treatment programs. Methadone dependence is substituted in individuals who are physiologically dependent on heroin, opium, or other opioids. The mechanism of action of methadone is similar to that of morphine, as are the pharmacokinetics. See Table 4-4. Side effects and adverse reactions are also similar to those for morphine, although methadone's miotic and respiratory depressant effects may be present for more than 24 hours. Excessive sedation is reported in some patients following a regular dosing schedule.

Levorphanol (Levo-Dromoran)

Levorphanol is an opioid analgesic used for moderate to severe pain. See Tables 4-4 and 4-5 for additional information.

Oxycodone (Percodan, Tylox, Percocet)

Oxycodone is approximately 10 times more potent than codeine. It is available alone and in combination with aspirin (Percodan) or acetaminophen (Tylox, Percocet). See Tables 4-4 and 4-5 for additional information.

Oxymorphone (Numorphan)

Oxymorphone is pharmacologically similar to morphine, with the following exceptions: (a) in equianalgesic dosages oxymorphone usually causes more nausea, vomiting, and psychic effects (euphoria) than morphine; and (b) it may be less constipating and cause less suppression of the cough reflex than morphine. Oxymorphone is a potent analgesic used for moderate to severe pain, for preoperative medication, for obstetric analgesia, or as adjunct therapy for the treatment of anxiety caused by dyspnea resulting from pulmonary edema associated with left ventricular failure. See Tables 4-4 and 4-5 for additional information.

Fentanyl

Fentanyl is an opioid analgesic available in a preservative-free solution (Sublimaze), in combination with droperidol (Innovar), and as a topical transdermal patch (Duragesic). Fentanyl solution and fentanyl with droperidol are used parenterally (IV) for analgesia during the premedication, as an adjunct to anesthesia, and in the immediate postoperative period, that is, in the recovery room if necessary. Fentanyl has also been used for the induction and maintenance of anesthesia for selected surgical patients (USP DI, 1994). Parenteral administration of fentanyl should be restricted to those experienced with this product and with the management of fentanyl-induced respiratory depression. Fentanyl and the fentanyl derivative sufentanil (Sufenta), if given rapidly in large doses, may cause chest wall muscle rigidity, which then requires supportive respiratory ventilation and perhaps a rapid-acting muscle relaxant. This depression is dose related (USP DI, 1994; Omoigui, 1992).

The transdermal patch releases fentanyl continuously by absorption through the skin, which aids in controlling pain around the clock for 72 hours. This product is used in the management of chronic pain as an alternative to the other opioids, especially for clients that have difficulty swallowing or complying with a schedule of oral medications. See the box on p. 107 for nursing tips.

Fentanyl is metabolized in the liver and excreted in urine. Drug interactions and side/adverse effects are similar to those for the other opioids. The patch is available in 25 μg/hr, 50 μg/hr, 75 μg/hr, and 100 μg/hr dosage forms. The manufacturer publishes an equianalgesic and morphine-to-fentanyl conversion chart, which should be utilized to determine the fentanyl dose.

Application instructions for fentanyl are as follows:

1. Use water to clean the skin area prior to application. Do not use soap, oils, lotions, alcohol, or other products because they may alter the absorption of this product.
2. Apply fentanyl transdermal to a nonhairy, dry area on a flat skin surface of the upper torso, front or back. Do not apply it to skin that is burned, cut, irritated, very oily, or recently shaved. If the skin area is hairy, cut the hair with a scissors.
3. When applying the patch to skin, press and hold it firmly on the skin for 10 to 20 seconds. Then check the system to make certain that skin contact is complete and the edges of the system adhere well to the skin.
4. Wash hands after each application of the patch. Use large amounts of water in washing, especially if the gel accidentally comes in contact with skin. Avoid use of soap, alcohol, or any other solvent.
5. Dosing
   a. In opioid-naive patients (that is, persons not taking any opioid medication), in elderly patients (60

FENTANYL TRANSDERMAL NURSING TIPS

- Fentanyl provides continuous opioid administration via the skin.
- It has a slow onset of action; therefore, other, shorter-acting analgesics should be administered as ordered when therapy is begun.
- Fentanyl has a long duration of action (up to 72 hours); therefore, side and adverse effects are not easily reversed.
- Fentanyl is *not* indicated for the treatment of mild, acute, postoperative, or intermittent pain.
- It should be applied intact (do not cut or damage the system) to a flat body surface, preferably the upper torso front or back. Avoid exposing the patch site to direct heat sources, such as heating pads, electric blankets, heat lamps, or hot tubs, because increased fentanyl release, absorption, and toxicity may result.
- Fentanyl serum concentrations may increase by one third in patients with body temperature of 40° C (102° F).
- Fentanyl should not be administered to children less than 12 years old or to patients less than 18 years old who weigh less than 50 kg (110 lb).
- Fentanyl should not be used in nursing women, because it is excreted in human milk (PDR, 1994).

years and older), and in cachectic or debilitated patients, the starting dose should not be higher than 25 μg/hr. For a patient taking an opioid product, calculate the patient's 24-hour opioid requirement and then determine the appropriate fentanyl dose using the manufacturer's charts.

b. Following application, fentanyl is absorbed and concentrated in the upper layers of skin. Serum levels increase slowly, usually reaching a plateau in 12 to 24 hours. It is recommended that during the initial application of the patch, a short-acting analgesic be prescribed for the first 20 to 24 hours, since peak serum levels of fentanyl usually occur between 24 and 72 hours. Thereafter the patient should have an order for a short-acting opioid (such as morphine sulfate) for breakthrough pain.

c. The average half-life of fentanyl is 17 hours (range 13 to 22 hours). Because it may take as long as 6 days to reach steady-state levels of a new fentanyl dose, dosage adjustments, after the initial 72-hour change, should be instituted on an every-6-day schedule.

d. Discontinuation of fentanyl

   1) If the transdermal system is removed because of an adverse reaction, monitor the patient closely because fentanyl may be absorbed from the skin for approximately 17 hours or more after the system is removed. Fentanyl serum levels drop slowly: a 50% decrease in serum level occurs approximately 17 hours after system removal. If the reaction was severe, monitor respiratory status and keep naloxone and resuscitative equipment available. Close supervision in an acute care hospital setting may be necessary.

   2) To switch to an alternative oral opioid, remove the fentanyl patch(es) and start treatment with the new opioid at 50% of the calculated equianalgesic dose 12 to 18 hours after the fentanyl is removed. The physician should prescribe a short-acting opioid for pain during this withdrawal time period and also later for breakthrough pain.

   3) When discontinuing fentanyl transdermal in a patient who no longer requires the product, withdraw the drug gradually to prevent a drug withdrawal reaction. For example, if the patient was receiving a high fentanyl dose, remove the system for 12 to 24 hours and then apply the next-lower-dose patch for several days. Three days later remove this patch, and 12 to 24 hours later apply the next-lower-dose patch. Continue

this procedure until the 25 μg patch has been applied for 3 days prior to removal. This type of procedure will usually reduce the potential for a severe withdrawal reaction.

6. Be aware that patients may have absorption variability, which can make dose selection and pain control difficult. Also, if this product is used for a non-opioid-sensitive pain, such as nerve damage pain, increasing the fentanyl dose will not enhance pain relief but may increase the potential for side or adverse effects.

   The manufacturer states, "Some patients will require a change to other methods of opioid administration when the DURAGESIC dose exceeds 300 μg/hr" (PDR, 1994, p. 1086). Patient reevaluation and assessment should be employed to determine the proper adjuvant medication or other interventions necessary to achieve the desired effect.
7. Fentanyl drug absorption may be increased up to 33% of the usual amount, in patients with fever of 102 °F or greater. Monitor patients with fever closely for opioid side or adverse effects; the physician may need to adjust the dosage.
8. Instruct the patient and family on the proper administration techniques reviewed in this section and on the suggested method for disposing of the transdermal units, that is, folding the adhesive sides together, wrapping the system in some toilet tissues, and then flushing it down the toilet. See the box for fentanyl nursing tips.

Propoxyphene (Darvon) and Propoxyphene Napsylate Combinations (Darvocet-N)

Propoxyphene is a synthetic analgesic structurally related to methadone that is indicated for the treatment of mild to moderate pain. It has been reported that 65 mg propoxyphene is equivalent to or less effective than 650 mg acetaminophen, 650 mg aspirin, 32 mg codeine, 30 mg pentazocine (Talwin), or 50 mg meperidine (Demerol) (McCaffery & Beebe, 1989). When combined with aspirin or acetaminophen, propoxyphene combinations usually provide analgesia greater than either medication alone.

Propoxyphene binds to opioid receptors and produces an analgesic effect similar to that of codeine and the opioids. The hydrochloride dosage form is more rapidly absorbed than the water-insoluble napsylate formulation, although peak serum levels are approximately equivalent. The bioavailability of 65 mg propoxyphene hydrochloride is equivalent to that of 100 mg propoxyphene napsylate. The duration of action of propoxyphene is 4 to 6 hours. Propoxyphene crosses into the CNS and is believed to cross the placenta. Metabolism occurs mainly in the liver, where approximately one fourth of the dose is metabolized to norpropoxyphene. Norpropoxyphene is a toxic metabolite (USP DI, 1994) with a half-life of 30 to 36 hours; propoxyphene is also more apt to cause convulsions than most of the other opioid analgesics. See Tables 4-4 and 4-5 for additional information.

Patient Management Strategies

General Information

1. Perform a thorough pain assessment, utilizing a pain rating scale whenever possible. This process will help the practitioner to develop a proper management plan (pharmacologic, nonpharmacologic, psychosocial, etc.) and, in many instances, to identify the appropriate drug for pain control. (Review the discussion of assessment in Chapter 1.)
2. Achieving optimal pain control is often the responsibility of various members of the health care team, although the nurse in an institutional or home setting is often the initiator or coordinator of the resources necessary for optimal pain relief.
3. The primary objectives for pain management are as follows:
   a. Actively seek patient involvement and satisfaction with the pain management plan.

TIME REQUIRED TO PRODUCE MAXIMAL RESPIRATORY DEPRESSION EFFECTS WITH OPIOID ANALGESICS

Approximate Time	Route of Administration
Within 7 minutes	IV
Within 30 minutes	IM
Within 90 minutes	SC

b. Monitor drug therapies and institute interventions to reduce or avert the potential for drug side or adverse effects, especially nausea, vomiting, constipation, urinary retention, and respiratory depression.

c. The fear of inducing addiction or respiratory depression in a patient in severe pain is not an acceptable reason for undertreatment. (See the box above for times when maximum respiratory depression effects are generally reported with parenteral opioids.) The risk of addiction after the use of opioids for pain control is very low.

   Be aware of the term *pseudoaddiction* (Weissman & Haddox, 1989) as it refers to patients who are inadequately treated for pain and develop a pattern of drug-seeking behaviors to achieve pain control. This pattern is often mistaken for opioid addiction (Carr et al., 1992a; Jacox et al., 1994).

d. Dosages should be adjusted according to pain severity and the patient's response to the medication. Utilize nonopioid and nonpharmacologic interventions in conjunction with, or in place of, other therapies as appropriate.

4. Tolerance, or the need to increase the dose of an analgesic to maintain the desired effect, may be of

concern. Tolerance is unusual in opioid-naive patients who are receiving opioids for severe acute or chronic pain for which there is a physical cause, such as trauma, tumor growth and invasion, or surgery. Patients in pain respond differently to an analgesic than drug-seeking individuals who crave opioids for a euphoric effect (psychologic dependence or addiction). One should not confuse physical or psychologic dependence with tolerance (Jacox et al., 1994).

Physical dependence is an altered physiologic condition in a long-term drug user who requires consistent use of the drug to avoid withdrawal symptoms. Studies have indicated that the increased need for opioid analgesia in cancer patients is usually due to disease progression. Patients with cancer may be titrated to large amounts of opioids to control pain without experiencing the adverse effects of respiratory depression or excessive sedation. Pain specialists believe this is the result of *selective tolerance,* that is, tolerance to some of the effects of the drug without interference with the opioid's analgesic effect (Jacox et al., 1994; Portenoy, 1990).

5. Serve as a patient advocate. Understand that pain management is unsuccessful for a reason: a missed diagnosis: the wrong drug, drug dosage, or dosing interval: complication of disease state or therapy; or some other cause. Strive to individualize pain management.

Specific Dosing Information

See Table 4-5 for equianalgesic dosages and usual starting doses for parenteral and oral opioids for children and adults (Carr et al., 1992a,b).

Tolerance and opioid dosing Some patients may not achieve pain relief even with an increase of a specific opioid to enormously high dosage levels. In such instances the physician should consider switching the patient to a different opioid analgesic. Cross-tolerance with the opioids is incomplete; therefore, the alternative opioid may be more effective. In converting a patient on high opioid doses to another opioid, it is recommended that therapy with the new analgesic be initiated at 50% of the calculated bioequivalent dose (American Pain Society, 1990; Woodruff, 1993), with appropriate accompanying orders for additional analgesic for breakthrough pain (Kinzbrunner & Salerno, 1994). If the opioid switch and titration does not achieve the desired pain control, a reevaluation and assessment of the patient, both physically and psychosocially, should be performed.

Opioid use in pregnancy, labor, and delivery Opioid analgesics cross the placenta, so routine use of such drugs in the mother may lead to physical drug dependence in the fetus. After birth, severe withdrawal reactions may occur in the neonate. Pregnant women in methadone maintenance programs may demonstrate fetal distress syndrome in utero and usually deliver an underweight baby.

Since opioid analgesics cross the placenta to enter fetal circulation, the potential for inducing respiratory depression in the fetus must be considered. If at all possible, such drugs should be avoided in the delivery of a premature infant because the respiratory depressant effect is enhanced. Because of its extended duration of action, methadone should not be used in obstetrics. Morphine, codeine, and perhaps other opioids reportedly prolong labor.

Meperidine (Demerol) IM or IV is the most commonly used opioid for the relief of pain for women in labor. See Table 4-4 for pharmacokinetics of meperidine. Meperidine should be used with caution in women with cardiac disease because it may induce tachycardia. Morphine has also been utilized in dosages of 1 to 2 mg IV. Neonatal respiratory depression is greater with morphine than with meperidine. Naloxone (Narcan) should be available to treat the mother or neonate in case excessive CNS depression occurs. If an opioid is administered to a woman who is nursing, she should wait 4 to 6 hours before the next scheduled feeding to minimize the amount of drug passed on to the infant (McKenry & Salerno, 1995).

Opioid use in the elderly Analgesic dosing in the elderly usually requires dosage and dosing interval adjustments based on the client's therapeutic response or the development of undesirable side effects (increased pain, confusion, excessive untoward CNS effects, respiratory depression). The elderly reportedly have enhanced medication responses and may not tolerate side or adverse drug effects as well as younger patients. Elderly persons often have multiple medical problems and may have additional medications prescribed for them (polypharmacy). Thus it is important to carefully assess, evaluate, and closely monitor the geriatric client to reduce the potential for undertreatment or overtreatment and adverse effects. Height, weight, and body surface area are not accurate measures for dosing analgesics in the elderly.

Because analgesic effects have been reported to last longer in the geriatric patient due to altered pharmacokinetics (Yoshikawa, Cobbs, & Brummel-Smith, 1993), lower dosages of analgesics have often been recommended. This approach, though, should not be the rule. Age is not a significant factor in determining analgesic dosage, but it is important in establishing the frequency of drug dosing. Liver or kidney impairment may reduce drug clearance; thus less frequent drug dosing may be necessary. Both dosage and frequency should be carefully adjusted to the individual's response to the analgesic medication. The presence of unwanted adverse effects will influence drug dosage and drug frequency.

The intramuscular and subcutaneous routes of analgesic administration may also be influenced by the aging process. The elderly may have diminished circulation, resulting in slower absorption of drugs administered by these routes. Administering additional dosages in such a situation may result in unpredictable or increased drug absorption, which increases the potential for adverse effects.

The elderly client may be less likely to request pain medication because of an acceptance of pain as a part of old age, not wanting to be a "bother," or denying discomfort as a cultural and ethnic issue. Nonverbal communication, such as irritability, anorexia, decreased activity, crying easily, or gripping an object, should be carefully assessed. The decreased activity resulting from pain increases the risk of complications of immobility. The stress of the pain experience leads to fatigue and anxiety, reducing the elderly patient's diminished physical and psychologic resources. Because the elderly client may be taking many drugs concurrently, health care providers should be aware of specific drug interactions with analgesic therapy. Careful nursing care should be used in working with the elderly person experiencing pain (McKenry & Salerno, 1995). (See Chapter 1 for assessment and Chapter 12 for additional information on geriatric pain management.)

Respiratory depression An additional concern of health care professionals is the risk of inducing respiratory depression with the use of opioids. With careful assessment, prescription, opioid titration and monitoring, the potential for this adverse effect is low.

In advanced cancer or terminally ill patients, very large amounts of opioids are often necessary to control pain. In such instances, tolerance develops to the respiratory depression effect but not to the analgesia; therefore, the patient in true pain may have opioid doses increased until pain control is achieved (Gossel & Wuest, 1993).

Treatment of an opioid overdose If an oral opioid overdose occurs, emesis or gastric lavage is employed. If respiratory depression or any other life-threatening adverse effect is present, the treatment for this effect takes precedence.

For respiratory depression, establish a patent airway and controlled respiration. Administer naloxone (Narcan), an opioid antagonist, intravenously to reverse the opioid-induced respiratory depression and sedation by displacing the opioids at the receptor site. In opioid-dependent individuals, naloxone can also induce acute drug withdrawal. The naloxone adult dose is 0.4 mg to 2 mg as a single dose or 0.1 to 0.2 mg for postoperative opioid depression. For continuous intravenous infusion, 2 mg of naloxone may be diluted in 500 ml of normal saline or 5% dextrose injection. Generally, its effects are seen within 2 minutes. It can also be given intramuscularly or subcutaneously, but the onset of action then is 2 to 5 minutes (USP DI, 1994). Naloxone is shorter acting than most opioids; therefore, to prevent the recurrence of respiratory depression, naloxone must be administered by a continuous infusion or by repeated injections.

Heroin During the past decade or so congressional legislation for the approval of diacetylmorphine (heroin) for intractable pain has been proposed and denied. The proponents of this bill have used the argument that heroin is an alternative therapy to other opioids that might be useful for persons in intolerable pain because of its analgesic and euphoric effects. Some advocates believe it is more potent, is faster acting, and produces a more prolonged analgesic and euphoric effect than other analgesics (McCarthy & Montagne, 1993).

The opponents of the analgesic use of heroin in the United States state that heroin approval is unnecessary because the opioids now available, if properly prescribed, are sufficient for the treatment of intractable pain. Pharmacologically, heroin is a prodrug; that is, when it is administered orally or intravenously, it is converted in the liver to morphine and morphine metabolites. Although rapid IV injection of heroin crosses the blood-brain barrier faster than morphine to cause the euphoric or high effect, a clouded sensorium is generally undesirable clinically. Most ill persons want pain relief but also want to communicate with friends and family during their illness.

Although heroin is legitimately available in Belgium, Canada, and England, it is rarely used in Belgium and Canada. Heroin is a popular illegal drug of abuse; thus an additional fear in legalizing it is that it may result in an increased risk of drug diversion, pharmacy burglaries, and crime (Lipman, 1993). If heroin offers few if any advantages over the already marketed opioids, then, as Lipman (p. 998) has succinctly stated, "legalization of heroin is not in the public interest."

OPIOID AGONIST-ANTAGONIST ANALGESICS

Although the exact mechanism of action of the agonist-antagonist agents is unknown, these agents have both analgesic agonist and antagonist effects on the opioid receptors. Butorphanol (Stadol), nalbuphine (Nubain), and pentazocine (Talwin) produce agonist effects at the κ-receptors (Twycross, 1994). Nalbuphine and pentazocine may displace agonists (opioids) from the μ-receptor sites, thus inhibiting their effects and perhaps inducing a drug withdrawal reaction in clients physically dependent on agonist opioids. Butorphanol has minimal effects on the μ-receptors.

Morphine and opioid agonists produce their analgesic effects at the μ- and κ-receptors. Buprenorphine has some agonist effect at the μ-receptor sites. Generally, these drugs have a lower dependency potential than opioids, and withdrawal symptoms are not as severe as those reported with the opioid agonist medications. They also have a ceiling dosage level with respect to their analgesic and respiratory depressant effects (Carr et al., 1992a). The opioid agonist-antagonist agents have pharmacokinetics, adverse effects, and significant drug interactions similar to those of morphine. See Table 4-5 for dosing information.

Dezocine (Dalgan), a parenteral analgesic indicated for short-term treatment of pain, is a partial agonist at the μ-receptor, but it can displace other μ-receptor opioid agonists (e.g., morphine) and can also induce a drug withdrawal reaction in opioid-dependent persons. This opioid agonist-antagonist is reported to be comparable to morphine in analgesic potency, onset, and duration of action (USP DI, 1994).

NONOPIOID ANALGESICS

Nonopioid medications are effective for mild to moderate pain and are often combined with opioid analgesics to enhance pain control in cases of severe pain. They correspond to step 1 on the WHO ladder (see Chapter 10) and, in combination with a weak opioid, are included in step 2. See Figure 4-1. Aspirin, acetaminophen, and the nonsteroidal antiinflammatory drugs (NSAIDs) represent the major drugs in this classification. These products are used for the treatment of pain and inflammation caused by rheumatoid arthritis, osteoarthritis, and various other acute and chronic musculoskeletal and soft tissue inflammations, as well as pain associated with the peripheral nerves (neuralgia). The NSAIDs are also used to treat metastatic bone pain, usually in combination with an opioid analgesic (Twycross, 1994). For dosing information on acetaminophen and the NSAIDs, see Table 4-6.

Ketorolac (Toradol) is an oral and parenteral NSAID drug used for short-term pain management. It has been

Table 4-6 Dosing Data for Acetaminophen and NSAIDs

Drug	Usual Dose for Adults ≥ 50 kg Body Weight	Usual Dose for Adults[a] < 50 kg Body Weight
Acetaminophen and Over-the-Counter NSAIDs		
Acetaminophen[b]	650 mg q 4 hr 975 mg q 6 hr	10-15 mg/kg q 4 hr 15-20 mg/kg q 4 hr (rectal)
Aspirin[c]	650 mg q 4 hr 975 mg q 6 hr	10-15 mg/kg q 4 hr 15-20 mg/kg q 4 hr (rectal)
Ibuprofen (Motrin, others)	400-600 mg q 6 hr	10 mg/kg q 6-8 hr
Prescription NSAIDs		
Carprofen (Rimadyl)	100 mg tid	
Choline magnesium trisalicylate[d] (Trilisate)	1000-1500 mg tid	25 mg/kg tid
Choline salicylate (Arthropan)[d]	870 mg q 3-4 hr	
Diflunisal (Dolobid)[e]	500 mg q 12 hr	
Etodolac (Lodine)	200-400 mg q 6-8 hr	
Fenoprofen calcium (Nalfon)	300-600 mg q 6 hr	
Ketoprofen (Orudis)	25-60 mg q 6-8 hr	

Table 4-6 Dosing Data for Acetaminophen and NSAIDs—cont'd

Drug	Usual Dose for Adults ≥ 50 kg Body Weight	Usual Dose for Adults[a] < 50 kg Body Weight
	Prescription NSAIDs	
Ketorolac tromethamine (Toradol)[f]	10 mg q 4-6 hr to a maximum of 40 mg/day	
Magnesium salicylate (Doan's, Magan, Mobidin, others)	650 mg q 4 hr	
Meclofenamate sodium (Meclomen)[g]	50-100 mg q 6 hr	
Mefenamic acid (Ponstel)	250 mg q 6 hr	
Naproxen (Naprosyn)	250-275 mg q 6-8 hr	5 mg/kg q 8 hr
Naproxen sodium (Anaprox)	275 mg q 6-8 hr	
Sodium salicylate (generic)	325-650 mg q 3-4 hr	
	Parenteral NSAIDs	
Ketorolac tromethamine[f,h] (Toradol)	60 mg initially, then 30 mg q 6 hr Intramuscular dose not to exceed 5 days	

From Jacox, A., Carr, D. B., Payne, R., Berde, C. B., Breitbart, W., Cain, J. M., Chapman, C. R., Cleeland, C. S., Ferrell, B. R., Finley, R. S., Hester, N. O., Hill, C. S., Leak, W. D., Lipman, A. G., Logan, C. L., McGarvey, C. L., Miaskowski, C. A., Mulder, D. S., Paice, J. A., Shapiro, B. S., Silberstein, E. B., Smith, R. S., Stover, J., Tsou, C. V., Vecchiarelli, L., & Weissman, D. E. (1994). *Management of cancer pain. Clinical practice guideline.* AHCPR Pub. No. 94-0592. Rockville, MD: Agency for Health Care Policy and Research, PHS, USDHHS.

[a]Acetaminophen and NSAID dosages for adults weighing less than 50 kg should be adjusted for weight.

[b]Acetaminophen lacks the peripheral antiinflammatory and antiplatelet activities of the other NSAIDs.

[c]The standard against which other NSAIDs are compared. May inhibit platelet aggregation for ≥ 1 week and may cause bleeding.

[d]May have minimal antiplatelet activity.

[e]Administration with antacids may decrease absorption.

[f]For short-term use only.

[g]Coombs-positive autoimmune hemolytic anemia has been associated with prolonged use.

[h]Has the same GI toxicities as oral NSAIDs.

Note: Only the above NSAIDs have FDA approval for use as simple analgesics, but clinical experience has been gained with other drugs as well.

q, Every; *tid,* thrice daily.

reported (AHFS, 1994) that a single dose of 30 mg ketorolac IM produced pain relief equivalent to that achieved by a single dose of 50 or 100 mg meperidine IM and 6 or 12 mg morphine IM. The duration of action for ketorolac is also longer than that for the opioids (Arzeno, 1990).

Aspirin is available in a variety of dosage forms, including oral tablets, chewing gum, ointments, extended-release tablets, buffered formulations, and rectal suppositories. It is also available in combination with other drugs, such as caffeine, and various formulations, such as choline salicylate, magnesium salicylate, salsalate, and sodium salicylate. Choline salicylate is the only liquid salicylate available. It is absorbed faster from the GI tract and produces less adverse gastrointestinal effect than aspirin. This form may be useful for clients experiencing difficulty in swallowing tablets.

Salsalate (salicylsalicylic acid) is converted to salicylate during absorption from the GI tract and in the liver. It has the advantage of producing little if any adverse gastrointestinal effect, and it does not affect platelet aggregation. Salsalate's analgesic effects are equivalent to those of aspirin.

Caffeine has been combined with aspirin in a number of oral preparations. Caffeine may provide a more rapid onset of aspirin action or an enhanced analgesic effect, allowing for lower doses of salicylates. According to the FDA, evidence to support the claim that caffeine is an effective analgesic adjuvant is lacking. Caffeine, though, does constrict cerebral blood vessels, which may help in headache relief (USP DI, 1994).

Buffered aspirin formulations have been promoted to produce a more rapid onset of effect with a decrease in the adverse gastrointestinal effect. Covington (1993) has reported that buffering can enhance aspirin's dissolution and absorption rate, but evidence that buffered aspirin produces greater or faster pain relief than unbuffered aspirin is lacking. The American Hospital Formulary System (AFHS, 1994, p. 1209), however, states, "all buffered aspirin tablets are dissolved and absorbed more rapidly than all uncoated plain aspirin tablets." In addition, there is evidence that buffered tablets do not cause less gastric irritation than the uncoated, plain aspirin tablets (AHFS).

Mechanism of Action

Aspirin and NSAIDs work by inhibiting the synthesis and release of prostaglandins peripherally. This effect in inflamed tissue is believed to be responsible for their analgesic and antiinflammatory action (see the discussion of pain pathophysiology in Chapter 8). Salicylates also block the generation of pain impulses and may have a central analgesic action (hypothalamus). The NSAIDs also inhibit leukocyte migration and the release of the lysosomal enzymes, which contributes to their antiinflammatory effect.

Acetaminophen appears to produce its analgesic effect by inhibition of prostaglandin synthesis in the CNS (predominant effect) and peripherally. Although the exact mechanism of action is unknown, antiinflammatory effects are minimal. The antipyretic effect for these agents is mediated centrally via the hypothalamus.

Pharmacokinetics

Aspirin is rapidly absorbed from the stomach and upper small intestine and reaches a peak serum level within 1 to 2 hours. Aspirin doses up to 600 mg have a half-life of approximately 3 to 5 hours, and larger, antiinflammatory doses of aspirin have a much longer half-life (up to 15 hours or even more) (Katzung, 1992). Salicylates are metabolized in the liver and excreted by the kidneys as free salicylic acid and various conjugated metabolites.

Enteric-coated aspirin has a delayed absorption, and aspirin chewing gum and rectal suppositories have a delayed and incomplete absorption.

Therapeutic analgesic and antipyretic salicylate plasma levels are between 25 and 50 μg/ml. The antiinflammatory or antirheumatic desired plasma level is 150 to 300 μg/ml. Attainment of a peak antirheumatic effect may require 2 to 3 weeks of chronic therapy. Salicylates may be transferred to breast milk, especially when peak serum levels are 173 to 483 μg/ml. Such levels have been reached after the maternal ingestion of only 650 mg (USP DI, 1994).

Oral acetaminophen is absorbed and reaches peak serum levels within $\frac{1}{2}$ to 1 hour. The half-life of acetaminophen is 2 to 3 hours; it is metabolized primarily by the liver to inactive metabolites and excreted by the kidneys. In overdosage, an intermediate active metabolite may accumulate, leading to hepatotoxicity and possibly nephrotoxicity. Peak plasma level is 5 to 20 μg/ml with acetaminophen doses up to 650 mg orally. It is transferred in breast milk, with peak concentrations of 10 to 15 μg/ml reported after a single 650-mg dose maternally (USP DI, 1994).

Drug Interactions

The patient's concurrent drug therapy should be assessed for potentially significant drug interactions.

1. If adrenocorticoids or mineralocorticoids are given chronically or in high doses with salicylates, increased salicylate excretion may occur, resulting in lower salicylate plasma levels. In addition, the risk for gastrointestinal ulceration, bleeding, and sodium and fluid retention is increased. Monitor for abdominal pain or distress, black or bloody stools, hematemesis, and other signs. Always advise patients to take aspirin with a full glass (8 oz) of water. If the stomach is upset, administration after meals may reduce GI irritation.
2. Chronic use of alcohol or hepatotoxic medications may increase the risk of hepatotoxicity with acetaminophen. Avoid concurrent use if possible, or, if it cannot be avoided, carefully monitor drug dosages and watch for signs and symptoms of liver toxicity.
3. Antacids (high doses, chronic use) and other urinary alkalizers administered with salicylates (aspirin, etc.) may result in an alkaline urine that leads to increased excretion of salicylates. Buffered aspirin does not contain sufficient buffering to induce this effect, but the buffered effervescent aspirin tablets, if used in large quantities, may produce this result. Avoid chronic high doses of alkalizers whenever possible.

4. Antibiotics (cefamandole, cefotetan, moxalactam, and plicamycin) administered with NSAIDs may induce hypoprothrombinemia or platelet aggregate inhibition, which can result in an increased potential for bleeding episodes. Avoid concurrent drug administration.
5. Anticoagulants (coumarin, heparin, or thrombolytic agents) with NSAIDs may result in an increased risk of bleeding caused by inhibition of platelet aggregation and an increased risk of GI ulceration or hemorrhage. Avoid concurrent drug administration.
6. Diuretics, especially triamterene or antihypertensives, may result in a decrease in diuretic or antihypertensive effect when given with NSAIDs. Monitor closely for fluid retention, such as weight gain of 1 lb or more daily and edema, or elevation of blood pressure.
7. An increase in serum levels of lithium may result when it is taken with NSAIDs. Monitor lithium levels closely during concurrent drug administration and after the NSAID is discontinued.
8. Methotrexate given with ibuprofen and possibly other NSAIDs may decrease methotrexate excretion, leading to elevated methotrexate serum levels and toxicity. Discontinue ibuprofen (and other short-acting NSAIDs) for at least 12 to 24 hours prior to, and 12 to 24 hours following, high-dose methotrexate infusion. For longer-acting NSAIDs such as piroxicam, the drug should be discontinued for up to 10 days prior to administration of the methotrexate infusion.
9. There is increased risk of GI side effects such as bleeding and ulceration when NSAIDs are given with salicylates. Aspirin is also reported to decrease the bioavailability of diclofenac, fenoprofen, flurbiprofen (50% reduction), indomethacin, meclofenamate, piroxicam, and the active metabolite of sulindac. There may also be a decrease protein binding, resulting in elevated serum levels and possible

toxicity of ketoprofen. Avoid concurrent drug administration.

10. Probenecid may decrease ibuprofen (and other NSAID) excretion, which can result in increased serum levels and increased potential for toxicity. NSAID dosage decrease may be necessary.
11. Salicylates given with vancomycin, aminoglycosides, or furosemide, for example, result in an increased risk of ototoxicity.

See the following box for additional information about NSAIDs.

ADDITIONAL INFORMATION ON NSAIDs

NSAIDs usually produce an improvement in arthritis within a few days to 2 weeks for most types of arthritis, but achieving the maximum effectiveness usually requires the following time periods:

Drug(s)	Usual Time Period
Diclofenac (Voltaren), diflunisal (Dolobid), flurbiprofen (Ansaid), ibuprofen (Motrin), phenylbutazone (Butazolidin), tolmetin (Tolectin)	Between 1 and 3 weeks
Fenoprofen (Nalfon), ketoprofen (Orudis), meclofenamate (Meclofen), sulindac (Clinoril)	Between 2 and 3 weeks
Indomethacin (Indocin), naproxen (Naprosyn)	Up to a month in selected cases
Piroxicam (Feldene)	Up to 3 months in selected cases

ADMINISTRATION RECOMMENDATIONS

For acute pain, the oral solid dosage forms of the NSAIDs are better absorbed on an empty stomach. For chronic use or in patients who report GI irritation or are taking indomethacin, mefenamic acid, phenylbutazone, or piroxicam, administer tablets or capsules with meals or antacids. To reduce the possibility of esophageal irritation, advise patients to take medication with a full glass of water (8 oz) and to sit up for 15 to 30 minutes afterward (USP DI, 1994). The additional water will also increase drug dissolution (enhance absorption), and although it is postulated that the GI toxicity reported with these drugs is due to a reduction in prostaglandin synthesis and activity of the prostaglandins, these highly acidic drugs may also produce a local irritating effect. Dilution of the drug may reduce the lcoal irritation of the mucosa.

WARNINGS

- Patients with aspirin or NSAID intolerance described as a hypersensitivity or allergy manifested by asthmatic attack, bronchospastic activity, nasal polyps, or angioedema should not be administered aspirin or the other NSAIDs.
- Aspirin platelet inhibition is irreversible for the life of the platelet (approximately 10 days), whereas for other NSAIDs platelet inhibition is reversible. Platelet function recovery time after discontinuation of the NSAID is within 1 day for ibuprofen, diflunisal, diclofenac, sulindac, and others; 4 days for naproxen; and approximately 2 weeks for piroxicam, a drug with a prolonged elimination half-life (USP DI, 1994).
- Elderly persons taking NSAIDs should be monitored more closely since they are more likely to develop adverse GI, hepatic, or renal effects because of accumulation of the drug due to age-related reduction in renal function. It has been recommended that elderly patients be given half the usual adult dose initially, followed by drug titration as necessary. Close monitoring for NSAID side and adverse effects is necessary.
- Careful consideration should also be taken before a NSAID drug is administered to persons with anemia, fluid retention, bleeding disorders, hepatic impairment, and those with a history of or active peptic ulcer as these conditions may be exacerbated.

ADJUVANT MEDICATIONS

Adjuvant (coanalgesic) medications are used in combination with other analgesics to enchance pain relief or to treat symptoms that exacerbate pain, or in some instances they are used alone to treat specifically identified pain. NSAIDs are often listed with the adjuvant analgesics, but with this exception the primary indications for adjuvant medications are not for the treatment of pain. Nevertheless, these agents have been reported to have an analgesic effect in some pain conditions.

Adjuvant analgesic medications include a variety of medications, such as anticonvulsants, antidepressants, antihistamines, corticosteroids, local anesthetics, antiarrhythmics, neuroleptics, psychostimulants, clonidine, and capsaicin.

Anticonvulsants, antidepressants, anesthetics, and antiarrhythmics are often prescribed for the treatment of neuropathic pain. They are often used in combination with opioids for cancer-associated nerve pain (Jacox et al., 1994). Corticosteroids are beneficial for cancer pain that originates in a fairly restricted area, such as intracranially; alongside a nerve root; or in pelvic, neck, or hepatic areas. Dexamethasone is prescribed for an increase in intracranial pressure and for relief of pain caused by pressure on a nerve. Corticosteroids may also relieve pain by suppressing the release of prostaglandins and thus inhibiting the inflammatory process. Hypercalcemia tends to reduce the pain threshold, but this effect may be reversed by the increased excretion of calcium induced by corticosteroids. Additional steroid effects of appetite stimulation and elevation of mood can also be useful in selected cases (Farr, 1990).

The neuroleptic (phenothiazine) methotrimeprazine (Levoprome) also has analgesic effects. Administered IM, it also has antiemetic, anxiolytic, sedative, and antipruritic properties. Its usage has been limited by its severe orthostatic hypotensive effects, which require patients to "remain in bed or be closely supervised for at least 6, but preferably 12 hours, after each of the first several doses" (AHFS, 1994, p. 1530). This limits the use of methotrimeprazine to nonambulatory patients, but it may also be used for obstetric analgesia when respiratory depression must be avoided (USP DI, 1994).

The antihistamine hydroxyzine (Vistaril) is reported to have some analgesic properties (Haddox, 1992). It also has anxiolytic and sedative effects that may be useful in some patients.

Psychostimulants, such as methylphenidate (Ritalin) and dextroamphetamine (Dexedrine), potentiate opioid analgesia and also help to increase alertness or reduce persistent, opioid-induced sedation in some patients. The analgesic effects are postulated to occur centrally and in the descending spinal inhibitory pathways. (See the discussion of the pathophysiology of pain in Chapter 1). Opioid-induced cognitive impairment in cancer and AIDS patients has improved with administration of a psychostimulant drug (Bruera & Watanabe, 1994). The usual approach to opioid-induced persistent sedation is to reduce the opioid dose and increase daily drug frequency; if the patient does not appropriately respond to this method, the opioid should be switched. If the sedation problem persists with these alternative strategies, a psychostimulant may be added to the opioid regime (Jacox et al., 1994).

Additional useful adjuvant analgesics include clonidine (Catapres) and capsaicin. Clonidine is a centrally acting, α_2-adrenergic agonist that has been used for the treatment of pain associated with reflex sympathetic dystrophy (RSD) (Rauck, Eisenach, Jackson, Young, & Southern, 1993), diabetic neuropathy, postherpetic neuralgia, spinal cord injury, phantom pain, and pain in cancer patients who were opioid tolerant (Portenoy, 1993).

Capsaicin, an alkaloid found in chili peppers, is formulated into a topical cream (Zostrix), which is indicated for the treatment of neuralgia (postherpetic and diabetic neuropathy) and arthritic pain. On application, it causes an initial release and then a depletion of substance P (SP) from nociceptive fibers. A decrease in SP decreases pain transmission (USP DI, 1994). See Table 4-7 for additional information on selected adjuvant medications.

Table 4-7 Adjunct Analgesic Medications

Drug	Usual Adult Daily Dose*	Route of Administration	Comments
		Anticonvulsants	
Carbamazepine	S 100 mg hs/bid R 200-1600 mg in divided doses	PO	May cause marrow toxicity For neuropathic pain, especially lancinating (shooting) pain
Phenytoin	S 100 mg hs/bid R 300-500 mg in divided doses	PO	For neuropathic pain May increase sedation Monitor phenytoin serum levels
		Antidepressants	
Amitriptyline Doxepin Nortriptyline Desipramine	S 10-25 mg hs R 25-150 mg hs or divided doses	PO	For neuropathic pain and pain complicated by depression or insomnia Desipramine and nortriptyline have the least sedative and anticholinergic properties
		Antihistamine	
Hydroxyzine	S 25-50 mg q 4-6 hr R 300-450 mg in divided doses	IM	Limited by need for parenteral dosing For short-term use No proven analgesic effect orally

	Corticosteroids		
Dexamethasone	S 4 mg qid R 16-96 mg in divided doses	PO	Dexamethasone usually the preferred agent because of low mineralocorticoid effects
	Local Anesthetics/Antiarrhythmics		
Lidocaine	S 1-1.5 mg/kg R 1-5 mg/kg	IV	For postherpetic neuralgia, chronic diabetic neuropathy, and other chronic pain conditions
Mexiletine	S 150 mg tid R 450-900 mg in divided doses	PO	For neuropathic pain
	Neuroleptic		
Methotrimeprazine	S 10 mg q 6-8 hr R 40-80 mg in divided doses	IM	Limited by need for parenteral dosing For short-term use No oral preparation available
	Psychostimulants		
Dextroamphetamine	S 2.5-5 mg q day R 10-40 mg	PO	Has analgesic effect in postoperative pain Administer as single or divided dose, before noon

Continued.

Table 4-7 Adjunct Analgesic Medications—cont'd

Drug	Usual Adult Daily Dose*	Route of Administration	Comments
Methylphenidate	S 2.5-5 mg q day R 10-40 mg	PO	Has analgesic effect in cancer pain Administer single or divided dose before noon
		Miscellaneous	
Clonidine	Available in 0.1 mg, 0.2 mg, 0.3 mg Dosing information limited	PO, epidural, transdermal	Oral and epidural used to treat pain from spinal cord injury, phantom pain, and peripheral nerve injuries Trial of oral or transdermal may be indicated for neuropathic pain refractory to opioids and other adjuvants in palliative care setting

From Ackerman, W. E., Phero, J. C., & McDonald, J. S. (1992). Analgesia with intravenous local anesthetics. In P. P. Raj (Ed.), *Practical management of pain* (2nd ed., pp. 851-855). St. Louis: Mosby; Jacox, A., Carr, D. B., Payne, R., Berde, C. B., Breitbart, W., Cain, J. M., Chapman, C. R., Cleeland, C. S., Ferrell, B. R., Finley, R. S., Hester, N. O., Hill, C. S., Leak, W. D., Lipman, A. G., Logan, C. L., McGarvey, C. L., Miaskowski, C. A., Mulder, D. S., Paice, J. A., Shapiro, B. S., Silberstein, E. B., Smith, R. S., Stover, J., Tsou, C. V., Vecchiarelli, L., & Weissman, D. E. (1994). *Management of cancer pain. Clinical practice guideline.* AHCPR Pub. No. 94-0592. Rockville, MD: Agency for Health Care Policy and Research, PHS, USDHSS; Portenoy, R. K. (1993). Adjuvant analgesics in pain management. In D. Doyle, G. W. C. Hanks, & N. Macdonald (Eds.), *Oxford textbook of palliative medicine.* New York: Oxford University Press; Portenoy, R. K. (1993). *3-step analgesic ladder for management of cancer pain.* Columbus, OH: Roxane Laboratories.

**S,* Usual starting dose; *R,* dosage range; *hs,* bedtime; *bid,* twice daily; *PO,* by mouth; *q,* every; *IM,* intramuscular; *qid,* four times daily; *IV,* intravenous; *tid,* thrice daily.

The use of a placebo for the treatment of pain to distinguish psychic and real pain is a deceptive practice that should be avoided (Fox, 1994; Payne, Thomas, & Raj, 1992). The American Pain Society guidelines (1992, p. 25) state, "Do not use placebos to assess the nature of pain. . . . The deceptive use of placebos and the misinterpretation of the placebo response to discredit the patient's pain report are unethical and should be avoided."

SUMMARY

Pain continues to be a universal health problem. It is more distressing and disabling than any other patient symptom and is probably the most common reason a person seeks health care. Few things that a nurse does are more important than alleviating pain. Knowledge of basic pharmacologic approaches is necessary for the nurse to accurately assess and intervene effectively to achieve pain relief for their patients.

References

AHFS (1994). *American Hospital Formulary Service drug information '94.* Bethesda, MD: American Society of Hospital Pharmacists.

American Pain Society (1990). Principles of analgesic use in the treatment of acute pain and chronic cancer pain. *Clinical Pharmacy, 9*(8), 601-612.

American Pain Society (1992). *Principles of analgesic use in the treatment of acute pain and cancer pain* (3rd ed.). Skokie, IL: American Pain Society, p. 25.

Arzeno, S. (1990). *Toradol.* Palo Alto, CA: Syntex Laboratories.

Bruera, E., & Watanabe, S. (1994). Psychostimulants as adjuvant analgesics. *Journal of Pain and Symptom Management, 9*(6), 412-415.

Carr, D. B., Jacox, A., Chapman, C. R., Ferrell, B., Fields, H. L., Heidrich, G., Hester, N. K., Hill, C. S., Lipman, A. G., McGarvey, C. L., Miaskowski, C., Mulder, D., Payne, R., Schechter, N., Shapiro, B. S., Smith, R. S., Tsou, C. V., Vecchiarelli, L. (1992a). *Acute pain management: Operative or medical procedures and trauma. Clinical practice guideline.* AHCPR Pub. No. 92-0032. Rockville, MD: Agency for Health Care Policy and Research, PHS, USDHHS.

Carr, D. B., et al. (1992b). *Acute pain management in infants, children and adolescents.* AHCPR Pub. No. 92-0020. Rockville, MD: Agency for Health Care Policy and Research, PHS, USDHHS.

Covington, T. R. (Ed.). (1993). *Handbook of nonprescription drugs* (10th ed.). Washington, DC: American Pharmaceutical Association.

Farr, W. C. (1990). The use of corticosteroids for symptom management in terminally ill patients. *American Journal of Hospice Care,* January-February, 41-46.

Fox, A. E. (1994). Ethical issues confronting the use of placebos for pain. *American Journal of Nursing, 94*(9), 42-45.

Gossel, T. A., & Wuest, J. R. (1993). Control of chronic cancer pain. *Florida Pharmacy Today, 57*(4), 21-30.

Haddox, J. D. (1992). Neuropsychiatric drug use in pain management. In P. P. Raj (Ed.), *Practical management of pain* (2nd ed., pp. 636-659). St. Louis: Mosby.

Jacox, A., Carr, D. B., Payne, R., Berde, C. B., Breitbart, W., Cain, J. M., Chapman, C. R., Cleeland, C. S., Ferrell, B. R., Finley, R. S., Hester, N. O., Hill, C. S., Leak, W. D., Lipman, A. G., Logan, C. L., McGarvey, C. L., Miaskowski, C. A., Mulder, D. S., Paice, J. A., Shapiro, B. S., Silberstein, E. B., Smith, R. S., Stover, J., Tsou, C. V., Vecchiarelli, L., & Weissman, D. E. (1994). *Management of cancer pain. Clinical practice guideline.* AHCPR Pub. No. 94-0592. Rockville, MD: Agency for Health Care Policy and Research, PHS, USDHHS.

Katzung, B. G. (1992). *Basic and clinical pharmacology* (5th ed.). Norwalk, CT: Appleton & Lange.

Kinzbrunner, B., & Salerno, E. (1994). *Vitas pain management formulary* (2nd rev. ed.). Miami: Vitas Healthcare.

Lipman, A. G. (1993). The argument against therapeutic use of heroin in pain management, *American Journal of Hospital Pharmacy, 50*(5), 996-998.

Mather, L. E., & Denson, D. D. (1992). Pharmacokinetics of systemic opioids for the management of pain. In R. S. Sinatra, A. H. Hord, B. Ginsberg, & L. M. Preble (Eds.), *Acute pain* (pp. 78-92). St. Louis: Mosby.

McCaffery, M., & Beebe, A. (1989). *Pain: Clinical manual for nursing practice.* St. Louis: Mosby.

McCarthy, R. L., & Montagne, M. (1993). The argument for therapeutic use of heroin in pain management. *American Journal of Hospital Pharmacy, 50*(5), 992-996.

McKenry, L., & Salerno, E. (1995). *Mosby's pharmacology in nursing* (19th ed.). St. Louis: Mosby.

Omoigui, S. (1992). *The anesthesia drug handbook.* St. Louis: Mosby.

Payne, R., Thomas, J., & Raj, P. P. (1992). Pain due to cancer. In P. P. Raj (Ed.), *Practical management of pain* (2nd ed., pp. 434-450). St. Louis: Mosby.

PDR (1994). *Physicians' desk reference* (48th ed.). Montvale, NJ: Medical Economics.

Portenoy, R. K. (1990). Drug therapy for cancer pain. *American Journal of Hospice and Palliative Care, 7*(6), 10-19.

Portenoy, R. K. (1993). Adjuvant analgesics in pain management. In D. Doyle, G. W. C. Hanks, & N. Macdonald (Eds.), *Oxford textbook of palliative medicine.* New York: Oxford University Press.

Rauck, R. L., Eisenach, J. C., Jackson, K., Young, L. D., & Southern, J. (1993). Epidural clonidine treatment for refractory reflex sympathetic dystrophy. *Anesthesiology, 79*(6), 1163-1169.

Sinatra, R. S., & Savarese, A. (1992). Parenteral analgesic therapy and patient-controlled analgesia for pediatric pain management. In R. S. Sinatra, A. H. Hord, B. Ginsberg, & L. M. Preble (Eds.), *Acute pain.* St. Louis: Mosby.

Twycross, R. (1994). *Pain relief in advanced cancer.* Edinburgh, Churchill Livingstone.

USP DI (1994). *Drug information for the health care professional* (14th ed.). Rockville, MD: U.S. Pharmacopeial Convention.

Weissman, D. E., & Haddox, J. D. (1989). Opioid pseudoaddiction—An iatrogenic syndrome. *Pain, 36*(3), 363-366.

World Health Organization (1990). *Cancer pain relief and palliative care. Report of a WHO expert committee.* Technical report 804. Geneva: WHO.

Woodruff, R. (1993). *Palliative medicine.* Melbourne: Asperula Pty Ltd.

Yoshikawa, T. T., Cobbs, E. L., & Brummel-Smith, K. (1993). *Ambulatory geriatric care.* St. Louis: Mosby.

5

Nonpharmacologic Approaches to Pain

Nancy Fleming Courts

        - Guidelines for Use
    - Music and Prayer
  - Behavioral Techniques
    - Relaxation
      - Clinical Indications and Contraindications
      - Guidelines for Use
    - Imagery
      - Clinical Indications and Contraindications
      - Guidelines for Use
- Summary

Key Points

- Nonpharmacologic pain interventions are never a substitute for appropriate medications.
- Successful use of nonpharmacologic pain interventions is dependent on a therapeutic nurse-patient relationship and understanding of the mechanism of action of the interventions and the mind-body connection.
- Nonpharmacologic interventions enhance patients' sense of perceived control and decrease the muscular tension and anxiety that accompany breakthrough pain.
- It is essential to communicate to patients, families, and staff that successful results from nonpharmacologic interventions do not mean that the pain is not real.
- Nonpharmacologic pain interventions require uninterrupted time, a commitment to and belief in the efficacy of the interventions, and patients who are willing and able to participate in the intervention.
- Careful patient assessment is required before the introduction of nonpharmacologic pain

interventions; not all patients are able or desire to use these techniques.

- More than one nonpharmacologic pain intervention can be used at one time.
- Nonpharmacologic pain interventions are based on learning new skills, require practice, and are implemented when the patient has mild to moderate pain, or are appropriately used in conjunction with analgesics for patients in moderate to severe pain.

Pain, as a universal, multidimensional, and subjective phenomenon (see Chapter 1), demands pain management interventions that are universally used and validated, multidimensional, and designed for each patient's subjective pain experience. Even when drug therapy is clearly the first choice for pain management, nonpharmacologic approaches enhance pain management and patients' perceived feelings of control. Nurses are the primary professional resource for patients' pain management, and failure to provide adequate pain management interventions can lead to legal and ethical liabilities (Jurf & Nirschl, 1993).

This chapter is based on a holistic nursing philosophy with emphasis on the interconnectedness and reciprocity of mind, body, and spirit. The main focus centers on patients with chronic pain; however, the interventions are frequently useful in acute pain situations. This chapter begins with the psychophysiology of pain and psychosocial pain assessment. Two psychologic pain models will be presented: the interpersonal influence model and the self-regulation model. The stages of psychologic intervention will be described. The specific nonpharmacologic interventions discussed are stimulation-induced analgesia, cognitive interventions, and behavioral interventions. The interventions and techniques in this chapter are those that (1) are within the practice scope of nursing, (2) do not require special equipment or physician's orders, (3) do not interfere with any medical treatment, and (4) do not require informed consent (Witt, 1984). Transcutaneous electrical nerve stimulation (TENS) is prescribed by physicians and is the only exception to these criteria.

PSYCHOPHYSIOLOGY OF PAIN

According to the gate control theory (GCT) of pain (see Chapter 1 for further discussion), a sensory message or stimulated nerve signal travels to the spinal cord. There the message is processed and sent through open gates to the thalamus. It is in the thalamus that pain is consciously perceived, synchronized, and transmitted to the cerebral cortex (Hall, 1994). The thalamus, limbic, and cortex areas are connected. Negative and positive emotions exist in the limbic-thalamic system (Dossey, 1992a). It is in the cortex, however, that information from these systems is monitored (Hall). The gates are then opened or closed depending on the patient's current emotional state, interpretation of the situation based on past experiences, and the amount of attention given to the pain stimulus (Turk & Nash, 1993). The response to pain stimulus, then, has cognitive and affective dimensions (McGuire, 1992). See Figure 5-1 for a schematic diagram of cortical influence on opening or closing the pain gates.

It is theorized that thoughts and images originating in the frontal cortex are sent to the limbic-hypothalamic system (a major mind-body link), which then communicates via neurotransmitters. The autonomic nervous system (ANS) neurotransmitters are epinephrine and norepinephrine from the sympathetic nervous system (SNS) and acetylcholine from the parasympathetic nervous system (PNS). Sympathetic nervous system stimulation increases heart rate (HR), respiratory rate (RR), blood pressure (BP), and metabolism. Parasympathetic nervous system stimulation slows down the functions increased by the SNS. These neurotransmitters determine a patient's psychophysiologic state.

Learning is dependent on the psychophysiologic state at the time of the experience. This is known as state-dependent

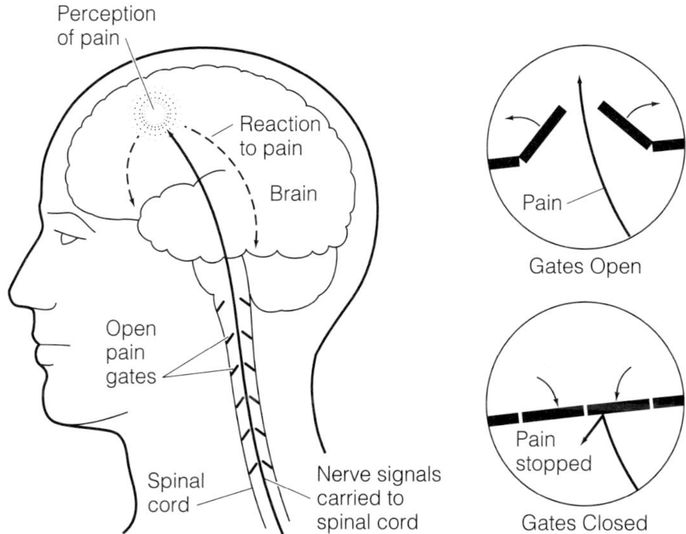

Figure 5-1 Representation of cortex and gating theory. (From Turk, D. C., & Nash, J. M. (1993). Chronic pain: New ways to cope. In D. Goleman & J. Gurin (Eds.), *Mind body medicine: How to use your mind for better health* (pp. 111-130). Yonkers: Consumer Reports.)

learning (Dossey, 1992a). Since the limbic-hypothalamic system contains positive and negative emotional patterns, stimulation of psychophysiologic responses evoke memories of joy, effective coping patterns, health, and well-being, as well as painful memories that need healing (Dossey).

Psychophysiologic stimulation can elicit painful experiences that can be reframed to change psychophysiologic responses. For example, the psychophysiologic state—beliefs, thoughts, and feelings—at the time of the pain stimulus shapes the pain experience (Turk & Nash, 1993). A past painful experience may have stimulated the SNS and resulted in muscle tension, rapid HR, and increased RR and led to feelings of helplessness and loss of control. Recollection of that experience or anticipation of a second painful episode can produce the same psychologic feelings and physiologic responses, even before the episode occurs. Thus the patient becomes more sensitive and fearful, and pain is more difficult to control.

Psychologic factors also influence pain perception indirectly by influencing coping responses (Turk & Nash, 1993). Feelings of helplessness and loss of control from pain or pain anticipation deplete available coping resources and initiate behaviors that may worsen pain. These feelings increase psychophysiologic responses, promote overreaction to painful stimuli, and lead to lack of physical activity, which further increases muscle tension and anxiety. Finally, people in pain may experience secondary gains, such as extra attention from family and friends, that shape pain perception and influence overt pain behaviors (Turk & Nash).

PSYCHOLOGIC PAIN MODELS

Dane and Kessler (1994) identify two models for psychologic intervention: the interpersonal influence model and the self-regulation training model. The interpersonal influence model incorporates the tenets of holistic nursing practice.

Interpersonal Influence Model

In the interpersonal influence model the willingness to listen and to be with troubled patients when there is nothing to be done provides relief of suffering. Patients need to talk and cry about losses as they work through the stages of grief. Nurses who display tolerance of uncomfortable emotions and can recognize when anger and affect displacement may constitute avoidance behavior for grieving are providing primary preventive interventions for pain and feelings of powerlessness (Dane & Kessler, 1994). Expression of painful feelings can decrease the requests for pain medication and increase the patient's perceived sense of control.

To be effective listeners, nurses must learn to deal with their own powerlessness to "fix" the problem. They must also recognize when the patient's pain triggers their own pain or feelings of helplessness to clearly delineate with whom the pain lies. Patients are hesitant to express painful or uncomfortable emotions to nurses who are unable, unwilling, or emotionally unavailable to listen or who cannot tolerate their pain. The effectiveness of this model is based on nurses' role modeling. When the nurse can tolerate patients' pain, patients are willing to share their pain, and through this process they obtain permission to grieve. When the nurse responds to inappropriate patient behaviors in appropriate ways, the behavior of the patient may change.

The interpersonal model of psychologic intervention is the treatment of choice for patients exhibiting emotional regression and experiencing a sense of powerlessness (Dane & Kessler, 1994). The following example describes this phenomenon.

> An oncology nurse approached the Pain Service psychologist with a sense of urgency concerning a female patient who was requesting inordinate amounts of pain medication because of inadequate relief. A brief discussion indicated that the patient had just been told that her cancer was terminal. ...[The psychologist] encouraged the nurse to ask the patient, "Which pain hurts worse, your cancer or what you have just been told?" The nurse subsequently reported that in response to her question, the patient had burst out crying and when provided further opportunity to ventilate, had no further requests for additional pain medication (Dane & Kessler, 1994, p. 66).

The interpersonal influence model is based on the skills of nurses, whereas the self-regulation training model involves teaching skills to patients.

Self-Regulation Training Model

The purposes of the self-regulation training model are to teach patients about the cognitive, affective, and physiologic aspects of pain perceptions and responses in order to enhance their pain management skills (Dane & Kessler, 1994). Cognitive self-regulation strategies include interventions such as imagery, music, and humor, all of which also act as distractions (Rowlingson, Kessler, Dane, & Hamill, 1994). Self-regulation interventions vary in the amount of time required for nurses to teach patients the skill; they also vary in impact (Rowlingson et al.).

Successful use of self-regulation or nonpharmacologic pain interventions require information and education, training and practice, follow-up, and environmental preparation. First, nurses need to be educated about nonpharmacologic pain interventions in order to teach them to patients. Although some nonpharmacologic interventions can be implemented based on reading about them, others require more specialized education (Owens & Ehrenreich, 1991). It is helpful if nurses experience the interventions to enrich their understanding and explanations to patients (Dossey, 1992a). The self-regulation interventions are discussed later in the chapter.

The next section will describe the process factors that shape the pain experience. The process factors include (a) affective and cognitive principles that affect pain awareness, (b) perceived control, and (c) location of the patient on the recovery continuum (Dane & Kessler, 1994).

AFFECTIVE AND COGNITIVE FACTORS AFFECTING PAIN

Subjective cognitive and affective factors that influence pain awareness include thoughts, beliefs, and emotions about the pain. Cognitive and affective responses are influenced by arousal of positive and negative emotions and the intrapsychic meanings of the pain. The level of suffering and emotional arousal associated with a painful stimulus increases or decreases pain awareness (Dane & Kessler, 1994).

The greater the significance of a pain event, the greater the meaning associated with that event. Thus, the meaning of pain events are shaped by personal history, prior learning, self-concept, goals, and values. For patients with cancer, pain may mean that the cancer is out of remission and their condition is worsening. Metastatic cancer pain is accompanied by low levels of perceived control and increased suffering. Childbirth pain, on the other hand, is often better tolerated because the outcome is positive and the duration is known to be limited.

Pain and suffering are not the same phenomenon (Fishman & Loscalzo, 1987). Suffering results from a threat to one's self-concept; it is distress caused by an actual or impending threat to personal integrity (Cassell, 1991). There is a sense of the future with suffering. Perceived suffering, then, is related to the meaning of the pain (Dane & Kessler, 1994).

Intrapsychic factors also influence the meaning of the pain. Pain may be viewed as punishment for past sins or punishment of others. It may be accompanied by high levels of guilt; patients may believe that they deserve to suffer. Current pain experiences may reactivate repressed or unresolved past, painful physical or emotional experiences such as physical or sexual abuse (Dane & Kessler, 1994). Patients who experience high levels of suffering have low levels of pain tolerance and often "act out" behaviorally.

Perceived Control

People who feel confident in their ability to manage or influence their pain experience a sense of control. Lack of perceived control contributes to feelings of inadequacy and anxiety (Dane & Kessler, 1994). Feelings of helplessness increase pain perception, deplete inner strength, and lead to overreacting (Turk & Nash, 1993). Therefore, nursing interventions are designed to allow patients as many choices and as much control as possible. Patients who feel that they have some control and some choices exhibit major shifts in cognitive, affective, and physiologic outcomes. The more of a sense of control patients experience, the more power they feel they have to affect outcome and the more willing they are to participate in self-initiated pain interventions.

Recovery Continuum

Location on the continuum of recovery involves both psychologic and physiologic factors and determines the amount of energy available for coping (which implies chronic pain). The recovery continuum has two components: (a) from "victim of injury" to "manager of recovery" and (b) successful grieving (Dane & Kessler, 1994, p. 58). When patients feel victimized by circumstances, they search for something or someone to blame. Even when patients are truly victims through no fault of their own, recovery does not begin until they shift to "managers of recovery." Until then, they are unable to participate in self-care management interventions and their energy is misplaced.

The second stage is movement through the process of grief. The loss of hopes, dreams, and goals may interfere with rehabilitation. For example, a mild cerebrovascular accident in a healthy individual represents both physical and psychologic losses. Although the physical recovery may be excellent, the inability to lift and hold grandchildren or to keep them overnight represents severe psychologic losses. Unless patients grieve over their emotional losses, they may be unable to incorporate effective nonpharmacologic pain management interventions. Patients who are dealing simultaneously with pain and unresolved grief exhibit unique behavioral characteristics (Dane & Kessler, 1994). See the box on p. 147 for a listing of the characteristics indicating possible arrested grief response. Understanding and assessing process factors in the pain experience provide psychosocial assessment data for planning nursing care.

PSYCHOSOCIAL PAIN ASSESSMENT

The multidimensional aspects of pain support a multidimensional assessment framework (McGuire, 1992). The goals of assessment are identified in Chapter 1. Each person's pain experience is unique and emerges from past experiences with pain, disease, and medical personnel. Pain is shaped by one's values, goals, fears, losses, and needs. Therefore, additional assessment data are needed to understand patients' personal

PATIENT CHARACTERISTICS INDICATING POSSIBLE ARRESTED GRIEF RESPONSE

1. Is unresponsive to reasonable reassurance about his or her condition
2. Continues to insist on the need for a clear diagnostic label for the etiology of the pain, even when one is not reasonably available, especially when potentially lethal or occult processes (e.g., cancer) have been ruled out (this may take the form of "doctor shopping" in the outpatient setting)
3. Exhibits unreasonable and unrelenting anger or hostility toward family, caregivers, and others who are supportive
4. Is obsessively preoccupied with the details of a particular medication or exercise regimen
5. Persists in focusing on the history and unfairness of the injury, pain, or illness rather than on the recovery process

From Dane, J. R., & Kessler, R. S. (1994). A matrix model for the psychological assessment and treatment of acute pain. In R. J. Hamill & J. C. Rowlingson (Eds.), *Handbook of critical care pain management* (pp. 53-81). New York: McGraw-Hill.

pain experiences so that appropriate nonpharmacologic pain interventions can be designed. Dimensions to be considered include the physiologic and sensory dimensions, which are discussed in Chapter 1. The affective, cognitive, and behavioral dimensions are discussed next.

The affective response to pain often results in anxiety and depression. Assessment begins with applying the process factors that shape the pain experience. This information may reveal that patients are experiencing more suffering than pain. Fear of the unknown outcome of medical problems may stimulate the SNS to produce physiologic anxiety and a negative psychophysiologic state, which require resolution before patients can absorb additional information or participate in self-care activities. In addition, pain intensifies anxiety, which stimulates the SNS and increases focus on pain, which in turn lowers the pain threshold and further intensifies the pain (Oates, 1993). Patients are assessed for placement on the recovery continuum and stage of grief so that individualized interventions can be designed.

The cognitive domain includes the meaning of the pain; the view of the self, which determines the level of suffering; previous treatment; and other influencing factors. Cognitions also include mental activities involved in coping, such as problem solving (Fishman & Loscalzo, 1987). Cognitions may be assessed through self-report and questioning, or inferred from observation of behavior (Fishman & Loscalzo).

Behavioral assessment includes physical actions or physiologic responses that can be objectively assessed (Fishman & Loscalzo, 1987). Physiologic responses to acute pain include those stimulated by the ANS, such as increased heart and respiration rates, which can be objectively measured. Other behaviors, such as limping, bracing, sighing, and grimacing, are respondent pain behaviors and are assessed by observation (Fishman & Loscalzo). These behaviors also occur in anticipation of pain. Pain behaviors frequently elicit support from family and are reinforced.

To select appropriate nonpharmacologic pain interventions for patients, assessment data are needed about problem-solving ability and coping style, emotional age, and hypnotic capacity. Patients who have resolved ongoing life crises and have been successful in other lifestyle areas such as work, education, and family generally demonstrate higher problem-solving skills and more positive attitudes about involvement in pain resolution (Dane & Kessler, 1994). However, if these patients are experiencing unresolved grief, are in the "victim of injury" mode, or are overwhelmed by their situations, they may have good problem-solving skills but be unable to use them.

Additional areas of patient assessment include level and style of coping. Identification of a patient's coping style determines the effectiveness of pain interventions (Faucett,

1991). Dane and Kessler (1994) characterize coping styles as "repressing avoiders" and "coping sensitizers." Repressing avoiders cope by minimizing problems or even denying the seriousness of their condition. They trust the caregiver's advice and are cooperative. Repressing avoiders may be threatened if they are given too much information or expected to assume too much control. Those with low levels of fear may experience increased anxiety if presented with too much information (Faucett, 1991). Staff work well with repressing avoiders since they generally are less demanding, are cooperative, and follow directions. Repressing avoiders probably have an external locus of control (LOC), meaning that they give power to others. Patients with an external LOC may be threatened by expectations that they actively participate in pain control or self-care management. In the initiation of nonpharmacologic pain interventions, those with an external LOC tend to take a passive stance and want specific instructions.

Coping sensitizers, on the other hand, desire information, ask questions, and seek reassurance to gain control and lower anxiety levels. They may even demand to "talk to the person in charge." They want information and choices, and they react to environments over which they have no control. For these patients, information can lower anxiety levels (Faucett, 1991). They are often seen by caregivers as demanding and troublesome patients. Coping sensitizers tend to have an internal LOC and prefer interventions that maintain their sense of control (Dane & Kessler, 1994). They are good candidates for most nonpharmacologic pain interventions.

Individuals who are able to focus their attention and become absorbed in daydreaming, reading, or watching television tend to exhibit hypnotic capacity. They exhibit high levels of responsiveness to suggestion from others or self (Dane & Kessler, 1994). The use of hypnosis can be an effective intervention for the 60% to 70% of the population who can benefit. (See Chapter 7 for a discussion of hypnosis.) The successful use of imagery also entails the patient's ability to concentrate and imagine what might be.

The successful use of nonpharmacologic pain interventions is founded on a therapeutic nurse-patient relationship. This relationship is enhanced when nurses encourage patients to tell their stories, accept without judgment what they say about their pain, and involve them in pain evaluation. Excellent patient assessment data, then, allow nurses to identify appropriate patients for nonpharmacologic pain interventions.

NONPHARMACOLOGIC INTERVENTIONS

Nonpharmacologic pain interventions can be classified as stimulation-induced analgesia and self-regulation techniques (Rowlingson et al., 1994) or as peripheral and central techniques (Edgar & Smith-Hanrahan, 1992). The GCT suggests that pain modulation occurs at four points: peripheral site, spinal cord, brainstem, and cortex (Herr & Mobily, 1992). Stimulation-induced or peripheral intervention techniques include those that stimulate the skin for pain reduction (Edgar & Smith-Hanrahan). They include heat and cold, acupressure, and massage. Self-regulation or central nervous system intervention techniques include cognitive, affective, and behavioral interventions and range from patient information and education to relaxation, mental imagery, music, distraction, humor, positive suggestion, biofeedback, psychotherapy, and hypnosis. In the following sections interventions will be defined, mechanisms of action discussed, and clinical indications and contraindications presented along with guidelines for use.

Stimulation-Induced Analgesia

Cutaneous stimulation, stimulation of the skin to relieve pain (McCaffery & Beebe, 1989), has physiologic and psychosocial outcomes. Physiologic effects result in a decrease of pain intensity and muscle spasm. The exact mechanisms of pain relief from cutaneous stimulation are unknown. The GCT, however, suggests that large-diameter fibers are stimulated with this technique, which closes the gate and prevents the transmission of pain impulses (see Chapter 1). Muscle spasms secondary to joint pathology (e.g., degenerative joint disease) are relieved by heat or cold or alternating heat and cold (McCaffery & Beebe, 1989). Some types of cutaneous stimulation may increase the production of endorphins, lowering pain sensations (McCaffery & Beebe).

There are also psychosocial benefits from cutaneous stimulation interventions. The muscle relaxation and distraction increase activity, which leads to a more relaxed state with decreased anxiety and more involvement with life. The use of touch in these interventions can improve body image, especially in those patients who have received a body image insult such as mastectomy or amputation (McCaffery & Beebe, 1989). Involving family and friends in the intervention increases social support for patients, and family and friends experience less helplessness.

Determination of which cutaneous stimulation intervention to use is dependent on knowledge of the patient's pathophysiology and the desired physiologic and psychosocial outcomes of the interventions. A given patient will frequently prefer one type over another. Patient education plays an important role because patients who understand the purposes of the intervention and the expected outcomes can make better choices and may be willing to accept some temporary discomfort. Patient education includes (a) information about how the interventions work, (b) conveying the need for trial and error to determine the most effective intervention, (c) assurance that successful outcome does not mean the pain is not real, and (d) emphasizing the importance of patient participation in ongoing evaluation.

The application sites for cutaneous stimulation are identified by trial and error but may be directly over the painful area; distal, proximal, or contralateral to the pain; or over acupuncture points (McCaffery & Beebe, 1989). See the box on p. 152 for terms that describe site selection. Stimulation at one site can produce a response at a distant site, which is known as consensual response or counterirritation (McCaffery & Beebe).

TERMS RELATED TO SITE SELECTION

Acupuncture point: A point or spot on the body associated with a conceptual (not anatomic) system of meridians. Between 500 and 800 points were identified centuries ago by cultures of the Far East. Some are related to pain syndromes, but others are not. Those related to pain are often located near or in the same place as trigger points.

Contralateral: On the opposite side of the body; opposed to ipsilateral.

Distal: Farthest from the center of the body; opposed to proximal.

Ipsilateral: On the same side of the body; opposed to contralateral.

Proximal: Nearest the center of the body; opposed to distal. May be referred to here as "between pain and the brain."

Trigger point: A point or area of hyperirritability in tissue such as myofascial (skeletal muscle and its fascia). When compressed it is tender and may give rise to referred pain, but after stimulation, e.g., with ischemic pressure, pain may be relieved. They are often located near or in the same place as acupuncture points.

From McCaffery, M., & Beebe, A. (1989). *Pain—Clinical manual for nursing practice.* St. Louis: Mosby.

Cutaneous stimulation can be modified by (a) increasing the intensity of stimulation, (b) alternating intervention, (c) interrupting the intervention every few minutes or even seconds, and (d) using different methods on two locations simultaneously (McCaffery & Beebe, 1989). Thus it is clear why patient participation is necessary to determine cutaneous stimulation technique and location.

The cutaneous stimulation interventions described in this section are low risk, inexpensive, effective, simple, and not time consuming. The interventions include massage, heat, cold, and transcutaneous electrical nerve stimulation (TENS), which is the only technique requiring a physician's order.

Massage

Massage is a natural, instinctive action when one experiences an ache or pain (Edgar & Smith-Hanrahan, 1992). It is the application of friction or pressure to an area of the body either superficially, deeply, or via vibrations (Jurf & Nirschl, 1993). Massage or mechanical pressure increases circulation and promotes capillary and arteriole dilation, which reduce edema and thus pain (Edgar & Smith-Hanrahan). Massage theoretically stimulates the large nerve fibers of the skin to close the gate and block transmission of pain messages (McCaffery & Beebe, 1989). There appear to be no randomized, clinical studies of the effects of massage (Edgar & Smith-Hanrahan). Massage can be superficial or deep.

Patients generally find superficial massage of the back, neck, shoulders, hands, or feet comforting, soothing, and relaxing. It is a form of nonverbal communication that can enhance nurse-patient communication and also assist patients in verbally expressing their concerns.

Pressure massage is the use of massage at trigger or acupuncture points. Acupuncture points can be stimulated by ischemic pressure or massage, with ice applied as firmly as can be tolerated, and with the sustained pressure of thumb, knuckle, or an object such as a rubber ball (McCaffery & Beebe, 1989). When massage is done with acupressure, contact is maintained with the skin while the muscles are massaged. Any patients with bleeding tendencies or who bruise easily should not receive acupressure. (See Chapter 7 for more information about acupuncture.)

Clinical indications and contraindications Although research data are absent, it is the experience of most nurses that a back rub has multiple therapeutic uses. First, it is relaxing for patients. Second, through touch it communicates a message of caring and thus improves the therapeutic nurse-patient relationship. Third, patients often talk about their worries and concerns during a back rub. Massage of the hands and feet is especially therapeutic. Massage is useful for patients who are restricted to bedrest, experiencing sleep difficulties, under excessive stress and tension, anxious or depressed, or "just need" a massage.

Although there are few contraindications to massage, patients who refuse should not be pressured. Patients who are potentially violent or who exhibit inappropriate sexual behaviors are not candidates for massage. It should not be used on inflamed areas or in the presence of phlebitis or open lesions (McCaffery & Beebe, 1989). Finally, nurses must be prepared to stay with patients if the massage stimulates emotional catharsis and the patient is upset.

Guidelines for use Scheduling the length of time of massage is dependent on the availability of the person performing the massage and the desires of the patient. The use of lotion for the massage is optional, but if used it can be carefully warmed in the microwave or a sink filled with hot water. For patients with dry skin, application of lotion is beneficial. Both the patient and the nurse should be in relaxed positions. Acupressure points should be stimulated from 7 to 10 seconds to a minute (McCaffery & Beebe, 1989).

Massage over the trunk and extremities is generally performed with the palms of both hands using enough pressure to prevent a sensation of tickling. Hands and feet are massaged with both hands with separate massages for each finger and toe. Patients are involved in the process by describing what feels good. This can increase patients' perceived sense of control. Nurses can explain that they will not talk during the procedure. This allows the patient to remain quiet or to talk about cares and concerns.

Superficial Heat Applications

The local application of moist or dry heat is a pain-relieving intervention that has been used for centuries (Edgar & Smith-Hanrahan, 1992). Superficial heat has physiologic and musculoskeletal effects that vary according to the type and duration of application. Physiologically, heat increases metabolic activity (Henahan & Baruch, 1994) two to three times with each 10° C increase (Cailliet, 1993). The vasodilation action of heat enhances blood flow, increasing tissue nutrition, eliminating cellular debris (Edgar & Smith-Hanrahan), decreasing the viscosity of fluids, and increasing the extensibility of collagenous tissue (Henahan & Baruch).

Heat affects gamma (γ) fiber activity in muscles, leading to a decrease in the sensitivity of muscle spindles to stretch and thus inducing muscle relaxation. In addition, heat reduces local tissue ischemia and stimulates endorphin release (Henahan & Baruch, 1994). It also triggers pain-inhibiting reflexes through temperature receptors. Heat increases the pain threshold, but not as much as cold.

Superficial heating methods include hot water bottles, wrapped to prevent burns; hot, moist compresses (towels that have been soaked in hot water); K-pads; hydrocollator packs heated in special containers; immersion in warm water, basin, sitz bath, or whirlpool; and the sun.

Clinical indications and contraindications Heat is used for muscle and joint pain to increase circulation, induce muscle relaxation, and decrease inflammation. Conditions that respond to heat include arthritis and phlebitis, swelling, joint stiffness, low back pain, and aching muscles. Heat applied to the abdomen reduces peristalsis and gastric acidity within 5 to 10 minutes (McCaffery & Beebe, 1989).

Applications of heat are contraindicated immediately after trauma because the vasodilation increases swelling. The elevated temperature increases metabolic demands and the need for oxygen; therefore it should not be used when circulation is compromised. Heat should not be applied over neuropathic areas since burns can occur without the awareness of pain. Do not apply heat where there is active bleeding or swelling (McCaffery & Beebe, 1989). Heat should not be used with patients who have sickle cell anemia, have been on long-term steroid use (Henahan & Baruch, 1994), or have an elevated temperature. Methods to deliver deep heat (shortwave diathermy, microwave diathermy, and ultrasound) should be used with caution in cancer patients and should not be applied directly over a cancer site (Jacox et al., 1994).

Guidelines for use Treatment should be limited to 30 minutes, three or four times a day (McCaffery & Beebe, 1989). The temperature of hot packs ranges from 104° to 113° F (40° to 45° C). The patient's skin is protected with a covering or towel to prevent burns.

Cold

Cold therapy (cryotherapy) takes little nursing time, is inexpensive, and is easily taught to patients and their families. The local application of cold may work via (a) vasoconstriction, (b) decreasing metabolism of local tissue, (c) neutralization of histamine from cell injury, (d) decreasing muscle sensitivity and spasms, and (e) raising the pain threshold (Cailliet, 1993). The vasoconstrictive action reduces blood flow. When cold is applied to recently injured areas, constriction of the blood vessels decreases cell permeability, thus preventing the release of pain-causing chemicals (lactic acid, kinins, serotonin, histamine); decreases production of lymph, thus decreasing edema; and slows conduction velocity of the small, unmyelinated pain fibers (McCaffery & Beebe, 1989). When acupuncture points are massaged with cold, afferent stimulations may activate the brainstem mechanisms that exert descending inhibitory influences on pain signals. Thus cold applications inhibit pain.

Clinical indications and contraindications Cold applications are useful in initial posttrauma conditions to reduce bleeding, swelling, and pain. Cold is also used with dental pain, bursitis, and muscle spasms caused by neurological disease such as degenerative joint disease (McCaffery & Beebe, 1989).

Applications of cold should be avoided in patients with vascular insufficiency, including patients with a diagnosis of peripheral arterial disease, Raynaud's phenomenon or disease, or other cold intolerance conditions. Patients with angina may experience a reflexive coronary artery constriction with cold application. Application of cold to the abdomen is contraindicated in patients with peptic ulcer disease since the cold may increase gastric acid secretion (McCaffery & Beebe, 1989).

Guidelines for use Cold applications provide more pain relief than heat but are used less often because patients generally prefer heat (McCaffery, 1990). Cold therapy is administered in a variety of ways. Commercial cold packs are available in most hospitals, but they are expensive. Cold packs can be made by placing wet washcloths or towels in the freezer or using ice. A nonsterile glove can be filled with crushed ice and wrapped in a washcloth. Cold applications also include immersion of a limb in cold water or a whirlpool.

Cold therapy may be more acceptable to patients if applied to a small area. Another technique is to cover the cold application so that the first sensation is cool, not cold. It is important to assess the skin before cold applications, to protect the skin during the application, and to assess the skin 20 to 30 minutes after the application. Alternating hot and cold applications is generally more effective than either hot or cold alone (McCaffery, 1990). Cold applications should not exceed 15 minutes. When ice or ice packs are used over acupoints, the time is reduced to 7 minutes per application.

Transcutaneous Electrical Nerve Stimulation

Transcutaneous electrical nerve stimulation (TENS) involves mild electrical stimulation to the skin using two carefully placed electrodes (Rowlingson et al., 1994). The GCT of pain provides a theoretical base for understanding how TENS relieves pain. Transcutaneous electrical nerve stimulation may activate the large-diameter, myelinated fibers to override stimuli from the A-delta (Aδ) and C fibers, thus closing the gate of pain transmission to the brain; or, it may increase endorphin release, thus activating the descending pathways and exerting an inhibition of pain transmission (Jurf & Nirschl, 1993; Rowlingson et al.;

Slack & Faut-Callahan, 1991). Chapter 8 discusses TENS in greater detail.

Clinical indications and contraindications Transcutaneous electrical nerve stimulation is used for both acute and chronic pain. Some examples are postoperative pain, angina, dysmenorrhea, orthopedic and neurologic pain, phantom limb pain, dental pain, headaches, lower back pain, peripheral nerve injuries, and labor pain (back only). Transcutaneous electrical nerve stimulation is noninvasive, is controlled by the patient, has no systemic effects, is nonaddictive and safe, and decreases the need for opioid administration, hence limiting the side effects (Rowlingson et al., 1994).

Transcutaneous electrical nerve stimulation should not be used for patients with contact dermatitis or in early pregnancy. Additionally, TENS is contraindicated in patients who have undiagnosed pain, are not psychologically disposed to want control of their pain, are experiencing skin numbness, or have demand pacemakers (Rowlingson et al., 1994).

Guidelines for use Transcutaneous electrical nerve stimulation must be prescribed by a physician and the electrodes placed by trained personnel. It can be used for only 3 to 5 days (Jurf & Nirschl, 1993). Patients require education about how to use TENS since they control the rate, amplitude, pulse width, and frequency of the stimulus (Rowlingson et al., 1994; Slack & Faut-Callahan, 1991). For deep, aching, chronic pain, electrodes are placed on acupressure points. The effectiveness of this mode is thought to result from the release of endorphins delaying the onset of pain relief but prolonging the duration (Rowlingson et al.). The burst mode delivers brief but intense stimulation for greater analgesia for such procedures as joint manipulation and debridement of wounds (Rowlingson et al.).

Stimulation-induced analgesia is effective and inexpensive and can be taught to patients and their support systems. These interventions may increase patients' perceived control since patients can design and implement them. The self-regulation techniques are also effective and inexpensive and can be taught to patients and their support systems, but they require longer periods of education and skill practice.

Cognitive Strategies

Cognitive strategies and behavioral techniques (discussed in the next section) have common outcomes, but cognitive techniques center on images, attitudes, and thoughts whereas biobehavioral interventions focus on changing physiologic and behavioral responses.

Cognitive interventions are based on the assumptions that (a) as individuals process information, thoughts modulate affect and physiology, thus influencing behavior; (b) behavior responds to environmental feedback; (c) patients can learn more effective ways of feeling, thinking, and doing; and (d) patients should be involved in the change process (Turk & Rudy, 1994). The main objectives of cognitive interventions are to identify and change distorted perceptions and to teach patients how to reconceptualize pain as manageable and themselves as competent and capable (Turk & Rudy). The cognitive strategies discussed here are self-talk, patient education, cognitive restructuring, distraction, music, and prayer.

Self-Talk

People constantly talk to themselves and respond physiologically. Self-talk that is optimistic and positive stimulates energy, whereas negative self-talk leads to physiologic anxiety (Dossey & Keegan, 1988). Cognitive strategies, then, include interventions that examine and evaluate self-talk and change negative self-statements to positive self-talk. Obviously, the first step is to listen to the patient's story (Turk & Rudy, 1994). It is vital to hear and understand patients' perspectives on their pain experience, to identify their misconceptions, and to determine how the pain affects their families and environment. Patient education affects self-talk.

Information about the disease, treatment, or pain can have major effects (Speigel, 1993). Patient preparation, an integral part of nursing care, permits patients to prepare themselves psychologically, reduces fear and threat, and increases their sense of perceived control, thus reducing anxiety and emotional distress. However, nurses must know their patients so that they can individualize the information, since too much information can increase the anxiety of patients with low levels of fear (Faucett, 1991). Relaxed patients experience less pain and are better able to participate in other interventions, such as breathing and relaxation techniques.

Patients also need education about cognitive interventions. It is important to emphasize that the success of these interventions does not mean that the pain is not real; it means that patients have additional techniques to handle the pain so that they can regain control (Burckhardt, 1990). Dispelling pain myths and misinformation is essential for these strategies to be effective. Specific cognitive strategies, such as cognitive restructuring, follow patient education.

Most people do not recognize how profoundly their thoughts affect their well-being, including physical state and mood (Turk & Nash, 1993). Thoughts, not facts, affect feelings (Edgar & Smith-Hanrahan, 1992). Patients may have little control over the facts, but they can have some control over what they think about the facts. Cognitive restructuring changes distorted ways of thinking and gives patients control.

Although this intervention sounds simple, it requires patient cooperation and time. The first step is for patients to identify when they begin to experience pain and anxiety. Second, they have to commit to examining what happened just before the pain and anxiety experience. What were they doing? What was being said? What was going on in the environment? After this assessment, patients must identify their self-statements. This is an ongoing process and requires that patients keep diaries or journals. Finally, with help from nurses, their thoughts can be restructured or reframed.

For example, a patient might think, "This bone marrow aspiration is so painful, I don't think I can take it." This can be reframed as a positive statement: "The pain from this bone marrow test will not last long. I can have some control over the pain if I use my relaxation exercise and listen to music." Reframing is a cognitive technique that helps people see their problems in another way (Stephens, 1993a).

This technique takes time. It is also dependent on the supportive attitude of the nurse since the nurse's beliefs and values affect pain management approaches (Griepp, 1992). In other words, nurses must appreciate the power of thoughts, believe in the competency of the patient, and, maybe more important, value patient control and independence. Depending on the assessment and extent of the problems, the nurse may want to negotiate a referral for the patient for more concentrated work. However, any time the patient makes a negative statement, the nurse can reframe the statement. This simple therapeutic intervention can have profound effects. The patient who incorporates the new statement may experience psychophysiologic changes.

Distraction

Pain intensity is increased when the individual concentrates on the pain. Therefore, a patient's pain perception can be modified by other sensory stimulation. Distraction is focusing the attention on something other than the sensation of pain (McCaffery & Beebe, 1989). The goals of distraction are to increase pain tolerance and perceived control and to decrease pain intensity. The disadvantages of distraction are that pain awareness, fatigue, and irritability may increase after the distraction (McCaffery & Beebe).

Distraction is more effective with mild pain but can be used with more severe pain that is treated with medications (Matassarin-Jacobs, 1993). Distracting interventions may even prolong the effects of the medication by redirecting patients' awareness. Distraction involves the senses of hearing, vision, movement, and touch, and interventions generally involve multiple sensory stimulation. Effective distraction techniques are interesting to patients, are consistent with their energy level and concentration ability, and provide increased stimulation when the pain intensity increases (McCaffery & Beebe, 1989).

Clinical indications and contraindications Distraction activities are appropriate for any patient who lacks sensory stimulation (McCaffery & Beebe, 1989), such as a patient in isolation or one with few visitors. Those who have limited mobility from casts or illness generally respond well to distraction interventions. Patients with high energy levels and no outlets not only respond but also enjoy distracting activities.

Patients who are experiencing overwhelming feelings of despair and depression may not be interested in participating in distracting activities. However, if it is possible to interest them in the environment even slightly, this can contribute to their healing. Patients who are fatigued are not good candidates.

Guidelines for use Distraction techniques are based on patients' interests. As pain increases, the intensity of the distraction must also increase. Multiple sensory distraction involves many senses concurrently. For example, patients can listen to music while they focus on a flower, plant, or visual image; have something to hold, touch, or rub; and tap or nod to the rhythm of the music (McCaffery & Beebe, 1989). Distraction is used for limited periods of time and works best if it is begun before the pain intensifies or before the painful experience (McCaffery & Beebe). Distraction is quite helpful for patients who are experiencing brief but intense pain, such as bone marrow aspirations or anxiety about an impending diagnostic test.

Music and Prayer

Music and prayer are distractions and can elicit the relaxation response. Therefore, these interventions are both cognitive-behavioral and biobehavioral. Used alone, they are effective, but they may also be used to prepare patients for other interventions such as relaxation techniques.

Listening to music is distracting and soothing for some patients. Music affects psychophysiologic responses (Guzzetta, 1994). Music that is soothing leads to a hypometabolic state similar to the relaxation response (Guzzetta). Since music preferences and responses vary and depend on the psychophysiologic state at the time of listening, better outcomes result from matching mind state and type of music (Guzzetta). Music can alter moods, with accompanying relaxing effects (Fishman & Loscalzo, 1987). It can lower systolic BP, reduce anxiety and depression, and change the pain experience (Updike, 1990).

Although music therapy involves a professionally trained therapist, it can be used effectively in a variety of settings and ways that nurses can implement in clinical settings. A type of nontraditional music has developed with no identifiable melody or central rhythm, and it allows patients to choose their responses based on their needs (Guzzetta, 1994). Music also provides an appropriate background for introducing other strategies, such as relaxation and imagery. Chapter 7 provides additional information about music therapy.

Prayer is used as a coping strategy by patients who have religious beliefs. Prayer may be silent or verbal, directed or nondirected, and is useful as a focusing technique (Dossey & Guzzetta, 1992). Repetitive prayer induces the same type of relaxation response as meditation, guided imagery, or hypnosis (Benson, 1993; Benson & McKee, 1993).

Behavioral Techniques

Behavioral techniques are methods of changing physiologic responses to pain (Fishman & Loscalzo, 1987). Imagery is a cognitive technique that induces psychophysiologic responses such as relaxation. This is an example of overlap between cognitive and behavioral techniques. Relaxation and guided imagery are independent nursing interventions (Tiernan, 1994) that promote the relaxation response.

The relaxation response is associated with low levels of psychophysiologic arousal identified by low SNS responses. A relaxed psychophysiologic state is one in which the parasympathetic system dominates and is marked by the absence of tension in physical, mental, and emotional states (Dossey & Guzzetta, 1992). It is characterized by a decrease in oxygen consumption, decreased muscle tone, decreased

HR and RR, lowered BP, and increased alpha wave activity (Benson & McKee, 1993). Nurses may observe a change in breathing patterns to slower and deeper breaths, eyelid fluttering, and jaw relaxation to the point of parting lips and drooping jaw (Dossey & Guzzetta). This reduction in anxiety may lead to a reduction in distressing feelings and thoughts (Edgar & Smith-Hanrahan, 1992). There are many procedures to induce the relaxation response and two phases.

Phase 1 includes the normal relaxation response resulting from decreased SNS stimulation or physiologic changes.

HOW TO ELICIT THE RELAXATION RESPONSE

Some general advice on regular practice of the relaxation response:

- Try to find 10 to 20 minutes in your daily routine; before breakfast is a good time.
- Sit comfortably.
- For the period you will practice, try to arrange your life so you won't have distractions. Put the phone on the answering machine, and ask someone else to watch the kids.
- Time yourself by glancing periodically at a clock or watch (but don't set an alarm). Commit yourself to a specific length of practice, and try to stick to it.

There are several approaches to eliciting the relaxation response. Here is one standard set of instructions used at the Mind/Body Medical Institute:

Step 1. Pick a focus word or short phrase that's firmly rooted in your personal belief system. For example, a nonreligious individual might choose a neutral word like *one* or *peace* or *love.* A Christian person desiring to use a prayer could pick the opening words of Psalm 23, *The Lord is my shepherd;* a Jewish person could use *Shalom.*

HOW TO ELICIT THE RELAXATION RESPONSE—cont'd

Step 2. Sit quietly in a comfortable position.

Step 3. Close your eyes.

Step 4. Relax your muscles.

Step 5. Breathe slowly and naturally, repeating your focus word or phrase silently as you exhale.

Step 6. Throughout, assume a passive attitude. Don't worry about how well you're doing. When other thoughts come to mind, simply say to yourself, "Oh, well," and gently return to the repetition.

Step 7. Continue for 10 to 20 minutes. You may open your eyes to check the time, but do not use an alarm. When you finish, sit quietly for a minute or so, at first with your eyes closed and later with your eyes open. Then do not stand for one or two minutes.

Step 8. Practice the technique once or twice a day.

From Benson, H. (1993). The relaxation response. In D. Goleman & J. Gurin, (Eds.), *Mind body medicine: How to use your mind for better health* (pp. 234-257). Yonkers: Consumer Reports.

Phase 2 follows immediately, and the key feature is that the mind is more open to new information (Benson, 1993). Therefore, eliciting the relaxation response enhances the receptivity of patients for other interventions, such as problem solving, imagery, and prayer.

Relaxation

Patient preparation is needed before beginning any type of relaxation technique; therefore, it is important to assess patient knowledge, experience, and feelings about relaxation. Knowledge about the mechanisms through which stress levels increase pain may encourage patients to participate (Edgar & Smith-Hanrahan, 1992). Relaxation techniques are a resource for pain management that increase patients' sense of control. However, it is essential that nurses and patients realize that relaxation can reduce the distress of pain but does not necessarily reduce the pain; therefore, relaxation is not a substitute for appropriate medication (McCaffery & Beebe, 1989). See the box on pp. 164-165 for an example of how to elicit the relaxation response. The prelude to relaxation techniques are breathing exercises.

Breathing exercises are an effective intervention that lead to relaxation and also prepare patients for additional relaxation strategies. Direct attention to the pace and depth of breathing helps patients focus, acts as a distraction technique, and relaxes superficial muscles (Faucett, 1991). Slow, rhythmic breathing can be used by patients anywhere and anytime for periods from 30 seconds to 10 minutes, and takes little time to teach (McCaffery & Beebe, 1989).

Another breathing exercise involves having the patient focus on each breath and count 1 on exhaling or count the breaths from 1 to 4 and repeat (Dossey & Guzzetta, 1992). When patients are comfortable with this simple exercise, the nurse can add imagery such as seeing the breath as a color and inhaling the color into the body. Another exercise is to imagine a hollow body that is filled with each breath or to breathe relaxation up one side or the front of the body and down the opposite side or back of the body (Dossey & Guzzetta). Breathing exercises are used to prepare patients for relaxation techniques. See the box on p. 167 for suggested techniques for focused breathing.

It is important to know the type and intensity of the patient's pain when using relaxation techniques. Those with very mild pain may be unwilling to learn the technique, whereas those with severe pain need more immediate relief; therefore, those with moderately severe pain for whom medications are not working or are presenting too many side effects may be ideal candidates (Edgar & Smith-Hanrahan, 1992). There are a number of relaxation techniques, ranging from jaw relaxation to remembering peaceful past experiences to progressive muscle relaxation.

PATIENT TEACHING FOR BREATHING TECHNIQUE INTERVENTIONS

Deep Breathe/Tense, Exhale/Relax, Yawn for Quick Relaxation

- Clench fists and take a deep breath and hold it.
- Breathe out slowly and go limp like a rag doll.
- Start yawning.

Heartbeat Breathing

- Take a deep, slow breath.
- Close your eyes or focus on your hands.
- Count radial pulse for two beats.
- Inhale on next two beats.
- Exhale on next three beats.
- Repeat several times.

Jaw Relaxation

- Drop your jaw as though starting a yawn.
- Let tongue rest in bottom of mouth.
- Let lips get soft.
- Breathe slowly and evenly.
- Stop thinking words and allow relaxation.

Slow Rhythmic Breathing for Relaxation

- Take a slow, deep breath.
- Imagine that you are in a warm, safe place.
- Breathe in and out slowly.
  Breathe in and say "in, two, three."
  Breathe out and say "out, two, three, four."
  or
  Breathe in silently, thinking "peace."
  Breathe out silently, thinking "relax."
- Repeat slow, rhythmic breathing from seconds to 20 minutes.

Modified from McCaffery, M., & Beebe, A. (1989). *Pain—Clinical manual for nursing practice.* St. Louis: Mosby.

Progressive muscle relaxation is a process of tightening muscle groups, focusing on and consciously experiencing the sensations, and then slowly releasing the tension (Kolkmeier, 1994). Progressive muscle relaxation provides a method for patients to be in control since it involves conscious, systematic, and progressive tensing and relaxing of the muscles (Dossey & Guzzetta, 1992). It helps draw attention away from thoughts that provoke anxiety by focusing on physical sensations (Faucett, 1991). Progressive muscle relaxation affects perceived control and also acts as a diversion technique since the patient is focused on tensing and relaxing the muscles and not on the stressful event. The instruction tempo is important since patients need time to focus on muscles but not enough time for the mind to wander (Faucett). See the box on pp. 169-171 for basic instructions for progressive muscle relaxation.

Clinical indications and contraindications Relaxation techniques are used for muscle tension and spasm, for chronic sympathetic arousal, and to decrease the fear and anxiety associated with the pain experience (Edgar & Smith-Hanrahan, 1992). Muscle tension, pain, and anxiety become a cycle; relaxation strategies can interrupt the cycle (McCaffery & Beebe, 1989). Relaxation used preventively can support sleep, improve other strategies such as problem solving and distraction, and positively affect the nurse-patient relationship (McCaffery & Beebe). Patients who are able to induce the relaxation response experience higher levels of control and are empowered to participate in their care.

Contraindications for relaxation interventions include patients who do not want to try or cannot muster the energy to try. Patients with a history of hallucinations, depression, or other psychiatric diagnoses may lose contact with reality if they focus internally. The elderly do not benefit as quickly or as much from relaxation interventions but often benefit from simple interventions (McCaffery & Beebe, 1989). Special care should be taken with cardiac patients since stimulation of the vagus nerve may increase the risk

BASIC INSTRUCTIONS FOR PROGRESSIVE RELAXATION

In progressive muscle relaxation, you methodically sweep through your body, tensing and then relaxing each major muscle group. This attunes you to the difference in feeling when your muscles are tensed or relaxed and is another way to elicit the relaxation response.

This technique can be done in any large chair that supports your head and neck, but is best done lying on your back on a firm but soft surface, such as a thick carpet or workout mat. (A bed is too soft—you're more likely to glide off to sleep.) Lie on your back with your arms along your sides. Loosen any clothing that's uncomfortably tight, and take off your shoes.

You can have someone read you the instructions, or make a tape for yourself. These should be read at a slow, easy-going pace:

First, tense the muscles throughout your body, from head to toe. Tighten your feet and legs, tense your arms and hands, clench your jaw, and contract your stomach. Hold the tension while you sense the feelings of strain and tightness. Study the tension and notice the difference between how the muscle feels when it is tensed and when it is relaxed. Then take a deep breath, hold it, and exhale long and slowly as you relax all your muscles, letting go of the tension. Notice the sense of relief as you relax.

Now you're going to tense and relax individual groups of muscles, keeping the rest of your body as relaxed as you can. You'll hold the tension for a few seconds in each part of your body while you get a clear sense of what the tension feels like; then breathe deeply, hold the breath for a moment, and let go of the tension as you exhale.

Start by making your hands into tight fists. Feel the tension through your hands and arms. Relax and let go of the tension. Now press your arms down against the surface they're resting on. Feel the tension. Hold it . . . and let go. Let your arms and hands go limp.

Continued.

BASIC INSTRUCTIONS FOR PROGRESSIVE RELAXATION—cont'd

Shrug your shoulders tight, up toward your head, feeling the tension through your neck and shoulders. Hold... then release, letting go. Drop your shoulders down, free of tension.

Now wrinkle your forehead, sensing the tightness. Hold ... release, letting your forehead be smooth and relaxed. Shut your eyes as tight as you can. Hold... and let go. Now open your mouth as wide as you can. Hold it... and gently relax, letting your lips touch softly. Then clench your jaw, teeth tight together. Hold... and relax. Let the muscles of your face be soft and relaxed, at ease.

Take a few moments to sense the relaxation throughout your arms and shoulders, up through your face. Now take a deep breath, filling your lungs down through your abdomen. Hold your breath while you feel the tension through your chest. Then exhale and let your chest relax, your breath natural and easy. Suck in your stomach, holding the muscles tight ... and relax. Arch your back... hold... and ease your back down gently, letting it relax. Feel the relaxation spreading through your whole upper body.

for dysrhythmias. Hypotensive patients who want to use relaxation techniques require careful monitoring (McCaffery & Beebe).

Imagery

Imagery is an ancient healing technique that uses the energy generated from mental images to perform specific tasks (Stephens, 1993b). It is an internal experience of dreams, memories, visions, and fantasies and uses the senses to enhance body-mind-spirit communication (Dossey, 1994). Patients often select an image in response to their unconcious physiologic processes (Stephens, 1993a; Tiernan, 1994). Imagery thus allows patients to gain access to their inner

BASIC INSTRUCTIONS FOR PROGRESSIVE RELAXATION—cont'd

Now tense your hips and buttocks, pressing your legs and heels against the surface beneath you...hold...and relax. Curl your toes down, so they point away from your knees... hold...and let go of the tension, relaxing your legs and feet. Then bend your toes back up toward your knees...hold... and relax.

Now feel your whole body at rest, letting go of more tension with each breath...your face relaxed and soft...your arms and shoulders easy...stomach, chest, and back soft and relaxed...your legs and feet resting at ease...your whole body soft and relaxed.

Take time to enjoy this state of relaxation for several minutes, feeling the deep calm and peace. When you're ready to get up, move slowly, first sitting, and then gradually standing up.

From Benson, H. (1993). The relaxation response. In D. Goleman & J. Gurin, (Eds.), *Mind body medicine: How to use your mind for better health* (pp. 234-257). Yonkers: Consumer Reports.

experiences by using the senses and produces dramatic psychophysiologic responses (Dossey). Since imagery increases communication between emotions and physiology, it can be used to create a milieu to support healing (Stephens, 1993b). It is a way for patients to gain some control.

There is no precise evidence for how imagery works; however, when the brain is monitored during imagery exercises with positron emission tomography, it has been found that the cerebral cortex is activated (Rossman, 1993). It is theorized that the cerebral cortex sends the image to the limbic system (emotional center), which then communicates with the endocrine and ANS, leading to physiologic changes (Rossman). During relaxation, the limbic system is stimulated to accept the image as reality (Tiernan, 1994).

Three major outcomes of imagery are increased emotional awareness, psychological insight, and physiologic changes (Rossman, 1993). Patients always have an image of the way their body is functioning and, with pain, images are often negative. Since a person can have only one thought or image at a time (Dossey, 1992b), changes resulting from imagery are the same whether one actually has an experience or only imagines it.

Clinical indications and contraindications Patients who have repeated contacts with nurses, read and use imagery in conversation, daydream, and express strong religious beliefs are ideal candidates for imagery (McCaffery & Beebe, 1989). However, most patients can remember past experiences that were pleasant, and these memories can help them begin to use imagery techniques (Faucett, 1991). Patients who have trouble visualizing may experience kinesthetic, auditory, or other images (Faucett).

Imagery is an important intervention in many clinical situations. It is a powerful technique to reduce anxiety and manage pain since it affects patients psychophysiologically. It supports a patient's adjustment to chronic illness and is helpful for mental rehearsal to prepare the patient for painful procedures (Stephens, 1993b). Leading patients through procedures such as wound debridement or chest tube removal provides them with sensory and factual information that supports coping. Imagery can also be used to support future adjustment of patients by helping them anticipate and prepare (mentally rehearse) for future experiences (Faucett, 1991).

Imagery may be contraindicated in psychiatric patients, those with severe emotional problems, and those who do not want to try or cannot concentrate (McCaffery & Beebe, 1989). Stop the imagery if the patient experiences guilt or distress (Stephens, 1993b). Patients who believe that imagery will cure them are often disappointed and experience great guilt feelings when healing does not occur. Free-flowing and unstructured imagery can evoke intense hidden feelings and must be stopped or modified (Stephens).

IMAGERY SCRIPT FOR BASIC PAIN ASSESSMENT

Imagery helps access and control both acute and chronic psychophysiologic pain. The following exercise can be done in 10 to 20 minutes.

Script: *Close your eyes and let yourself relax. . . . Begin to describe the pain in silence to yourself. Be present with the pain. . . . Know that the pain may be either physical sensations . . . or worries and fears. Let your pain take on a shape . . . any shape that comes to your mind. Become aware of the dimensions of the pain. . . . What is the height of your pain? . . . the width of the pain? . . . and the depth of the pain? Where in the body is it located? . . . Give it color . . . a shape . . . feel the texture. Does it make any sound?*

And now with your eyes still closed, . . . let your hands come together with palms turned upward as if forming a cup. Put your pain object in your hands. [Once again, the nurse asks these questions about the pain, preceding each question with this phrase: "How would you change the size, etc.?"]

Let yourself decide what you would like to do with the pain. There is no right way to finish the experience . . . just accept what feels right to you. You can throw the pain away . . . or place it back where you found it . . . or move it somewhere else. Let yourself become aware . . . of how pain can be changed. . . . By your focusing with intention, the pain changes.

It is not unusual for the pain to go completely away or at least lessen after this exercise. The client also learns to manipulate the pain so that it is not the controlling factor of his or her life. The exercise is also effective with severe pain. After giving pain medication, the nurse can have the client relax during the imagery process.

From Dossey, B. M. (1994). Imagery: Awakening the inner healer. In B. M. Dossey, L. Keegan, C. E. Guzzetta, & L. Kolkmeier (Eds.), *Holistic nursing: A handbook for practice* (3rd ed., pp. 573-605). Gaithersburg, MD: Aspen.

Guideline for use It is important for nurses to have an understanding of patients' pathophysiology to help patients choose an image that is healing for them. For example, the immune system in rheumatoid arthritis is overactive, with the body unable to distinguish self from nonself, whereas it is underactive in the patient with metastatic cancer. Therefore, images of the immune function are modified to meet patients' needs. Ongoing assessment and evaluation of patients are essential to ensure that images are appropriate and healing. Imagery is a learned skill that must be practiced (Edgar & Smith-Hanrahan, 1992). Patients are encouraged to use imagery two to three times a day for 20 minutes each time (Dossey & Guzzetta, 1992). See the box on p. 173 for dialogue for a pain assessment imagery.

SUMMARY

Nonpharmacologic approaches to pain are based on a holistic philosophy of nursing that emphasizes the interconnectedness and reciprocity of mind, body, and spirit. The pain experience is based on a patient's emotions at the time of the first pain experience and also on past painful experiences and emotions. The physiologic responses to pain, such as increased heart and respiratory rates, become associated with the pain experience. Subsequent pain experiences elicit these same psychophysiologic responses. Thus, moods, emotions, and past experiences with pain, and goals, values, and beliefs combine to form positive or negative emotional pain patterns. Careful psychosocial assessment is thus needed for the design of effective and appropriate nonpharmacologic nursing interventions.

Both psychologic pain models emphasize the opportunities and challenges nurses possess for helping patients and their families cope effectively with pain. The nonpharmacologic pain interventions identified in this chapter are independent nursing interventions (except for TENS), based on a therapeutic nurse-patient relationship, and include stimulation-induced analgesia, cognitive behavioral techniques, and biobehavioral strategies. Nurses are encouraged to continue to pursue experiences to enhance their learning and skill with these techniques, to use them in their own lives, and to teach patients to use them effectively.

References

Benson, H. (1993). The relaxation response. In D. Goleman & J. Gurin (Eds.), *Mind body medicine: How to use your mind for better health* (pp. 234-257). Yonkers: Consumer Reports.

Benson, H., & McKee, M. G. (1993). Relaxation and other alternative therapies. *Patient Care* 27(20), 75-90.

Burckhardt, C. S. (1990). Chronic pain. *Nursing Clinics of North America* 25, 863-870.

Cailliet, R. (1993). *Pain: Mechanisms and management. Physical intervention in pain* (pp. 64-81). Philadelphia: Davis.

Cassell, E. J. (1991). Recognizing suffering. *Hastings Center Report 21*(3), 24-31.

Dane, J. R., & Kessler, R. S. (1994). A matrix model for the psychological assessment and treatment of acute pain. In R. J. Hamill & J. C. Rowlingson (Eds.), *Handbook of critical care pain management* (pp. 53-81). New York: McGraw-Hill.

Dossey, B. M. (1992a). The psychophysiology of bodymind healing. In B. M. Dossey & C. E. Guzzetta (Eds.), *Cardiovascular nursing: Holistic practice* (pp. 17-25). St. Louis: Mosby.

Dossey, B. M. (1992b). Psychophysiologic self-regulation. In B. M. Dossey & C. E. Guzzetta (Eds.), *Cardiovascular nursing: Holistic practice* (pp. 27-39). St. Louis: Mosby.

Dossey, B. M. (1994). Imagery: Awakening the inner healer. In B. M. Dossey, L. Keegan, C. E. Guzzetta, & L. G. Kolkmeier (Eds.), *Holistic nursing: A handbook for practice* (2nd ed., pp. 609-666). Gaithersburg, MD: Aspen.

Dossey, B. M., & Guzzetta C. E. (1992). Biobehavioral interventions. In B. M. Dossey & C. E. Guzzetta (Eds.), *Cardiovascular nursing: Holistic practice* (pp. 98-122). St. Louis: Mosby.

Dossey, B. M., & Keegan, L. G. (1988). Holism and the circle of human potential. In B. M. Dossey, L. M. Keegan, C. E. Guzzetta, & L. G. Kolkmeier (Eds.), *Holistic nursing: A handbook for practice* (pp. 3-21). Gaithersburg, MD: Aspen.

Edgar, L., & Smith-Hanrahan, C. M. (1992). Nonpharmacological pain management. In J. H. Watt-Watson & M. I. Donoan (Eds.), *Pain management: Nursing perspective* (pp. 162-199). St. Louis: Mosby.

Faucett, J. (1991). Care of the critically ill patient in pain: The importance of nursing. In K. A. Puntillo (Ed.), *Pain in the critically ill* (pp. 115-136). Gaithersburg, MD: Aspen.

Fishman, B., & Loscalzo, M. (1987). Cognitive-behavioral interventions in management of cancer pain: Principles and applications. *Medical Clinics of North America, 71*(2), 271-287.

Greipp, M. E. (1992). Undermedication for pain: An ethical model. *Advances in Nursing Science, 15*(1), 44-53.

Guzzetta, C. E. (1994). Music therapy: Hearing the melody of the soul. In B. M. Dossey, L. Keegan, C. E. Guzzetta, & L. G. Kolkmeier (Eds.), *Holistic nursing: A handbook for practice* (2nd ed., pp. 667-698). Gaithersburg, MD: Aspen.

Hall, J. L. (1994). Anatomy of pain. In C. D. Tollison, J. R. Satterthwaite, & J. W. Tollison (Eds.), *Handbook of pain management* (2nd ed., pp. 11-17). Baltimore: Williams & Wilkins.

Henahan, K., Baruch, L. D. (1994). Physical and occupational therapy in the prevention and management of pain in the intensive care unit. In R. J. Hamill & J. C. Rowlingson (Eds.), *Handbook of critical care pain management* (pp. 251-268). New York: McGraw-Hill.

Herr, K. A., & Mobily, P. R. (1992). Interventions related to pain. *Nursing Clinics of North America, 27*(2), 347-369.

Jacox, A., Carr D. B., Payne R., Berde, C. B., Breitbart, W., Cain, J. M., Chapman, C. R., Cleeland, C. S., Ferrell, B. R., Finley, R. S., Hester, N. O., Hill, C. S., Leak, W. D., Lipman, A. G., Logan, C. L., McGarvey, C. L., Miaskowski, C. A., Mulder, D. S., Paice, J. A., Shapiro, B. S., Silberstein, E. B., Smith, R. S., Stover, J., Tsou, C. V., Vecchiarelli, L., & Weissman, D. E. (1994). *Management of cancer pain. Clinical practice guideline.* AHCPR Pub. No. 94-0592. Rockville, MD: Agency for Health Care Policy and Research, PHS, USDHHS.

Jurf, J. B., & Nirschl, A. L. (1993). Acute postoperative pain management: A comprehensive review and update. *Critical Care Nursing Quarterly, 16*(1), 8-25.

Kolkmeier, L. G. (1994). Relaxation: Opening the door to change. In B. M. Dossey, L. Keegan, C. E. Guzzetta, & L. G. Kolkmeier (Eds.), *Holistic nursing: A handbook for practice* (2nd ed., pp. 573-605). Gaithersburg, MD: Aspen.

Matassarin-Jacobs, E. (1993). Pain assessment and intervention. In J. M. Black & E. Matassarin-Jacobs (Eds.), *Luckmann and Sorensens' medical-surgical nursing* (pp. 311-358). Philadelphia: W. B. Saunders.

McCaffery, M. (1990). Nursing approaches to nonpharmacological pain control. *International Journal of Nursing Studies, 27*(1), 1-5.

McCaffery, M., & Beebe, A. (1989). *Pain: Clinical manual for nursing practice.* St. Louis: Mosby.

McGuire, D. B. (1992). Comprehensive and multidimensional assessment and measurement of pain. *Journal of Pain and Symptom Management,* 7(5), 312-319.

Oates, H. B. (1993). Non-pharmacologic pain control for the CABG patient. *Dimensions of Critical Care Nursing, 12*(6), 296-304.

Owens, M. K., & Ehrenreich, D. (1991). Literature review of nonpharmacologic methods for the treatment of chronic pain. *Holistic Nursing Practice,* 6(1), 24-31.

Rossman, M. L. (1993). Imagery: Learning to use the mind's eye. In D. Goleman & J. Gurin (Eds.), *Mind body medicine: How to use your mind for better health* (pp. 234-257) Yonkers: Consumer Reports.

Rowlingson, J. C., Kessler, R. S., Dane, J. R., Hamill, R. J. (1994). Adjunctive therapy for pain. In R. J. Hamill & J. C. Rowlingson (Eds.), *Handbook of critical care pain management* (pp. 229-249). New York: McGraw-Hill.

Slack, J., & Faut-Callahan, M. (1991). Pain management. *Nursing Clinics of North America, 26*(2), 463-476.

Spiegel, D. (1993). Social support: How friends, family and groups can help. In D. Goleman & J. Gurin (Eds.), *Mind body medicine: How to use your mind for better health* (pp. 331-349). Yonkers: Consumer Reports.

Stephens, R. L. (1993a). Imagery: A strategic intervention to empower clients. Part I: Review of research literature. *Clinical Nurse Specialist,* 7(4), 170-174.

Stephens, R. L. (1993b). Imagery: A strategic intervention to empower clients. Part II: A practical guide. *Clinical Nurse Specialist,* 7(5), 235-240.

Tiernan, P. J. (1994). Independent nursing interventions: Relaxation and guided imagery in critical care. *Critical Care Nurse, 14*(5), 47-51.

Turk, D. C., & Nash, J. M. (1993). Chronic pain: New ways to cope. In D. Goleman & J. Gurin (Eds.), *Mind body medicine: How to use your mind for better health* (pp. 111-130). Yonkers: Consumer Reports.

Turk, D. C., & Rudy, T. W. (1994). A cognitive-behavioral perspective on chronic pain: Beyond the scalpel and syringes.

In E. D. Tollison, J. R. Satterthwaite, & J. W. Tollison (Eds.), *Handbook of pain management* (2nd ed., pp. 136-151). Baltimore: Williams & Wilkins.

Updike, P. (1990). Music therapy results for ICU patients. *Dimensions of Critical Care Nursing, 9*(1), 39-45.

Witt, J. R. (1984). Relieving chronic pain. *Nurse Practitioner, 1,* 36-38, 78.

6

TEAM APPROACH TO PAIN MANAGEMENT

Barbara Miller

Susan M. Bruno

Barry Kinzbrunner

Key Points

- A team is a group of individuals who work together in a coordinated effort to achieve a unified outcome
- The team leader is an individual who ensures that the members of the group work as a unit to achieve the common goals of the team
- An interdisciplinary team is one in which each member conducts individual evaluations of the patient, and then the assessments are coordinated to develop a single treatment plan with integrated goals
- A multidisciplinary team is individuals functioning as separate consultative professionals within a group setting to develop individual plans of care
- The pain team is composed of specialists from a number of different health care disciplines with expertise in the treatment of the physical, emotional, psychosocial, and spiritual challenges that contribute to a patient's perception of pain
- Patient-family includes the individual under medical care and his or her immediate and extended family members plus significant others

Other chapters in this book have reviewed the different types and causes of pain and various pharmacologic and non-pharmacologic approaches to its treatment. This chapter will focus on the composition and types of teams and the rationale for utilizing a team approach in the management of pain.

MULTIFACTORIAL NATURE OF PAIN

To understand why it is important for a team of health care professionals from different disciplines to work together to manage pain, it is necessary to understand that pain is multifactorial in nature. A number of models have been developed that illustrate how a patient's perception of pain is influenced by a combination of physical, environmental, emotional, and spiritual factors. Three of these models—Welk (1991); Portenoy (1988); and Ferrell, Grant, Rhiner, & Padilla (1992)—will be reviewed in this section.

Welk (1991) views pain as one of four elements influencing what he describes as total suffering. Pain is viewed as physical suffering, whereas emotional suffering is termed fear, social suffering is manifested as conflict, and spiritual suffering is seen as despair.

Portenoy (1988) proposes a more complex model, in which *total pain* is separated into the components of pain and suffering (see Figure 6-1). In this model a patient's perception of pain is influenced by nociceptive and neuropathic physical stimuli combined with psychosocial, physical, and environmental factors that include the patient's psychologic state, potential physical disability and loss of work, the

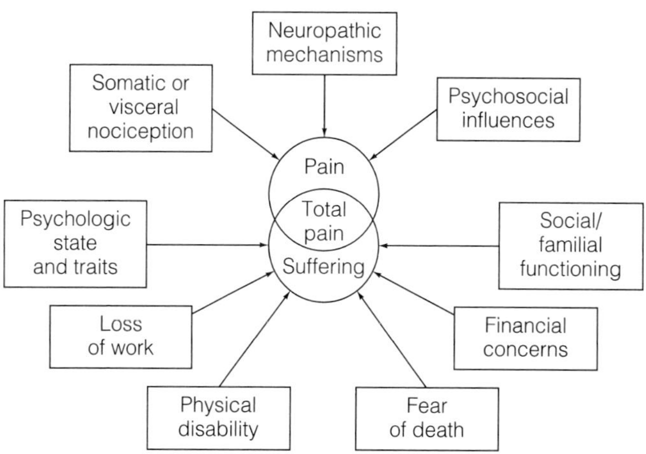

Figure 6-1 Multifactorial nature of pain. (From Portenoy, R. K. (1988). Practical aspects of pain control in the patient with cancer. *CA: A Cancer Journal for Clinicians, 38,* 327-352.)

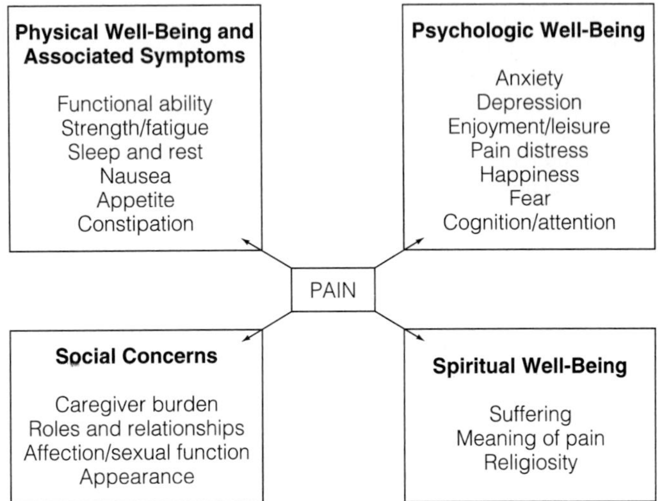

Figure 6-2 Effects of cancer pain. (From Ferrell, B. R., Grant, M. M., Rhiner, M., & Padilla, G. V. (1992). Home care: Maintaining quality of life for patient and family, *Oncology, 6*(suppl.), 136-140. By permission of S. Karger AG, Basel.)

financial concerns of chronic illness, changes in the social and functional structures of the family, and, in the case of pain secondary to cancer, the fear of disease progression and death.

Ferrell and colleagues (1992) propose that the presence of pain adversely affects the physical, psychologic, social, and spiritual well-being of the patient (see Figure 6-2). In this model patients with pain experience physical symptoms such as anorexia and fatigue; psychologic disturbances such as depression, anxiety, and fear; social concerns related to changing roles and relationships; and spiritual issues related to the meaning of pain and suffering.

Whichever model one chooses to adopt, the common factor in all three is the great influence that psychologic, spiritual, and social issues have on a patient's perception of what is commonly believed to be primarily a physical phenomenon. Therefore to properly manage a patient's pain, health care providers need to have expert skills in the management of the physical, psychologic, social, and spiritual challenges that contribute to a patient's pain. Equally clear is the fact that no single health care professional—whether physician, nurse, social worker, chaplain, pharmacologist, or any of a host of others—possesses the expertise necessary to manage the complexities of pain. It is only by combining the expertise and skills of all these disciplines to form a pain management team that inroads in the management of pain can be made.

TEAM APPROACH TO HEALTH CARE

The treatment of patients by a team of professionals from different disciplines is a concept significantly influenced by the evolving health care reform of the 1990s. Within the team the various specialists make recommendations regarding a particular challenge from their own unique points of view. Once all team members, including the patient and family, have agreed on a plan of action, they collectively implement the plan to attain the desired outcome. The team then meets at regular intervals to evaluate progress and make sure they are moving toward the original goal or to make appropriate adjustments in the plan of action as necessary.

The momentum of the team approach to health care in the 1990s is evidenced by changes in the education of health care providers. The student is introduced to focused collaboration and the team approach to care through both didactic and experiential approaches. In nursing schools, for example, faculty and students collaborate with other members of the health care team. The team delivers health care services within the community and shares planning, teaching, and research responsibilities and experiences (Oermann, 1994). In this way teamwork becomes the process with which the health care student is most familiar and comfortable, so that this process is likely to be the one that is preferentially utilized in health care in the twenty-first century.

Team

A team is a group of individuals who work together with the patient and family in an effort to achieve a unified outcome. Such a group is much more than a collection of individual personalities, attitudes, values, and beliefs; it is a composite of these characteristics from each individual on the team and their interactions. Gibson, Ivancevich, and Donnelly (1991) view a group in terms of perception, organization, motivation, and interaction. The members of the group, being parts of the whole, must perceive the existence of the group.

As in any group, there are parameters within which the team must function. By collectively setting organizational standards for role relationships and norms for the team, team members can establish an environment in which they can function effectively. Techniques utilized by teams to establish and maintain effective functioning include open communication between members, formalized regular interaction, and individual and group motivation.

Open communication is key to the successful functioning of the team and is characterized by the following qualities:

1. Communication is direct, clear, and specific.
2. The rules governing team behavior are flexible.
3. There is freedom within the team to communicate and comment on team rules with the goal of changing rules that no longer serve a purpose for the team members.

For open communication to be effective, formal and informal interactions between members of the team must be established in a frequent and timely fashion. These interactions may include regularly scheduled meetings in which members share information pertinent to achieving the goals of the team, and more informal conversations between members whenever an event occurs that may affect the outcome of the team's work. To provide the proper motivation for an individual to participate effectively as a team member, and to provide motivation to the group as a whole, recognition must be given to individuals for their participation and to the team as a whole when it achieves its established goals. Combining the techniques of open communication, formal and informal interaction, and individual and group motivation helps to ensure effective team function. Each member of the team acknowledges himself or herself as an integral part of the whole while remaining cognizant of individual contributions to the team's success.

One of the by-products of efficient team functioning is "role blurring" (Amenta & Bohnet, 1986). An individual on a team generally has functions clearly delineated by a job description, which defines roles and limitations. However, as a team develops into a cohesive unit, each member of the team becomes keenly aware of the responsibilities of the other team members as well. In so doing, team members learn various techniques from one another, strengthening their own personal and professional skills.

As an illustration, Mr. Koffer, a home care patient, is visited by a social worker at his own request. During the visit, the patient expresses concerns regarding his discharge from the acute care facility only days following his surgical procedure. Mr. Koffer appears anxious, seems to hold his breath, and tightens his abdominal muscles with some frequency. During the discussion Mr. Koffer explains that he doesn't want to be considered a complainer or a burden. Continuing to display signs of discomfort or pain, he states that although he is happy to be back at home, he does experience more pain than while he was in the hospital. The social worker asks Mr. Koffer if his pain is in the incisional area or if he feels he merely needs to be "straightened out in bed." The social worker notes that Mr. Koffer is not in proper anatomic alignment but does not want to rule out incisional pain without Mr. Koffer's own input. Mr. Koffer states that he is certain that the pain is not incisional but that he feels quite uncomfortable. In addition he knows that he cannot tell his wife about the pain because every time he does, she becomes overly concerned and worries. The social worker telephones the home health nurse in charge of Mr. Koffer's care and states that Mr. Koffer appears to have slipped down in his bed and therefore seems to be out of the proper body alignment in which he was maintained while hospitalized. The nurse replies that she will be at Mr. Koffer's home shortly for her regular visit and will then explain positioning to both Mr. and Mrs. Koffer.

In this case, the social worker assessed the patient's body alignment and immediately reported the findings to the nurse. Although social workers do not generally assess body alignment, they learn through team work that patient positioning often diminishes pain. Noting that the patient had slipped down in bed, this social worker responded effectively by notifying the patient's nurse of the situation. This "role blurring" would not have occurred had the social worker focused solely on her specific work assignment.

No matter how cohesively a team functions, the potential for dysfunction and conflict always exists. This is especially true if there is a lack of open communication between team members, either during the team meeting or between meetings. Individuals who interfere with open communication find it increasingly difficult to function as a part of the whole and weaken the team's organization, motivation, and interaction. Therefore to ensure that the team functions in a smooth and efficient manner, it is necessary for the team to have a leader.

Team leaders may be formally appointed or may rise from the ranks of the team in an informal fashion. The formal leader is generally hired by the team's employer or, less often, selected by the group. This individual is invested with the formal responsibility of ensuring that the members of the group work as a unit to achieve the common goals of the team. The formal leader challenges the team to consider alternative solutions to various challenges presented and encourages collaboration by ensuring that all ideas brought to the team are considered valid and worthy of consideration by the group. The informal leader, on the other hand, is a team member who is not appointed by anyone on the team but who takes a leadership role by actively and enthusiastically participating in team functions, fostering open and direct communication and interaction with team members, and setting an example of how the ideal team player functions. Despite the lack of formal recognition, the informal leader may have as much or more influence on the ultimate success of the team than the formal team leader.

Types of Teams

Two distinct types of teams are widely utilized: the multidisciplinary team and the interdisciplinary team. Although these terms are often used interchangeably, implying a case management approach to the delivery of patient care, they do have significant differences in meaning.

Multidisciplinary teams function through the use of separate consultations, with little or no communication occurring among the various specialists (Gage, 1994). In essence, each team member has a unique specialty and, within the scope of this specialty, develops a plan to address one or more specific goals of the patient. The goals being addressed may be independent of those of other team members or coordinated with them. Regardless of the level of team coordination, each member proceeds with his or her plan of care without regard to the treatment plans of other members. In multidisciplinary teams, therefore, the goals established by individual members supersede the goals of the team as a whole. Generally, the overall plan and goals of care are presented to the patient and family by one team member (usually the physician), although in some cases individual members will present their treatment plans and goals to the patient and family without collaborating with other members of the team.

The way a multidisciplinary team functions is illustrated by the following case. A patient enters an emergency room complaining of lower chest and upper abdominal pain. The emergency room physician evaluates the patient and orders an electrocardiogram (ECG), a chest x-ray, cardiac enzyme levels, and several other diagnostic tests. The tests are nondiagnostic, but the physician is impressed by the patient's complaints and remains concerned about potential cardiac or gastrointestinal causes for the pain. The physician then requests separate examinations by both a cardiologist and a gastroenterologist. Both specialists evaluate the patient, eliciting a history of alcohol abuse and heavy cigarette smoking as well as the current complaint of substernal chest pain. The cardiologist reveals to the patient suspicions that there is a problem with the heart, and in a separate conversation the gastroenterologist discusses the potential gastrointestinal etiology of the symptoms. The results of emergency room evaluation and tests and the consultative reports would either be shared with the referring physician or be recorded in the patient's chart. Then the patient may be admitted and undergo further cardiac and gastrointestinal diagnostic studies. Responsibility for the information shared with the patient and coordination of the hospital stay then lies with the patient's physician. This process can seem somewhat haphazard and disturbing to the patient and family.

In contrast to the lack of communication that sometimes characterizes multidisciplinary care, the interdisciplinary team functions by having each member conduct an individual evaluation of the patient and then coordinating these assessments to create a single treatment plan with integrated goals. If conflict among the treatment plans or goals of different disciplines exists, the team members negotiate to develop a unified and coordinated treatment plan. In the emergency room case just discussed, if the physicians were functioning in an interdisciplinary fashion, they would have conferred with each other, discussed their findings together with the patient, and developed a treatment plan providing for coordinated evaluation of both the cardiovascular and gastrointestinal systems.

According to Gage (1994), the interdisciplinary model is the most appropriate means of ensuring that patients receive consistent information and integrated care. She further discusses the various complications that may develop within an interdisciplinary team approach and uses Hirokawa's explanation of team interplay:

> There is little doubt that group decision-making is conducted by individual decision makers, each of whom possesses particular values, attitudes, beliefs, motives, knowledge, and skills. What is equally clear, however, is that the decisions of these individuals are subject to the constraints of a variety of system-level features, for example, norms, roles, decision rules, and so forth (Gage, p. 27).

Gage verifies, using her social work expertise, that decision making must be established based on the best interests of the patient rather than any particular discipline. This prevents a representative of any one discipline from commandeering the group toward one particular decision and creates an atmosphere of equal input from all specialists toward a unified outcome.

TEAM APPROACH TO PAIN MANAGEMENT

In view of the multifactorial nature of pain, it is easy to recognize the benefits of managing pain through a coordinated team effort. No matter which model of pain is used, it takes the combined efforts of many health care professionals as an interdisciplinary team to provide effective management of the multitude of factors that contribute to the patient's perception of pain.

Members of the Pain Team

Only by understanding the functions of each discipline represented on a team can one truly understand how each discipline contributes to achieving the team goals. It would be impossible to review the roles of every potential member of a pain management team, so the key disciplines that are necessary to develop a focused and unified plan of care to achieve the outcome of freeing the patient from pain will be briefly reviewed here.

Patient and Family

A patient and his or her family generally have numerous challenges that no one team member can take responsibility for defining and managing (Amenta & Bohnet, 1986). Thus it is appropriate to begin by establishing the patient and family as the focal point of the team. Too often the team excludes the patient and family from the decision-making process. In the effective management of pain it is crucial to involve the patient and family as equal partners in the development of a treatment plan. They should be involved in determining which members of the interdisciplinary team to include in the pain management process and in the formulation of treatment goals. Involving the patient and family as active participants in care planning contributes to successful outcomes for the patient-family unit and for the team.

Nurse

The role of the nurse is generally considered central to the pain management team. Although nurses at any level, including licensed practical nurses and licensed vocational nurses, may participate as members of a pain team, it is the registered nurse (RN) who is generally given responsibility for all nursing activities on the team and is often designated as the team's formal leader. In many instances RNs who lead the team have additional training and certification in nursing specialties such as diabetes, hospice, oncology, or pediatrics.

Nursing activities on the pain management team are quite broad and include:

1. The comprehensive assessment of the patient, including a full pain history, physical exam, and psychosocial history

2. Ensuring direct patient involvement in the management of the pain
3. Documentation of current medications, drug allergies, and drug sensitivities
4. Obtaining a comprehensive medical history
5. Administration of medications
6. Reassessing response to treatment
7. Monitoring the patient for side effects or complications of treatment
8. Collaborating with the physicians on the pain management team regarding the patient's response to treatments and obtaining any necessary alterations in therapy
9. Collaborating with other members of the pain team, such as social workers, chaplains, and pharmacists, in providing comprehensive pain management to the patient

As pain management teams become more commonplace, RNs will find ample opportunities for professional growth and development, including the education of colleagues in pain management skills and the ability to function in a supervisory role.

Physician

Physicians from a variety of specialty areas may participate as members of the pain management team. Due to the difficulty of treating patients with neuropathic pain, neurologists often are given leadership positions on the pain team. Since many of these challenging patients require administration of analgesia directly into the central nervous system, anesthesiologists are also often involved. (See Chapter 14). Nerve blocks require the expertise of the anesthesiologist as well, and for more difficult neuropathic pain challenges the participation of the neurosurgeon may be indicated. Various forms of cancer pain may respond to radiation therapy, necessitating the involvement of the radiation oncologist. With increased interest in the general management of cancer pain and forms of chronic nonmalignant pain, medical oncologists, rheumatologists, general internists, and family physicians are also becoming more common participants on the pain management team. Finally, with the ever-increasing recognition of the importance of psychologic factors on the perception of pain, psychiatrists are playing much more significant roles in the management of patients in pain.

Pharmacist

The role of the pharmacist has become appreciated as integral to an effective pain team. In addition to dispensing medication, pharmacists collect, organize, and evaluate information; formulate a course of action; provide medications and counseling; and monitor and manage patient outcomes (Meszaros, 1994). The pharmacist's knowledge of the patient's current prescriptions, over-the-counter medications, previous medication history, and drug allergies and prior adverse reactions permits immediate identification of potential drug interactions and other polypharmacy problems. Pharmacists provide education to the patient, family, and other team members on proper drug dosage and utilization, route of administration, scheduling, and appropriate precautions. They also provide professional education to team members regarding newly available therapies, possible alternative therapies, and the most cost-effective therapeutic approaches available to manage a particular patient's pain. Additionally, the pharmacist plays an integral role in developing pharmacy policies and procedures and establishing protocols for the use of various pharmaceutical agents by other members of the pain management team.

Social Worker

The social worker is generally viewed as having two functions: liaison and counselor. As the liaison between the patient-family and the social community network, the social worker can recommend the use of health care resources and support agencies to help the patient and family maintain their level of function and independence. The social worker facilitates the coordination of the various organizations on behalf of the patient and family. The social worker's goal is to minimize the bureaucratic stress (often resulting in social pain) encountered by the patient and family from lack of knowledge about how to access financial, housing, insurance, legal, health care, and practical assistance. For example, when a patient goes home from an inpatient facility there may be a continued need for medications, treatments, equipment, nursing follow-up, and physical therapy. The social worker helps to coordinate these aspects of care and assists the patient in gaining an understanding of each resource. Through this process, the patient-family learns what will be covered by insurance and what type of assistance is available from organizations such as the American Cancer Society or the American Lung Association.

As a counselor, the social worker provides a necessary source of support to the patient and family as they consider treatment options, changes in family roles, and opening communication within the family and between providers of care. Social workers are also invaluable in helping the patient cope with the psychosocial and emotional components of total pain and suffering.

Psychologist

Although the social worker provides much psychologic support, there are occasions where the professional skills of the psychologist are needed to manage the complex psychosocial aspects of a patient's pain. A patient suffering from pain may have a history of a psychologic or psychiatric disorder. If the disorder was severe and required medical intervention, a psychiatrist may be a necessary addition to the team. For many patients, however, the nature of the dysfunctional process does not call for a psychiatrist; for these patients a well-trained psychologist is a critical member of the pain management team.

Chaplain

Many patients, especially those suffering from cancer pain, wonder if their pain is something they must endure as a form of divine punishment for something they did in this life. For these patients, questions revolving around the possible religious meaning of their pain often affect how well that pain is controlled. For those who attach no overt spiritual or religious meaning to their pain, the need for spiritual guidance may exist or the services of a chaplain may be offered as an option. For these patients, the chaplain on the pain management team may be the professional best suited to answer spiritually based questions.

The chaplain's religious affiliation will not be important to some patients; however, many patients prefer the counsel of clergy of their own faith even if they have never been observant of the customs of their religion in the past. If a patient is reluctant to accept pain management due to religious beliefs, the chaplain is best suited to assure the patient that pain relief is the proper goal and that pain is something that they do not have to endure.

Certified Nursing Assistants

Certified nursing assistants (CNAs) are essential, often overlooked members of the pain management team. They assist patients in activities of daily life and may spend more time with the patient than any other member of the team. Whereas patients may put up a facade of adjustment for professional team members to avoid disappointing them, they are more willing to remove that facade with the CNA. This allows the CNA to learn much about the patient's feelings, fears and concerns, changes in body image, and other issues that patients are often reluctant to discuss with other care givers. The CNA can then bring this information to the attention of other team members at meetings or through informal interaction, thereby facilitating the assessment of physical and psychologic needs of the patient.

Therapists

Therapists are professionals skilled in specific treatments that correct a patient deficit or contribute to maintaining function.

1. An occupational therapist works to restore self-care and work-related skills in the patient who experiences performance deficits. For example, a stroke patient who can no longer feed himself or herself can learn to do so through practice and assistive devices.
2. A music therapist works to create an atmosphere that will reduce a stress-filled patient's anxiety or enhance mental stimulation in a comatose patient.
3. A physical therapist examines and treats individuals with physical limitations to correct or alleviate those disabilities.
4. A respiratory therapist is skilled in the treatment and management of patients with respiratory deficits. They administer aerosol or humidified treat ments, breathing treatments, and pulmonary function tests.

CASE STUDIES

The following case studies are included to illustrate how an interdisciplinary pain management team might function. In reviewing each case, it is important to note symptoms or situations that are uncovered by individual team members, and how they communicate their findings and involve other team members with the necessary expertise to manage the patient's complaints.

Case 1

Mrs. Strong has been under the treatment of Dr. Abbot for approximately 10 years. Approximately 7 years ago Dr. Abbot diagnosed multiple sclerosis (MS), which has progressed to the point that she needs a walker to ambulate for short distances. She has a visual deficit of nystagmus and has experienced a continual decline in visual acuity. Dr. Glass, her ophthalmologist, sees Mrs. Strong approximately every 3 to 4 months.

Eight days ago Dr. Abbot admitted Mrs. Strong to the hospital for the administration of ACTH due to the progressing symptoms of MS. She had received this treatment approximately one year ago and responded favorably to it. Dr. Abbot felt that it was time to repeat the treatment, and Mrs. Strong consented.

Following the admission process the nursing assistant, John, noticed Mrs. Strong wincing and rubbing the left side of her face. He asked her if something was bothering her face. She said she thought she had been "bitten by something." John looked at her face and did not see an insect bite. Even though no insect bite was visible, John told the RN about the situation.

Several hours later John took a food tray to Mrs. Strong and noticed that she was still grimacing and rubbing the left side of her face. He said, "Is that cheek still bothering you? Let me look at it again." He inspected her cheek and again failed to find an insect bite. He reported this interaction to the RN.

The nurse spoke with Mrs. Strong and learned that her left cheek was burning and painful although there was no insect bite visible. She contacted Dr. Abbot, who stated that it sounded like she was experiencing nerve pain and that it should be monitored overnight.

By morning observation and documentation indicated that Mrs. Strong seemed to complain about the left cheek and wince from discomfort only when she was up in the chair and not when she was in bed. The next morning, upon visiting Mrs. Strong, Dr. Abbot noted that she was uncomfortable. He asked her what was wrong and she stated that every time she sat up she felt discomfort, but when she laid down the pain subsided.

Dr. Abbot examined her and found nothing on her face or in her mouth. He left the room and met with the nurse and the CNA to discuss the findings. Through the team discussion it was discovered that the cheek discomfort had been developing for 2 days prior to hospital admission. Mrs. Strong reported that it was always left cheek pain and that it seemed to originate from the outside of her face and not from the inside of her mouth, although sometimes chewing or drinking cold liquids seemed to initiate irritation. Interestingly, John stated that he noticed that she only complained when she was sitting up and facing the door, and not when she was lying down and facing into the room. That caused Dr. Abbot to walk back into the room and assess the room layout. The air conditioner was located on the left side of the chair and therefore blew on the left side of Mrs. Strong's face. Dr. Abbot then fanned the left side of Mrs. Strong's face, which caused her to grimace. Dr. Abbot further assessed the patient and ordered Tegretol, which is often used to treat tic douloureux.

All members of this team worked together to diagnose a pain experienced by Mrs. Strong that was not a part of her original reason for admission. Together they discovered a pain that the patient had not mentioned prior to or during the admission process.

Case 2

Mr. Bold is an 84-year-old rheumatoid arthritis patient who suffers from chronic pain. He has been disabled for 20 years due to the severity of the pain. In the waking hours of the morning he suffers from severe stiffness due to lying still during sleep. After waking he is accustomed to stretching his extremities, although this is painful, to enable him to get out of bed without assistance. He then takes a warm shower and stretches his extremities again to gain mobility. Once dressed, he moves into the kitchen to prepare his breakfast and begin his day.

Three days ago, Mrs. Bold noticed that her husband was not eating as usual. He had oatmeal for breakfast and hot tea for lunch and totally refused dinner, explaining that he felt as if he might be coming down with the flu. The following morning Mr. Bold had hot tea for breakfast and liquids the remainder of the day. Yesterday Mr. Bold complained of abdominal discomfort and was admitted for a diagnostic workup.

Dr. Smith ordered an outpatient upper GI series followed by a liquid diet. The testing indicated that Mr. Bold had developed an ulcerative stomach and would require a diet change and medication to heal the ulcers. Upon explaining the results to Mr. and Mrs. Bold, Dr. Smith realized that a consulting dietitian would be needed to educate the family in meal planning and preparation practices to aid in healing. He ordered home health care with a dietary emphasis.

The home health team included Mr. and Mrs. Bold, Dr. Smith, the dietitian, a social worker, a chaplain, the pharmacist, the occupational therapist, the physical therapist, an RN, an LPN, and a CNA. Other specialists were available within the organization but were not in attendance at the first meeting. During the initial review of Dr. Smith's medical orders to be followed by the patient at home, the team identified a need for the physical therapist to visit, at least once, to ensure that Mr. Bold was performing the appropriate exercises for his morning stiffness. In addition, the team felt it would benefit the patient-family and the staff if the pharmacist reviewed the current medications to ensure that the ulcerative condition would not be exacerbated by interactions with any prescribed or over-the-counter drugs. This team was led by the RN, who contacted Dr. Smith to discuss the measures identified by the team. Dr. Smith was grateful for the input and agreed that the team should proceed with the unified plan just as they had developed it.

That afternoon the pharmacist reviewed the medication lists with the RN, who contacted Mrs. Bold to identify the over-the-counter medications taken by Mr. Bold in conjunction with the medications prescribed by Dr. Smith. After a review of the list no interactions or contraindications were noted. The review was documented within the medical record of Mr. Bold, and the team was notified.

The physical therapist (PT) arrived the next morning, as was planned with Mr. and Mrs. Bold, to observe the stretching exercises performed as a part of Mr. Bold's daily routine. Mr. Bold performed his exercises well, and they required very few modifications. The PT planned to return within a week for a follow-up visit to ensure that the modifications were followed as taught. This information was relayed to the team, and the unified plan of care was updated accordingly.

The dietitian arrived with pamphlets to assist in the explanation of the diet changes to which Mr. Bold would be asked to adhere. During the visit Mr. Bold fidgeted with apparent discomfort. The dietitian asked, "Why the discomfort?" Mr. Bold explained that without his usual antiinflammatory medications (discontinued because of the ulcerative condition of his stomach) used to reduce his usual stiffness and pain, his arthritis was just about unbearable in the early morning hours. The dietitian called the office and explained the situation to the team leader. The team leader contacted the PT and explained the new situation to him. They agreed on the need for a repeat visit by the PT to teach Mr. Bold about the benefits of an early morning warm shower with some stretching exercises immediately afterward to enable Mr. Bold to perform the other daily exercises he was accustomed to. The team leader telephoned Dr. Smith, who agreed to have the PT reevaluate the situation.

The physical therapist arrived that afternoon, evaluated Mr. Bold, and recommended several measures that would be immediately helpful: moist heat, stretching exercises that could be done while Mr. Bold sat in his favorite chair, and watching humorous television shows. Follow-up visits led to the introduction of various other exercises that resulted in an increased range of motion, decreased pain and stiffness, and a more positive attitude.

As it turned out, Mr. Bold had never received professional advice on the management of his arthritic condition. With the keen observations of the dietitian, Mr. Bold received the professional intervention that enabled him not only to return to normal activities but to exceed that which had been normal for him. With diet changes the ulcerative stomach condition subsided. With the aid of the dietitian and the PT,

Mr. Bold's condition required less medication and he experienced a greater quality of life.

SUMMARY

To properly manage a patient's pain, health care providers need expert skills in the management of the physical, psychologic, social, financial, spiritual, and other challenges that may be contributing to the pain. A strategy that includes collaboration and development of a plan of action; that considers the observation, evaluation, and skills of a variety of disciplines (preferably an interdisciplinary team approach); and that enlists the active participation of the patient-family unit will ultimately result in the desired outcome: pain management.

References

Amenta, M. O., & Bohnet, N. L. (1986). The interdisciplinary team. In *Nursing care of the terminally ill* (pp. 273-289). Boston: Little, Brown.

Ferrell, B. R., Grant, M. M., Rhiner, M., & Padilla, G. V. (1992). Home care: Maintaining quality of life for patient and family. *Oncology, 6*(suppl.), 136-140.

Gage, M. (1994). The patient-driven interdisciplinary care plan. *Journal of Nursing Administration, 24*(4), 26-35.

Gibson, J. L., Ivancevich, J. M., & Donnelly, J. H. (1991). Group-behavior. In K. Brockmann & J. Roberts (Eds.), *Organizations: Behavior, structure, process* (pp. 265-297). Homewood, IL: Richard D. Irwin.

Meszaros, E. C. (1994). Cognitive services: What are they worth? *Managed Healthcare, 4*(8), S18-S22.

Oermann, M. (1994). Reforming nursing education for future practice. *Journal of Nursing Education, 33*(5), pp. 215-218.

Portenoy, R. K. (1988). Practical aspects of pain control in the patient with cancer. *CA: A Cancer Journal for Clinicians, 38,* 327-352.

Welk, T. A. (1991). An educational model for explaining hospice services. *American Journal of Hospice and Palliative Care, 8*(5), 14.

7

Alternative Approaches to Pain Management

Lynda Peeler

- Physical Approaches
  - Acupuncture
  - Acupressure
  - Shiatsu
  - Myofascial Therapy
  - Qigong
  - Therapeutic Massage
  - Craniosacral Therapy
  - Chiropractic
  - Rolfing or "Structural Integration"
  - Bonnie Prudden Pain Erasure
  - The Feldenkrais Method of "Functional Integration"
  - The Trager Approach
  - Reflexology
- Mind-Body Approaches
  - Biofeedback
  - Guided Imagery
  - Humor Therapy
  - Hypnotherapy
  - Meditation
  - Music Therapy
  - Neurolinguistic Programming
  - Therapeutic Healing Touch
  - Yoga

Key Points

- Pain is seen not as an isolated entity, but as a symptom of imbalance of the integrity of the whole person; pain is physical, mental, and emotional.
- Promotion of healing rather than curing is the intent of alternative approaches
- Healing comes from within; all therapies or modalities merely act as triggers to activate the person's innate ability to heal.
- Many approaches have histories that support their efficacy, but they are not in the realm of our present knowledge base or research capabilities.
- No one modality is a panacea or is intended to replace present methods.
- No approach can claim instantaneous, total relief of symptoms.

The presentation of the material in this chapter is in no way intended to suggest that the many proven methods presently used to treat pain be discarded and replaced with any or all of these alternative therapies; that would be throwing out the baby with the bathwater. According to *Consumer Reports* (Alternative Medicine, 1994, p. 54), "Western medicine approaches disease or dysfunction by isolating the precise cause and attempting to control or eliminate it.... Most systems of alternative medicine claim to treat the... 'whole person' in a way conventional medicine may not." This alternative approach appears to appeal to a large portion of Americans; according to a 1993 study (Eisenberg et al., p. 246), one third of Americans surveyed had used at least one "unconventional therapy," defined as "uncommonly used interventions neither taught widely in U.S. Medical Schools nor generally available in U.S. hospitals."

The National Institutes of Health Office of Alternative Medicine (NIHOAM) funded the sum of $12,922,217 for alternative medicine research for 1994 (see Table 7-1) to provide an opportunity for practitioners to demonstrate the validity of their practices—not an easy task, perhaps, since present research methods and nomenclature may not apply.

The approaches to pain management that lie outside allopathic regimes are numerous and varied; only those therapies presently being taught and used in the United States are discussed here. Training can vary from a weekend workshop to a 5-year certification program; no practice should be implemented without specific training. Some of these systems should be viewed with an open mind; many may work as adjuncts to the routines presently in use. Some may require giving up the need to understand, and others may need to be seen to be believed.

The approaches reviewed in this chapter are broadly divided into the categories of physical, mind-body, and herbal medicine. Each therapy is described and research and resources are summarized.

PHYSICAL APPROACHES

Acupuncture

This 2500-year-old (or older) therapy is based on the belief that optimal health is directly connected to a balance of flow of the life force known as qi or chi (pronounced *chee*) along 12 energy pathways called meridians; each meridian is connected to specific organs, body structures, and systems. As Figure 7-1 illustrates, there are approximately a thousand

Table 7-1 NIHOAM Grants, 1994

Category	Number of Awards	Amount
Acupuncture	5	$2,527,025
Combination therapy	11	2,109,736
Biologics/pharmacologics	16	2,212,815
Antioxidants		
Bee venom		
Chelation therapy		
Dimethyl sulfoxide (DMSO)		
Drugs		
Homeopathy		
Hyperbaric oxygen		
Diet/nutrition	1	29,964
Herbs	3	243,100
Manual healing methods	9	579,902
Massage		
Chiropractic		
Therapeutic touch		
Medical systems	4	294,687
Ayerveda		
Traditional Chinese medicine (TCM)		
Mind-Body	38	4,458,616
Biofeedback		
Bioenergetics		
Hypnosis		
Meditation		
Music therapy		
Prayer/spirituality		
Qigong		
Relaxation		
T'ai chi		
Miscellaneous	3	466,372
Doulas		
Electrochemical therapy		
Energetic therapy		
Light therapy		
TOTAL	90	$12,922,217

From National Institutes of Health, Office of Alternative Medicine, *1994 Fact Sheet #2,* Appendix III.

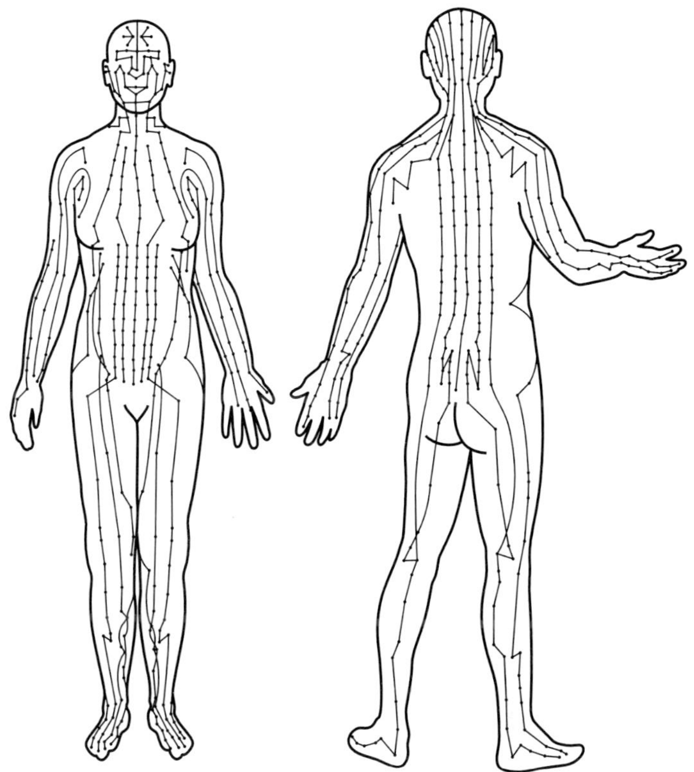

Figure 7-1 Meridian acupoints.

acupoints along these meridians that can be stimulated to balance the circulation of energy, which influences the health of the entire being. Acupuncture is performed using very fine (about the size of a thick hair) solid, sterile needles that create different sensations such as warmth or pressure, but not pain; patients describe it as almost pleasant and relaxing.

In an attempt to scientifically link this energy-based procedure to Western systems of substantiating existence and effectiveness, Kim Bong Han of Korea in 1960 (Gerber, 1988) used microdissection to establish the existence of an independent series of fine tubules corresponding to the paths of the traditional acupuncture meridians. These ducts differ from the vascular and lymph systems, as identified by Western medicine, but it was thought the ducts might exist within these systems. A French researcher, Pierre de Vernejoul, confirmed Kim's findings and differentiated the meridian system from blood vessels by injection of radioisotopes into both, determining that the isotopes did not travel in the same manner at all (Gerber). It was also determined that acupoints along the superficial meridians in the skin demonstrate unique electrical properties that distinguish them from the surrounding skin. Disease or imbalance of the system can produce characteristic disturbances in electric potential along particular meridians, making it possible to measure changes at the acupoints and allowing for diagnostic evaluation.

According to *Consumer Reports* (Alternative Medicine, 1994, p. 53):

> More than a decade of research provided scientists with a reasonable explanation of acupuncture's role in pain relief. There is evidence that acupuncture prods sensory nerves in the skin and muscles to signal the spinal cord, which enlists the midbrain. At each level, . . . endorphins are released. Acupuncture may also mobilize the pituitary gland to discharge pain blockers, and to trigger a process that releases anti-inflammatory agents into the bloodstream. According to Bruce Pomeranz, a professor of zoology and physiology at the University of Toronto, "We know more about analgesic acupuncture than about the mechanism of action of most anesthetic gases."

Acupuncture is listed as an independent category for NIHOAM grants, and awards totaled $2,527,025 (see Table 7-1).

Resource American Association of Acupuncture and Oriental Medicine
433 Front Street
Catasauqua, PA 18032-2506
(610)433-2448

Acupressure

Reportedly older than acupuncture, acupressure, as indicated by the name, is pressure of varying degree and duration ation applied with fingers and hands at acupoints, producing much the same effect as acupuncture. Self-acupressure techniques include Acu-Yoga, which uses the whole body through breathing, meditation, yoga postures, and stretches. Another method, Do-In, incorporates body awareness, stretching, breathing, and vigorous techniques to stimulate the body through the points and meridians (Goldberg, 1993).

Shiatsu (Finger Pressure)

Shiatsu, a Japanese synonym for acupressure, is a firm sequence of rhythmic pressure applications at specific points for 3 to 10 seconds, making use of charted points that, when stimulated, lead to reflex relaxation (Weintraub, 1992).

Moxabustion

Moxabustion is a method of producing analgesia or altering the function of a system that is accomplished by holding an ignited, slow-burning substance, such as an herb called moxa (mugwort) on a slice of ginger, over acupoints as close to the skin as possible until it feels too warm to the patient. This is best used on delicate parts of the body where needles cannot be used (Gerber, 1988; Anderson, 1994).

Myofascial Therapy

Myofascial therapy, or myotherapy, combines acupressure with a technique called tuina (tweena). This may be viewed as a transition from specific-point therapy to soft tissue rehabilitative therapy, and for this reason myotherapy may appear under other headings and possibly be used in combination with other therapies.

Qigong

The intent of Qigong, another multidimensional approach, is to mobilize and harmonize the flow of energy (qi, or chi) through peaceful, slow exercises that can be done standing, sitting, or lying down. One goal is to enhance the quality of breathing while stimulating the qi and the organs of the body, thus increasing circulation of oxygen- and nutrient-filled blood to the brain, organs, and tissues.

Qigong is a traditional practice in China, where approximately 200 million reportedly practice it on a daily basis, and it is gaining popularity in America. Goldberg (1993, p. 423) states, "In the United States, qigong is now being taught by qualified instructors at innovative hospital programs, at adult education centers, and in community fitness programs."

This is becoming a popular form of exercise for the elderly and the infirm as it helps maintain range of motion, circulation, and energy. It would be wise to learn this under the direction of a trained instructor to prevent injury.

Resource Academy of the Healing Arts
450 Sutter Street, Ste. 916
San Francisco, CA 94108
(415)788-2227

Therapeutic Massage

Therapeutic massage consists of kneading, stroking, and manipulating soft tissue of the body—skin, muscles, tendons, and ligaments—with varying rhythm, rate, pressure, and direction of movement. Physical rewards include muscle relaxation, increased circulation, decreased swelling, pain relief, softening and stretching of scars, and reduced adhesions. Psychological benefits include relieved stress, improved state of mind, and fulfillment of the need for human touch. Other benefits include the prevention of soft tissue adhesions, trigger points, scar tissue, and chronic postural distortions. Relaxation of soft tissue allows unimpaired motion in any direction, and massage works on the premise that anything one can do more easily, one can do longer.

Massage is contraindicated in patients with open wounds, skin infections, phlebitis, and some cancers.

Dr. Tiffany Field of the Touch Research Institute at the University of Miami has numerous projects under way to determine the effects of massage. Applications specifically related to physical pain include infant colic, pediatric oncology, juvenile rheumatoid arthritis, fibromyalgia syndrome, and arthritis (Kastner, 1994).

Craniosacral Therapy

There are three different approaches to craniosacral therapy: the sutural approach, the meningeal approach, and the reflex approach.

The sutural approach was developed at the turn of the century by Dr. William Sutherland, an osteopathic physician. He spent years experimenting and, although ridiculed for his belief that the sutures of the skull are not fixed, developed a system of diagnosis and treatment called cranial osteopathy.

The meningeal approach is the result of Dr. John Upledger's realization that the meninges have a rhythmic motion in keeping with the flow of cerebrospinal fluid. Dysfunction of the CNS or brain occurs when one or more of the cranial nerves are compressed, restricting the natural movement of the cranial bones and meninges. The technique he developed, craniosacral therapy, is a very gentle, noninvasive manipulative technique used to assess the cerebrospinal fluid flow and fluctuation to identify a lack of symmetry, tension, or restriction in the meninges. The therapist monitors the rhythmic movement and, upon detecting abnormal motion in the craniosacral system (skull, face, spine, and sacrum), uses gentle pressure (about the weight of a nickel) to assist in restoring flow.

The reflex approach utilizes a combination of techniques, such as kinesiology, with specific cranial adjustment to locate and treat distortions of the craniosacral system.

Upledger and a multidisciplinary team of anatomists, physiologists, biophysicists, and bioengineers working with patients 7 to 57 years old, found that the capacity for motion was present within the cranial sutures. They found that the suture line contains an abundance of collagen and elastic fiber, vascular networks that communicate with haversian canals of the bone, and nonmyelinated nerve fiber networks and receptors. Sutures from living patients were not calcified, in contradiction to the beliefs of anatomists. The appearance of calcification occurred postmortem and with the use of preservative chemicals. Nine publications resulted from this work. These and an additional extensive bibliography may be obtained from the following address.

Resource Upledger Institute
11211 Prosperity Farms Road
Palm Beach Gardens, FL 33410
(407)622-4706

Chiropractic

Basic chiropractic employs the principle that the nervous system, because it controls and coordinates all systems of the body, holds the key to the body's potential to heal itself. The spinal column acts as a switchboard, and it is believed that pressure on a nerve interferes with messages traveling between the brain and body systems, leading to malfunction and subsequent impairment. This interference is known as subluxation and may or may not be accompanied by symptoms. Inflammation, nerve pain, and muscle spasm are signs of the body's innate healing mechanism striving to pull the misaligned vertebra back into proper position.

The primary technique used to deal with pain is adjustment or manipulation of the spine to bring it into alignment. Methods of accomplishing this include the following:

1. Gently and precisely stretch the joint beyond its normal range of motion, at which point one or more clicks may be heard. The sounds, thought to be caused by gases escaping from the joints, are more uncomfortable than the procedure.
2. Apply gentle pressure along the spine, skull, and pelvis by hand or use of a rubber-tipped instrument to painlessly move the vertebrae.
3. Use network chiropractic as a stand-alone process or in conjunction with the other forms of chiropractic. The major difference among the procedures lies in the sequence and timing of adjustment, which, for this type of chiropractic, involves light touches to the body where vertebrae attach to the meningeal system. It is believed that this tissue bears imprints caused by physical, emotional, and chemical stress. If actual "bone crunching" chiropractic adjustment is warranted, it is performed after the network procedure. Emotional release, which can be manifested as crying, screams, or painful moaning, occurs as the past traumas stored in the nervous system and body are tapped. Care is taken to ensure that the client is quieted and able to leave the office safely. These patients should be under the care of a mental health practitioner for processing what surfaces (Krier, 1992).

An independent study funded by the Ministry of Health of the Government of Ontario, Canada, reports that there is a constellation of evidence for (a) the effectiveness and cost-effectiveness of chiropractic management of low-back pain; (b) the untested, questionable, or harmful nature of many current medical therapies; (c) the economic efficiency of chiropractic care for low-back pain compared with medical care; (d) the safety of chiropractic care; and (e) the higher satisfaction levels expressed by patients of chiropractors. This evidence constitutes an overwhelming case for the increased use of chiropractic services in the management of low-back pain (Magna, Angus, Papadapoulos, & Swan, 1993).

Resources

Association for Network Chiropractic
444 N. Main Street
Longmont, CO 80501
(303)678-8101

American Chiropractic Association
1701 Clarendon Boulevard
Arlington, VA 22209
(703)276-8800

Rolfing or "Structural Integration"

The goal of Rolfing* is to align the body (head, torso, pelvis, legs, and feet) to bring about a fluid, light balance and freedom from pain, stiffness, and chronic stress; the body is made at ease with itself and the earth's gravitational field. This method also improves performance in professional and daily activities and can facilitate a connection with one's emotional conflicts.

Rolfing movement integration focuses on developing balance and support in the gravitational field, moving harmoniously with gravity, and evoking an open and responsive body characterized by inner strength and centeredness instead of outer tension and armoring. Nearly everyone can benefit from Rolfing. Figure 7-2 shows the Rolfing movement integration.

The UCLA Department of Kinesiology (Connolly, 1977) concluded that as a result of Rolfing the movements of patients were increased, more fluid, and less constrained; fewer extraneous body movements were noted, with actual body movements being more dynamic and energetic; and the body carriage was more erect, requiring less strain to hold a position.

Cottingham, Porges, and Richard (1988) indicate that Rolfing reduces chronic stress, promotes change of body structure, and enhances neurologic functions. There was also a reduction in curvature of the spine due to lordosis or sway-back in those studied.

---

*The words Rolfing and Rolfer and the little boy logo (Figure 7-2) are registered service marks of the Rolf Institute of Structural Integration.

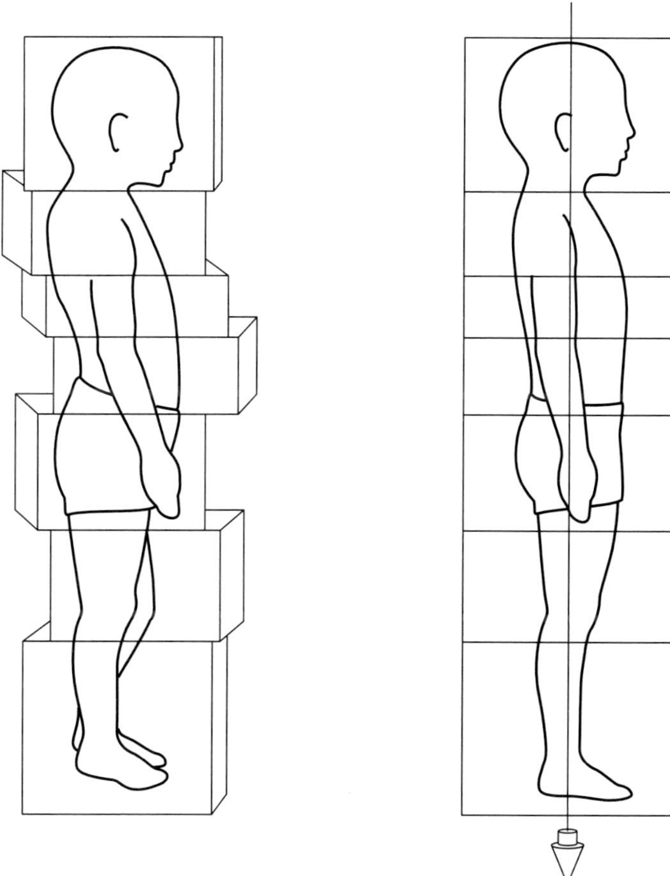

Figure 7-2 Rolfing movement integration.

Resource The Rolf Institute of Structural Integration
P.O. Box 1868
Boulder, CO 80306
(800)530-8875

Bonnie Prudden Pain Erasure

Trigger points are highly irritable spots in muscle resulting from routine recurring strain, a sprain, a blow, or overuse. Past trigger point therapy has involved locating the painful focal point and injecting it with saline or Procaine. Bonnie Prudden, while locating a trigger point in a patient, extended pressure that provided instant relief without the need for an injection. This accidental experience, combined with Prudden's open mind to "justifying springboard events," led to what is known as myotherapy today.

The process of Bonnie Prudden's pain erasure is initiated professionally through a written medical clearance from a physician, or a dentist where temperomandibular jaw or facial pain exists. With the interview concerning symptoms and previous treatment completed, the patient receives hands-on pressure to designated points. This is accomplished by fingertips, knuckles, or elbows, depending on the depth of the trigger point. The level of discomfort can be vocalized on a scale of 0 (no pain) to 10 (pain as bad as it can be). Although there can be intense, sometimes piercing discomfort, at the same time, as with acupuncture, the experience can be pleasant and relaxing.

The process does not end with release of muscle trigger points. The therapist works to increase mobilization of the affected muscles and of those connecting and distant that could have a bearing on the malfunctioning area. The result is a release of physical tension as if "the world was lifted off one's shoulders."

A primary goal is to keep the patient from becoming therapist dependent. This program has a built-in educational component that breaks the cycle of spasm and tension, empowering the patient to take care of his or her own problem. Families are encouraged to be part of the therapy as a support system in reinforcing techniques and principles.

An excellent therapy for reducing the stress-related aching of tight muscles through trigger point release and retraining postures and movements, myotherapy helps the individual control position-induced pain, such as pain resulting from long periods of telephone use, golf, and other sports that overuse specific muscle groups. The Oakland A's have used Bonnie Prudden's pain erasure myotherapy as part of their routine training and injury prevention education.

This is a program that lends itself to practice by nurses as it entails knowledge of anatomy and excellent teaching and communication skills.

Resource Bonnie Prudden Pain Erasure
7800 E. Speedway Blvd.
Tucson, AZ 85710
(800)221-4634

The Feldenkrais Method of "Functional Integration"

Another approach related to the interaction between sensory pathways carrying messages to the brain and the motor network carrying messages from the brain to the muscles to improve movement, the Feldenkrais method is based on the premise that when the brain is presented with a choice, it will pick the path of least resistance. Another assumption is that all the body's malfunctions are the result of faulty learning or "distortions." These include paralysis, pain, injury, fear, and stress and are incorporated into one's self-image as well as one's skeletal structure. Each time a movement is repeated, it is also repeated in the mental distortion. Eventually, through repeated improper movements such as allowing weaker muscles to do more than necessary or contracting muscles that have nothing to do with the desired movement, a strain is placed on the body.

The Feldenkrais therapist is a trained practitioner whose hands are sensitive enough to merely touch the body and feel exactly what is wrong and where. Communicating with the distorted portion of the nervous system, the therapist physically shows the body a more effective way of moving. This allows the brain to cancel the old image and transmit a new one. Throughout the session, work is done on troubled areas and the patient is shown alternative movements.

Dr. Feldenkrais is an internationally published author of books and articles. A bibliography of his works can be obtained from the following address.

Resource The Feldenkrais Guild
P.O. Box 489
Albany, OR 97321
(800)775-2118

The Trager Approach

"Approach" is a good descriptor for this method, because in a technical sense there are no rigid procedures connected to the desired results. Rather, it is a way of learning and teaching movement reeducation. The goal is not the use of particular muscle groups or joints but the use of motion in muscles and joints to produce positive sensory stimuli that enter the central nervous system and trigger tissue changes by means of sensory-motor feedback loops between the body and the mind. "Tragering" consists of gently and methodically moving the body as a whole and its individual parts, producing the sensation of being able to move the body freely, effortlessly, and gracefully on one's own. Trager practitioners don't change the condition of tissues, as in massage, but rather communicate the quality of feeling that ultimately makes the body stand and move as if it were lighter.

Post–touch therapy work includes instruction in "Mentastics," simple, effortless movement sequences developed to maintain and enhance the lightness, freedom, and flexibility instilled by the touch work. This appears to be similar to the Feldenkrais method but is intuitively based.

Because tension, tightness, pain, and many other physiologic conditions are based in the mind, the Trager approach is effective as a body-mind therapy.

Resource The Trager Institute
10 Old Mill Street
Mill Valley, CA 94941-1891
(415)388-2688

Reflexology

Taught in the United States since the 1930s, reflexology is an age-old science depicted on the wall of the tomb of Ankhmahor of the sixth Egyptian dynasty, about 2330 BC (Byers, 1994). It is based on the principle that there are foot reflexes corresponding to all organs and parts of the body. Figure 7-3 shows the reflexes in the foot, and Figure 7-4 shows the reflexes in the hand.

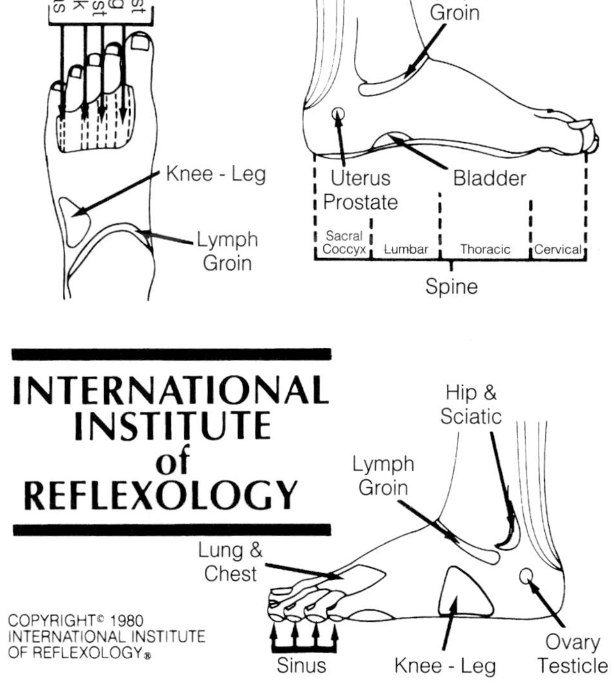

Figure 7-3 Foot reflex sites.

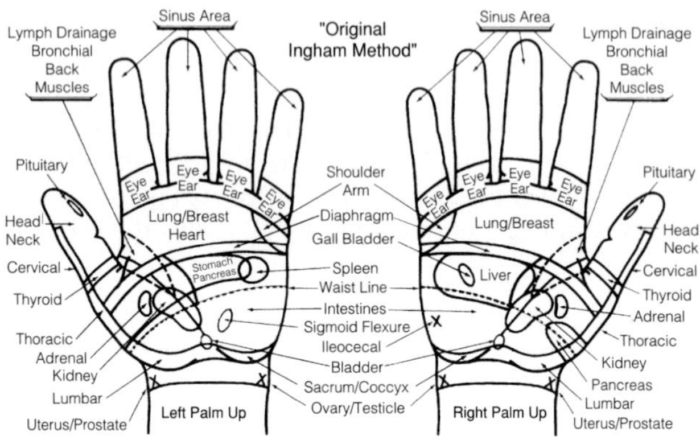

Figure 7-4 Hand reflex sites.

The purpose of reflexology is not to diagnose or treat medical disorders but to promote better health, such as through exercise or diet. There is no history of untoward effects resulting from the use of this therapy. Tools are limited to fingers and hands, with simple and safe pressure used to improve nerve and blood supply to help the body normalize itself.

Reflexology is used most effectively by nurses since it not only requires a knowledge of anatomy and physiology but relies on the ability to observe reactions and adjust to patient needs while employing the procedure. It is effective in pain management even in work with the terminally ill because it improves the psychologic response to pain as well as the physical. Anyone can benefit from reflexology.

In a premenstrual syndrome study Oleson and Flocco (1993) reported a 46% decrease in physical and psychologic symptoms after 2 months of true reflexology; the control group showed only 19% reduction in symptoms.

Resource International Institute of Reflexology
5650 1st Avenue North P.O. Box 12642
St. Petersburg, FL 33733
(813)343-4811

MIND-BODY APPROACHES

Biofeedback

The therapeutic approach known as biofeedback uses electronic instruments to accurately measure, process, and feed back signals about the patient's neuromuscular and autonomic activity. These feedback signals are obtained through sensors strategically attached to the patient to measure temperature, perspiration, and muscle contractility. The signals may be auditory, in the form of beeps of varying pitch and tone, or visual, consisting of computer graphics or manipulatable elements to be brought into alignment. The biofeedback therapist acts as a coach or teacher, assisting in the interpretation of the feedback with the goal of helping the patient develop greater awareness and voluntary control of physiologic processes. Stress, muscle pain, headache, and bladder control are only a few conditions helped by biofeedback. The success of this process depends largely on the personality, skills, and attention of the therapist.

This is a medically accepted though not thoroughly understood therapy that has been heavily researched (Schwartz, 1987). Certification requires extensive training through the following organization.

Resource Association for Applied Psychophysiology and Biofeedback
10200 W. 44th Avenue, Ste. 304
Wheatridge, CO 80033-2840
(303)422-8436 (800)477-8892

Guided Imagery

Guided imagery is a method of hypnosis in which the patient is guided to form mental images of sensory qualities (seeing, feeling, hearing, tasting, or smelling) in connection with an event. An example is getting hungry and thinking about a favorite food. This allows the patient to reinvent the whole picture, seeing more than the restrictive view of life that can result from pain, stroke, or a coronary incident. The images are elicited from the client through questioning techniques.

The client then makes emotional connections, reframes information, and initiates changes in behavior that heal emotional wounds and allow the visualization of more pleasant, alternative rewards.

There are limitations to effective imagery. The intensity and vividness of the imagery—be it auditory, tactile, olfactory, or gustatory (a combination of sensory approaches is best)—depends on one's ordinary level of imagery. Few people can generate imagery that is as vivid as their external perception; most use internal images that are more ethereal. The important point is that one accept what comes, free of expectations.

People who have difficulty imagining can still do very useful healing work (Rossman, 1993). It is a misconception that imagery is simply wish fulfillment, fantasy, or of no consequence. It is a powerful tool, but it would be an unsafe practice to employ the power of imagination in isolation, without other therapies—medical, surgical, or psychologic—that might be required for effective healing. Guided imagery is useful for relaxation and stress reduction; relief of headache, back and neck pain, and anxiety; decreasing blood pressure; and stimulating the healing response. Even though it is used to alleviate or significantly reduce these symptoms, it is best used as an adjunct therapy. It is a tool of healing, not a cure.

Resource The Academy for Guided Imagery
P.O. Box 2070
Mill Valley, CA 94942
(800)726-2070

Humor Therapy

The therapeutic value of humor has been appreciated over the centuries, from the time of Plato and Socrates, who used laughter as a remedy for colds and depression, to court jesters, who were expected to add mirth to meals and thus aid digestion. Freud and Darwin saw the benefit of laughter in releasing tension and reducing anxiety (Lee, 1990).

In these days of accountability, clear documentation, a process for this and a mandate for that, it is no wonder that the seriousness of one's work filters into his or her personal perspective. Humor comes in many disguises; some forms of humor reduce tension, whereas others chip away at self-esteem. Sarcasm, for instance, is a form of expressing anger, not mirthful humor. To keep humor on the positive side it is important that while taking one's work seriously, one does not take oneself too seriously. This is not a new concept, but it sometimes requires a conscious choice and a willingness to laugh at oneself.

Eustress is a healthy state of stress that can include mirthful laughter. Laughter is probably as important a preventive measure as a therapeutic one. Several organizations in the United States have dedicated their energies to putting on workshops and acting as clearinghouses for information and research, all geared to help people "lighten up."

Berk (1994) delivered a paper entitled "Eustress of Humor Associated Laughter Modulated Specific Immune System Components," which described a definitive study in which those exposed to humor showed an increase in activated T cells, in the number of killer cells, in immunoglobulin A, and in gamma (γ)-interferon, as well as other positive effects.

Resources

Humor & Health Letter
Joseph R. Dunn, PhD
P.O. Box 16814
Jackson, MI 39236

The HUMOR Project
Joel Goodman, EdD
110 Spring St.
Saratoga Springs, NY 12866
(518)587-8770

Hypnotherapy

Hypnosis, like most of the therapies covered here, depends to a large extent on the establishment of initial therapist-patient rapport created by dispelling anxiety, providing a comfortable environment, and developing trust. Once a comfortable setting is established, the client enters hypnosis in a natural way, of his or her own accord, simply by following the suggestions of the hypnotherapist.

A possible definition of hypnosis is an artificially induced state of consciousness characterized by a heightened receptivity to suggestion. Note the word *consciousness* rather than *unconsciousness;* it is a misconception of the general population that one is put to sleep when placed in a hypnotic state. The process of hypnosis includes relaxation, attention fixation, narrowing of the field of external influences, and achievement of a deep state of relaxation. No matter what method of induction is used, the goal is to quiet the conscious mind of distractions so that the portion of the mind we call the unconscious becomes more accessible, for the reason that the unconscious is less critical and analytical and thus more accepting of suggestion.

Hypnosis is both an art and a science and is a powerful tool for pain management. Studies have shown that physiologic changes—lowered blood pressure, pulse, and respiration—occur in the hypnotic state. For this reason it must be taken seriously and should be utilized only by trained therapists. It is not difficult to learn but carries a great responsibility for professionalism. Contraindications include patients with psychoses, organic psychiatric conditions, or antisocial personality disorders.

Resource The American Institute of Hypnotherapy
16842 Von Karman, Ste. 475
Irvine, CA 92714
(714)261-6400

Meditation

At least several thousand years old, the process of meditation focuses on the here and now to access the relaxation response and, with deeper focus, to reach the inner physician, where the healing body-mind connection lies. Meditation can assist the user in learning self-regulation, much like biofeedback, in the areas of anxiety, hypertension, stress management, and pain management and can increase quality of life, sensitivity, and compassion.

However one practices meditation—using Transcendental Meditation (TM) with a mantra (an intonation that makes one comfortable), visual focus, or musical induction—it is necessary to tune out distractions in the environment to reach the peace of the quiet within.

As with biofeedback, TM studies (Goldberg, 1993) have shown that the healthy state of relaxation causes a general reduction of physiologic and biochemical markers including decreased heart rate, pulse, respiration, and plasma cortisol (a major stress hormone) and increased alpha wave on the EEG, which denotes relaxation.

Resource Institute of Transpersonal Psychology
P.O. Box 3049
Stanford, CA 94309
(415)327-2066

Music Therapy

Music and sound are a form of vibrational energy that can help correct imbalances in the body, including stress. Imagery is a natural partner of music; specific kinds of music can enhance creation of images, bring clarity of mind, and release emotional blocks.

Matching the right type of music to the patient is a case-by-case decision. The therapist's goal is to elicit spontaneous healing images unique to the individual, not supplied by suggestion or script, by activating the subconscious. The synergy of music and imagery assists in activating a broad range of responses, sensory enhancements, memory images, and feelings.

Music therapy is beneficial as an adjunct therapy and in assisting people in general to develop inner trust, reframe personal perspectives, manage pain or other physical symptoms, practice healthy decision making, and cultivate patience. This is a professional modality requiring extensive training to make an effective match.

Empirical research is reported annually in the Music Therapy (AAMT Journal).

Resource American Association for Music Therapy
P.O. Box 80012
Valley Forge, PA 19484
(610)265-4006

Neurolinguistic Programming

Neurolinguistic programming, or NLP as it is popularly called, is a process of determining a person's limiting belief system and "reprogramming" it. The NLP practitioner interviews the patient about life and presenting problem(s) while observing eye movement, muscle tone, gestures, language patterns, and postures. These cues represent conscious and unconscious patient perceptions and indicate his or her limiting beliefs.

This process is very helpful as an adjunct therapy for the terminally ill, for posttraumatic disorders, and for chronic pain, to name a few areas. The outwardly healthy can also benefit from the enrichment of quality of life and increased productivity that NLP makes possible. It is an overall wellness tool.

Resource Western States Training Associates
346 South 500 East, Ste. 200
Salt Lake City, UT 84102-4022
(801)534-1022

Therapeutic Healing Touch

Therapeutic or healing touch is based on the assumption that the body is made up of energy in a solid form and is surrounded by an invisible energy field in constant interaction with the energy in our environment. This meditative therapy involves control of body energy centers known as chakras (wheels of subtle energy). Chakras appear to be physiologically involved with the flow of higher energies into the cellular structure of the body (Krieger, 1992).

During therapy the healer becomes quiet, passively listening with his or her hands and gently attuning self to patient. The hands are used to assess the body for areas of "accumulated tension" and to redirect the energies of the patient. One does not have to touch the person physically to obtain the intended result, making this therapy especially suited to work with burn patients and delicate premature infants. It works through clothing, casts, and rubber gloves. The exchange of energy from healer to healee is intended to (a) accelerate healing and enhance the body's natural ability to "self-correct," (b) reduce and possibly eliminate pain, and (c) relieve anxiety and bring about a state of well-being and relaxation (Chiappone, 1993).

A benefit of this approach is that it can be taught to anyone. A few moments spent teaching a loved one the simple techniques can reduce the feeling of helplessness and empower the person to feel part of the effort.

Resource American Holistic Nurses' Association
4101 Lake Boone Trail, Ste. 201
Raleigh, NC 27607
(919)787-5181
(800)278-AHNA

Yoga

Yoga is difficult to categorize because it involves physical and mental energies. Because it is connected to the chakra system, it is included in this section. The practice of yoga ranges from the deeply meditative somatic transformation of the yogis to aerobic physical exercise. Keeping the chakras open and balanced for optimal flow of energy is the primary focus. Yoga encompasses practices intended to develop sound morals and basic life habits, specific postures to enhance psychophysiologic functioning, breathing exercises to promote vitality, internal focus and withdrawal of attention from outside distractions, and concentration and contemplation. Pain is seen as an obstacle that can be eased through meditation, breathing away the discomfort, and also through stretching to one's full capacity to keep muscles nourished with oxygenated blood.

Resource International Association of Yoga Therapists
109 Hillside Avenue
Mill Valley, CA 94941
(415)383-4587

HERBAL APPROACHES

Aroma Therapy

Essential oils extracted from plants and herbs have been used for centuries for hygiene and to treat nausea, bites, and burns. "Aroma" therapy is something of a misnomer because fragrance properties, although beneficial for conditions such as asthma, are secondary to the benefit of the molecular structure of the oils, which enhances penetration of body tissues. These oils are purported to be effective as bacteriostatic agents and in stimulating, pacifying, and detoxifying different areas or organs of the body.

Because of the caustic nature of some of the oils, and to ensure that the oils used are of sufficient quality to produce the desired result, it is imperative that one seek a highly trained aroma therapist. This modality is a useful adjunct therapy for anything from health maintenance to traumatic illness. It is pleasant to the senses and is recommended for the general population.

Resource Pacific Institute of Aroma Therapy
P.O. Box 6723
San Rafael, CA 94903
(415)479-9121

Herbal Medicine

Herbs have been used for medicinal purposes since early human existence, when their use was overseen by the shaman or medicine woman or man who collected, dried, distilled, or otherwise refined and dispensed them according to need. This history of one person being solely responsible for the preparation of herbs based on the individual's specific condition suggests the importance of taking herbs seriously, with the proverbial statement borne in mind that he who treats himself treats a fool.

Preparations available for self-medication include herbal tablets or capsules, herb teas, and transdermal (as in aroma therapy) tinctures and extracts. Some preparations to be used for pain relief contain as many as 13 herbs in combination. Many of the most powerful medications currently available by prescription today are herbal derivatives.

An herbal tea can change from a pleasant repast to a powerful carminative simply by letting it steep longer. For instance, a combination of hops, blueberry, and alfalfa steeped 3 minutes is a gentle cleansing solution; steeped longer than 5 minutes it becomes a potent product that can increase stomach secretions and bile flow and decrease the normal flora of the bowel.

What can appear to be a benign treatment to a patient seeking self-cure can turn out to cause severe reactions such as pain, nausea, goiter, sodium retention, anticoagulation, depression, abnormal platelet count, uterine contractions, and dermatitis. The concern here is not the person who uses oil of cloves for toothache, takes peppermint tea for indigestion, or rubs wintergreen over sore muscles. The potential problem is self-treatment with herbal medications that can cause any of the preceding signs and symptoms. More and more patients are seeking alternative therapies and not reporting this to their primary caregiver in the allopathic arena. Failure to report the use of alternative treatment methods can be hazardous because of the resulting difficulty in diagnosing problems related to the self-remedy regime. Consulting a reference on herbs that details their healing qualities, evidence of effectiveness, safety, and potential side effects (e.g., Tyler, 1993) might be of benefit during an intake interview when symptoms are of undetermined origin.

Resources

American Herbalist Guild
P.O. Box 1683
Soquel, CA 95073
(408)464-2441

California School of Herbal Studies
9309 Highway 116
P.O. Box 36
Forestville, CA 95436
(707)887-7457

SUMMARY

Alternative approaches to pain management are commonly utilized in the United States. The nurse should be informed on these methods, and their efficacy, safety, and potential for injury and side effects. As public interest in natural health care and self-treatment increases, the use of unconventional methods will also increase. Additional funding for research and studies may help to validate the safety and efficacy of the various alternative therapies.

References

Alternative medicine: The facts. (1994, January). *Consumer Reports, 59*(6), 51-53.

Anderson, K. N., Ed. (1994). *Mosby's medical, nursing and allied health* (4th ed.). St. Louis: Mosby.

Berk, L. (1994). New discoveries in psychoneuroimmunology. *Humor and Health Letter, 3*(6), 1-7.

Byers, D. (1994). *Better health with foot reflexology: The original Ingham method.* St Petersburg, FL: Ingham, p. xxiii.

Chiappone, J. (1993). *The light touch.* Centerville, VA: Holistic Reflections, p. 19.

Connolly, L. (1977). Ida Rolf. *Human Behavior, 6*(5), 17-23.

Cottingham, J., Porges, S., & Richard, K. (1988). Shifts in pelvic inclination angle and parasympathetic tone production by Rolfing soft tissue manipulation. *Physical Therapy, 68,* 1364-1370.

Eisenberg, D., Kessler, R., Foster, C., Norlock, F., Calkins, D., & Delbance, T. (1993). Unconventional medicine in the United States: Prevalence, costs, and patterns of use. *New England Journal of Medicine, 328,* 246-252.

Gerber, R. (1988). *Vibrational medicine.* Santa Fe, NM: Bear, pp. 122-123.

Goldberg, B. (1993). *Alternative medicine: The definitive guide.* Puyallup, WA: Future Medicine.

International Institute of Reflexology, St. Petersburg, FL.

Kastner, M. (1994). Researching massage as real therapy. *Massage Therapy Journal, 33*(3), 56-74, 112-114.

Krieger, D. (1992). *The therapeutic touch: How to use your hands to help or heal.* New York: Prentice Hall, p. 155.

Krier, M. (1992, April 9). A lighter touch: "Network" chiropractors tap gently to release pain in the body and the mind. *Los Angeles Times,* p. E1.

Lee, B. (1990). "Humor relations" for nurse managers. *Nursing Management, 21*(5), 86-92.

Magna, P., Angus, D., Papadapoulos, C., & Swan, R. (1993). *A study to examine the effectiveness of chiropractic management of low-back pain* (monograph). Richard Hill, Ont.: Kenilworth.

National Institutes of Health. Office of Alternative Medicine. (1994). *Fact sheet #2: Research programs.* Bethesda, MD: NIH, Appendix III.

Oleson, M., & Flocco, W. (1993). Reflexology relieves PMS distress. *Obstetrics and Gynecology, 82,* 906.

Rossman, M. (1993). Imagery and visualization: An overview. In *Fresh perspectives on psychological health: A practitioner's guide to mind/body medicine* (pp. 400-430). Mansfield, CT: National Institute for Clinical Application of Behavioral Medicine.

Schwartz, M. (1987). *Biofeedback: A practitioner's guide.* New York: Guilford, pp. 488-506.

Tyler, V. E. (1993). *The honest herbal* (3rd ed.). New York: Pharmaceutical Products Press.

Weintraub, M. (1992). Alternative medicine: Shiatsu, Swedish massage, and trigger point suppression in spinal pain syndrome. *American Journal of Pain Management, 2*(2), 574-576.

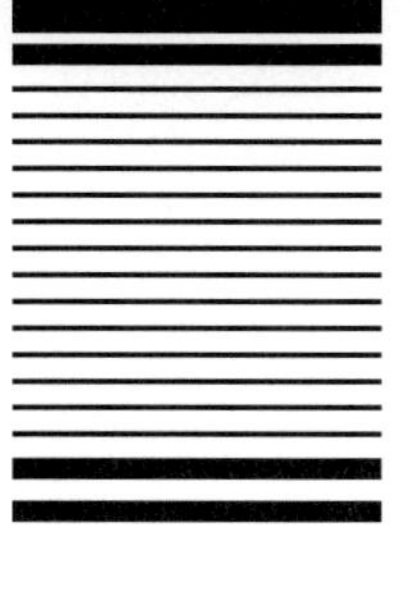

SECTION THREE

Clinical Application of Pain Management

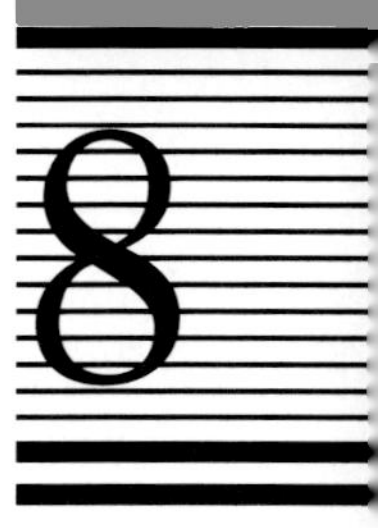

Acute Pain

Julie A. Stanik-Hutt

Characteristics of Acute Pain
Basic Principles and Pathophysiology
- Acute Pain Stimuli
- At-Risk Populations
- Consequences

Therapeutic Management
- Assessment
  - Comprehensive Pain Measurement
  - Systematic Pain Assessment
- Pharmacologic Interventions
  - Opioids
  - NSAIDs
  - Routes of Administration
  - Patient-Controlled Analgesia
  - Clinical Decision Making
- Nonpharmacologic Interventions
  - Physical Interventions
  - TENS
  - Psychologic Interventions

Team Approach
Summary

Key Points

- Prevention is better than treatment.
- Systematic assessment and documentation is crucial to adequate management.
- Analgesic medications are the primary interventions used to control acute pain.
- Medications used to treat acute pain should be administered around the clock for at least the first 48 hours.
- Therapies based on peripheral mechanisms of action should be used in combination with those based on central mechanisms.
- Therapies should be titrated to patient response rather than based on standardized protocols.

Pain is the "unpleasant sensory and emotional experience associated with actual or potential tissue damage" (IASP, 1979, p. 250). It is an internal experience that may be manifested by externally observable verbal, behavioral, and physiologic responses.

Pain is commonly characterized as acute or chronic. Acute pain is often described as a protective mechanism associated with tissue injury or destruction (Curro, 1987). It is a nearly universal human experience, and its occurrence is the most common reason cited for seeking medical treatment.

Seventeen million Americans are hospitalized annually for the treatment of traumatic injuries (Cousins, 1989; Fought, 1988), and an additional 23.3 million undergo surgical procedures (Carr et al., 1992). More than 70% of patients with acute tissue damage, such as that occurring with traumatic and surgical injuries, recall experiencing severe pain (Puntillo, 1988).

Intramuscular injections of standardized doses of narcotics every 3 to 4 hours prn is the most commonly prescribed therapy for acute pain. Many authors have described the cycle

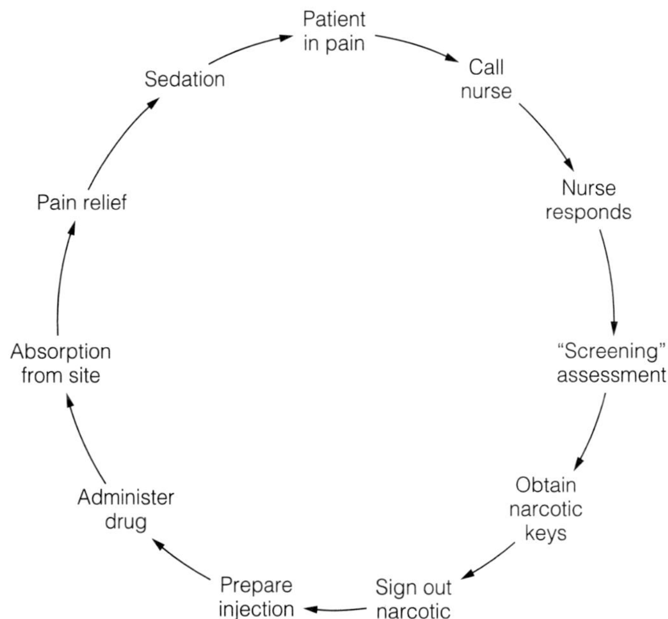

Figure 8-1 The pain cycle. (From Graves, D. A., Foster, R. L., Batenhorst, R. L., Bennett, R., & Baumann, T. (1983). Patient-controlled analgesia. *Annals of Internal Medicine, 99*, 360-366. American College of Physicians.)

of pain (Figure 8-1), and studies have documented the overall undertreatment of pain that can accompany reliance on this approach to pain management (see Chapters 1 and 2). Contrary to popular belief, most acute pain can be effectively managed using available methods of pain relief.

Nurses are in an ideal position to assess and treat patients in pain. They are in almost constant contact with patients and provide assistance with the most basic life functions. They also perform many procedures that are recognized as causing pain. "Nurses, as primary care providers, should recognize the importance of their role as pain managers" (Wells, 1984, p. 51).

This chapter will provide a review of acute pain and its nursing management. Information describing specific characteristics and pathophysiologic processes related to acute pain will be discussed. Basic principles of acute pain management and methods of assessing acute pain in clinical settings will be described. The administration of pharmacologic agents, including opioid and nonsteroidal antiinflammatory drugs, will be reviewed with recommendations for dosages and routes of administration. Utilization of nonpharmacologic pain relief therapies will be described as well. Invasive therapies such as peripheral nerve blocks and intrathecal and epidural analgesics will not be described here; information on these medical therapies is included in Chapter 14.

CHARACTERISTICS OF ACUTE PAIN

Acute pain serves a useful purpose, alerting us to the presence of potentially harmful conditions, and leads to constructive action (Davis, 1989a). It is a defense mechanism responsible for a cascade of voluntary and involuntary behaviors that prepare us to meet or escape a physical danger.

Critical features of acute pain are that it (a) is associated with an identifiable injury, disease, or medical procedure; (b) is accompanied by anxiety and sympathetic nervous system (SNS) activation; (c) is less than 6 months in duration; (d) subsides as healing occurs; and (e) is not associated with psychopathology (Ackerman & Stevens, 1989). Acute pain is an expected occurrence after any tissue injury. It can usually be successfully controlled using traditional analgesic methods (American Pain Society, 1992).

BASIC PRINCIPLES AND PATHOPHYSIOLOGY

The experience of acute pain is a psychologic, perceptual phenomenon initiated by nociception (Puntillo, 1991). Nociceptors are the nerve receptors that, when stimulated, transmit afferent impulses that are ultimately interpreted as pain. (Pain receptors have not been found to exist.)

Tissue injury results in specific pathophysiologic responses, whether the injury is caused by disease, trauma, or a medical procedure. These pathophysiologic responses produce changes in the local tissue environment, causing the release of pain-producing substances that directly stimulate or sensitize nociceptors (Armstrong, Jepson, Keele, & Stewart, 1957; Drain & Cain, 1981; Mense & Meyer, 1981; Rosenthal, 1977; Schmitt, 1977). The inflammatory mediators produced after an injury, including prostaglandins and leukotrienes, further reduce the normally high threshold of nociceptors. All of these changes cause a hyperalgesic state (Pflugg & Bonica, 1977). In this state, previously innocuous stimuli are able to stimulate nociceptors and may elicit a pain response because of the lowered nociceptive threshold.

When a nociceptor is stimulated, an excitatory afferent impulse (action potential) is created and transmission of pain is begun. (See Chapter 1 for details of the pain pathway.)

Acute Pain Stimuli

Reflex responses act as noxious stimuli. Vasospasm, for example, in response to liberated substances can lead to ischemia, tissue hypoxia, and local acidosis and can cause further nociceptive stimulation (Pflugg & Bonica, 1977).

As nociceptive impulses pass through the spinal cord, motor reflex responses are initiated that result in withdrawal from the noxious stimuli and are accompanied by generalized increased muscle tension (Edwards & Breed, 1990). This increased muscle tension, called splinting, may further contribute to nociceptive stimulation.

Some forms of tissue injury, such as surgery and trauma, act as mechanical stimulants to nociceptors. Hemorrhage and edema increase extravascular hydrostatic pressure and also directly stimulate nociceptors. Surgical drains, intravenous catheters, urinary drainage catheters, and nasogastric tubes act as continuing noxious stimuli (Harrison & Cotanch, 1987). In view of the changes in nociceptor threshold and the occurrence of reflex vasospasm and increased muscle tension, it is important to remember that the occurrence of pain is not dependent on the presence of exogenous noxious stimuli.

At-Risk Populations

Acute pain is commonly associated with medical conditions and diseases, injuries, and medical procedures. Medical conditions that are accompanied by acute pain include acute appendicitis, dental abscess, gout, migraine headache, acute myocardial infarction, sickle cell crisis, deep vein thrombosis, and kidney stones. Injuries such as burns, fractures, lacerations, sprains, and contusions are also associated with acute pain.

Many medical procedures, such as surgery, dental work, and diagnostic procedures, although necessary for diagnostic and therapeutic purposes, actually cause acute pain. Commonly performed nursing procedures—endotracheal suctioning, nasogastric intubation, turning and mobilizing postoperative patients, dressing changes, and parenteral injections, for example—can also cause pain.

The need to perform potentially pain-producing procedures is in direct conflict with the health care provider's natural desire to avoid inflicting pain. Nurses are put in the position of being responsible for inflicting pain, as well as assessing and managing pain. Conflicts in values and roles lead health care providers to become relatively desensitized to the patient's pain or to the potential for a procedure to cause pain.

Consequences

Unrelieved acute pain has a significant detrimental effect on an individual's physical recovery from illness or injury and interferes with psychologic well-being (Collins, 1992; Levine, 1984; Puntillo, 1988). Inadequate pain relief contributes to complications in many hospitalized patients (Parkhouse, Lambrechts, & Simpson, 1961). Pulmonary complications of postoperative pain include atelectasis, inability to deep breathe and cough, intrapulmonary shunting, and hypoxemia (Hughes, 1983; Masson, 1971). Pain-induced hemodynamic instability, increased metabolic rate, and stress-mediated release of cortisol delay healing (Cooper & Schumann, 1979).

Acute pain can induce and prolong the stress response (Cooper & Schumann, 1979; Murry, 1975; Torda, 1983). The inability to ingest sufficient nutrients or acquire adequate sleep due to pain can delay recovery from illness (Fordham, 1982). Pain is a major deterrent to movement (Stanik-Hutt, 1994), predisposing patients to contractures, skin breakdown, and pulmonary emboli (Fordham; Masson, 1971).

Acute pain can affect psychologic status. It wastes energy, narrows one's perspective, and demands total attention (Schmitt, 1977). It can deny a patient a sense of progress and cause minor irritations to be exaggerated (Andrews, 1983; Fordham, 1982; Masson, 1971).

THERAPEUTIC MANAGEMENT

Knowledge gained from the multitude of research studies, years of clinical practice, and recently published clinical practice guidelines (Carr et al., 1992) has identified several essential principles for effective management of acute pain (see the following box).

BASIC PRINCIPLES OF ACUTE PAIN MANAGEMENT

Perform regularly scheduled pain assessments.

The patient's self-report is the best measure of pain.

Establish pain levels that trigger further treatment.

Individualize analgesic prescriptions and titrate based on response and side effects.

Administer analgesics initially on a regular, around-the-clock schedule rather than as needed.

Established pain is more difficult to manage; therefore institute treatment early.

Use drug and nondrug therapies based on peripheral and central mechanisms.

From Stanik-Hutt, J. (1993). Strategies for pain management in traumatic thoracic injuries. *Critical Care Nursing Clinics of North America, 5*(4), 713-722. Reprinted with permission.

Systematic assessment and documentation of pain is crucial to adequate management. Many simple pain measurement methods are available and should be used on a regular basis to quantify this subjective phenomenon. Assessment should begin with the patient's own description of the pain and may take into account a variety of other relevant data.

The experience of pain is unique to the individual and can even vary for the same individual between occurrences. Treatments and dosages that relieve pain in one person may not be effective for another individual under similar circumstances. Therapies should be titrated according to observed therapeutic response and side effects rather than using standardized protocols. Nurses are accustomed to titrating medications to effect in treating various conditions and should do likewise with therapies for acute pain.

Prevention of acute pain is better than treatment. Patients who receive preprocedural analgesia complain of less postprocedural pain. Analgesic therapy initiated at the first sign of pain is more effective than the same therapy administered after the pain becomes severe (Wall, 1988; Woolf & Wall, 1986). In fact, recent neurophysiologic research has shown that unrelieved pain can lead to changes in cell functioning within the spinal cord (Bullit, 1989; Fitzgerald, 1990). These changes could affect processing of impulses from painful stimuli. Therefore it is important to establish an around-the-clock plan to prevent and, if possible, preempt pain, for example, preoperatively (Figure 8-2).

Pain can be altered by any therapy that affects nociceptive impulse generation, transmission, or interpretation. Impulse generation therapies include those that act at the site of injury to prevent stimulation of nociceptors. Therapies that reduce inflammation, block production of prostaglandin, or prevent the release of substance P and serotonin (e.g., application of heat or cold, NSAIDs) can be classified as altering impulse generation (Aimone, 1992).

Treatments that affect impulse transmission act within the primary afferent neuron (peripheral nerve), at synapses within the spinal cord, or at higher nerve centers. Therapies that inhibit the release of excitatory neurotransmitters from

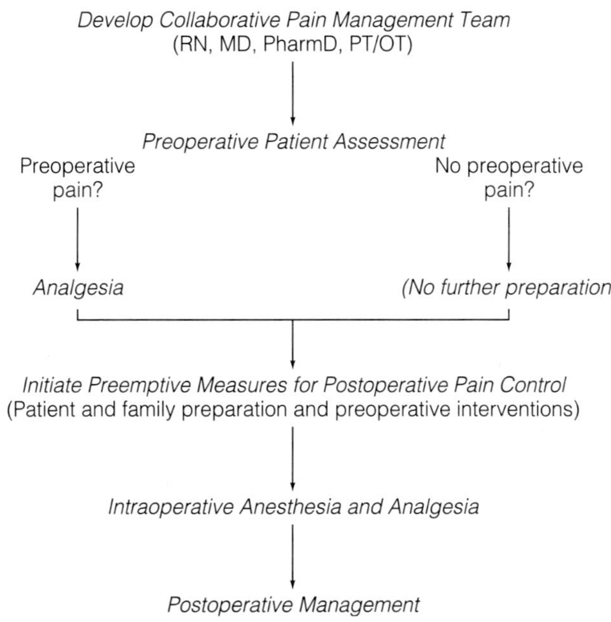

Figure 8-2 Acute pain treatment flow chart: preoperative and intraoperative phases. (Modified from Carr, D. B., Jacox, A., Chapman, C. R., Ferrell, B., Fields, H. L., Heidrich, G., Hester, N. K., Hill, C. S., Lipman, A. G., McGarvey, C. L., Miaskowski, C., Mulder, D., Payne, R., Schechter, N., Shapiro, B. S., Smith, R. S., Tsou, C. V., Vecchiarelli, L. (1992). *Acute pain management: Operative or medical procedures and trauma. Clinical practice guideline.* AHCPR Pub. No. 92-0032. Rockville, MD: Agency for Health Care Policy and Research, PHS, USDHHS.)

presynaptic neurons or that prevent excitation and firing of postsynaptic neurons will prevent the transmission of afferent nociceptive impulses. Opioid medications are known to inhibit the release of substance P presynaptically (Hirota et al., 1985) and to interfere with the firing of postsynaptic neurons primarily within the spinal cord (Sabbe & Yaksh, 1990). Endorphins are thought to cause the same changes in spinal cord processing of nociceptive impulses. Cutaneous stimulation of large-fiber mechanoreceptors is also thought to interfere with the transmission of nociceptive impulses within the dorsal horn (Wall & Sweet, 1967). Opioids, endorphin-stimulating interventions, and transcutaneous electrical nerve stimulation (TENS) are examples of therapies that can interfere with impulse transmission.

Therapies designed to alter the interpretation of nociceptive impulses work in higher centers. Opioids, hypnosis, and relaxation therapy are therapies that can affect how the limbic system, sensory cortex, and memory centers of the brain process and interpret these impulses and thus alter the pain experience.

Therapies based on peripheral mechanisms of action should be used in combination with those based on central mechanisms. Plans for pain management should incorporate interventions involving multiple sites of action that combine to interrupt the pain experience.

Assessment

A key to effective pain management is the routine, systematic assessment of pain. Pain is a complex, multidimensional phenomenon. Because of the subjective nature of pain, health care workers must remember that patients are the experts on their pain. A good assessment therefore begins with the patient's description of the pain. Chapter 1 discusses measures commonly used for the rapid assessment of pain. Instruments used for comprehensive pain measurement are discussed here.

Comprehensive Pain Measurement

Two multidimensional pain scales, the McGill Pain Questionnaire (MPQ) and the short-form McGill Pain Questionnaire (SFMPQ), have been used in clinical settings to quantify pain. The McGill Pain Questionnaire (Melzack, 1975) has been widely used in clinical practice and is considered the "gold standard" for pain measurement (Davis, 1989b) (Figure 8-3). It assesses pain as the expression of the complex psychophysiologic processes postulated in the gate control theory.

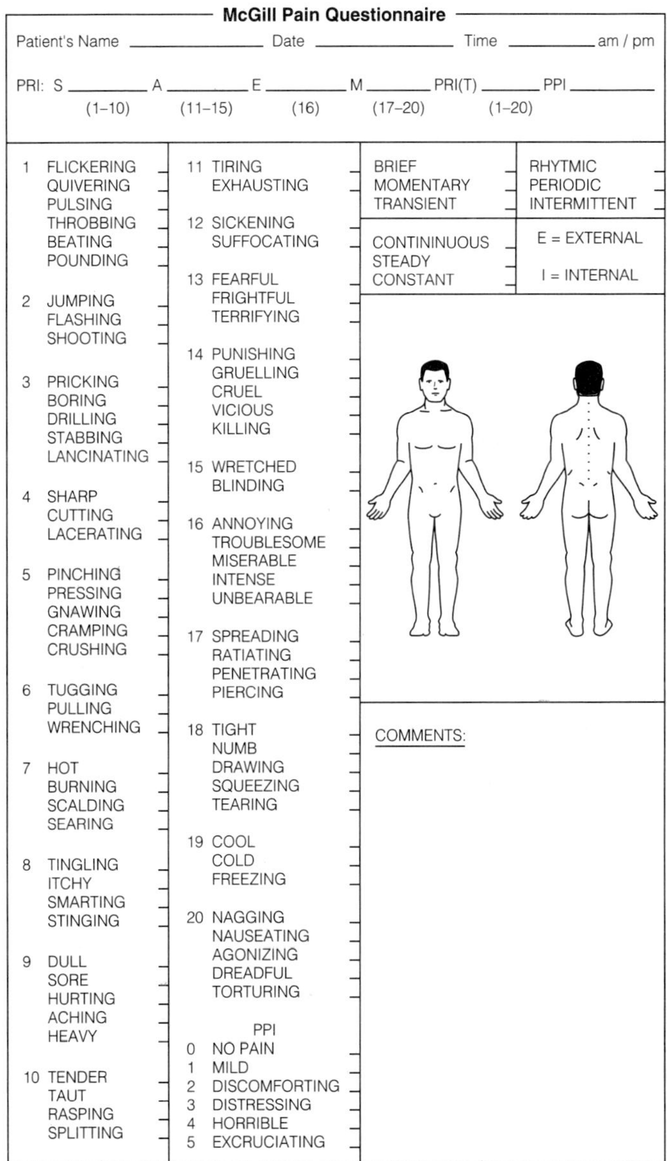

McGill Pain Questionnaire

Patient's Name ______ Date ______ Time ______ am / pm

PRI: S ______ (1–10) A ______ (11–15) E ______ (16) M ______ (17–20) PRI(T) ______ (1–20) PPI ______

1 FLICKERING
QUIVERING
PULSING
THROBBING
BEATING
POUNDING

2 JUMPING
FLASHING
SHOOTING

3 PRICKING
BORING
DRILLING
STABBING
LANCINATING

4 SHARP
CUTTING
LACERATING

5 PINCHING
PRESSING
GNAWING
CRAMPING
CRUSHING

6 TUGGING
PULLING
WRENCHING

7 HOT
BURNING
SCALDING
SEARING

8 TINGLING
ITCHY
SMARTING
STINGING

9 DULL
SORE
HURTING
ACHING
HEAVY

10 TENDER
TAUT
RASPING
SPLITTING

11 TIRING
EXHAUSTING

12 SICKENING
SUFFOCATING

13 FEARFUL
FRIGHTFUL
TERRIFYING

14 PUNISHING
GRUELLING
CRUEL
VICIOUS
KILLING

15 WRETCHED
BLINDING

16 ANNOYING
TROUBLESOME
MISERABLE
INTENSE
UNBEARABLE

17 SPREADING
RATIATING
PENETRATING
PIERCING

18 TIGHT
NUMB
DRAWING
SQUEEZING
TEARING

19 COOL
COLD
FREEZING

20 NAGGING
NAUSEATING
AGONIZING
DREADFUL
TORTURING

PPI
0 NO PAIN
1 MILD
2 DISCOMFORTING
3 DISTRESSING
4 HORRIBLE
5 EXCRUCIATING

BRIEF
MOMENTARY
TRANSIENT

RHYTMIC
PERIODIC
INTERMITTENT

CONTININUOUS
STEADY
CONSTANT

E = EXTERNAL

I = INTERNAL

COMMENTS:

Figure 8-3 McGill Pain Questionnaire: one-page version. (From Melzack, R. (1975). The McGill Pain Questionnaire: Major properties and scoring methods. *Pain, 1,* 277-299.)

The one-page version of the MPQ includes a list of 78 pain descriptors (Pain Rating Index, or PRI), a 6-point descriptive rating scale (Present Pain Intensity, or PPI), and a body diagram (qualitatively evaluated).

In administering the questionnaire, the list of 78 descriptors is given or read to the patient. Patients are asked to select the descriptors that describe their pain. These words are quantified with intensity ratings during scoring by the practitioner. The total scale range is 0 to 83.

It takes from 10 to 60 minutes to administer and score the MPQ. Complexity and length severely limit the use of the MPQ, particularly with acutely or critically ill patients (Chapman, 1985). "Clearly a shortened version of the MPQ is desirable for studies which require more rapid acquisition of data than is possible using the standard MPQ" (Melzack, 1987, p. 192).

The SFMPQ (Melzack, 1987) was developed for clinical use with acute pain syndromes (Figure 8-4). It is considerably shorter and easier to use than the original. The questionnaire includes a list of 15 pain descriptors, the PPI, and a horizontal Visual Analog Scale (VAS). Patients are asked to select from the list of 15 descriptors those that describe their pain. They also rate the intensity of each selected descriptor (mild = 1, moderate = 2, severe = 3), for a possible total score of 45. The PPI score (0 to 5) and the VAS score (0 to 100 mm) can be added to the descriptor score, for a total scale range of 0 to 150.

It takes less than 5 minutes to administer and score the SFMPQ. The scale has been used successfully with a variety of medical-surgical patient populations, including critically burned and traumatically injured individuals. Scores from the SFMPQ and MPQ are significantly correlated (r = .70 to .93) (Melzack, 1987; Stanik-Hutt, 1994) with reportedly adequate internal consistency (α = .72 to .94) (Ulmer, 1991; Stanik-Hutt).

Either of these pain questionnaires can be used in clinical settings to quantify acute pain. The SFMPQ is much easier for nurses and patients to use than the MPQ. The SFMPQ

SHORT-FORM McGILL PAIN QUESTIONNAIRE (SF-MPQ)

RONALD MELZACK

PATIENT'S NAME ____________ DATE ________

	NONE	MILD	MODERATE	SEVERE
THROBBING	0) ____	1) ____	2) ____	3) ____
SHOOTING	0) ____	1) ____	2) ____	3) ____
STABBING	0) ____	1) ____	2) ____	3) ____
SHARP	0) ____	1) ____	2) ____	3) ____
CRAMPING	0) ____	1) ____	2) ____	3) ____
GNAWING	0) ____	1) ____	2) ____	3) ____
HOT-BURNING	0) ____	1) ____	2) ____	3) ____
ACHING	0) ____	1) ____	2) ____	3) ____
HEAVY	0) ____	1) ____	2) ____	3) ____
TENDER	0) ____	1) ____	2) ____	3) ____
SPLITTING	0) ____	1) ____	2) ____	3) ____
TIRING-EXHAUSTING	0) ____	1) ____	2) ____	3) ____
SICKENING	0) ____	1) ____	2) ____	3) ____
FEARFUL	0) ____	1) ____	2) ____	3) ____
PUNISHING-CRUEL	0) ____	1) ____	2) ____	3) ____

PPI

0 NO PAIN ____

1 MILD ____

2 DISCOMFORTING ____

3 DISTRESSING ____

4 HORRIBLE ____

5 EXCRUCIATING ____

NO PAIN |————————————| WORST POSSIBLE PAIN

Figure 8-4 Short form McGill Pain Questionnaire. (From Melzack, R. (1987). The Short-form McGill Pain Questionnaire. *Pain, 30,* 191-197.)

may be used once per shift to obtain a more in-depth assessment of the pain than is possible with simple pain measures. This may also be useful in situations in which a patient's pain is particularly difficult to assess and manage. It would give a better sense of the qualities of the patient's pain and how he or she is perceiving it. This information would be helpful in tailoring interventions to better relieve pain.

Systematic Pain Assessment

Pain management should be systematically incorporated into care routines. The first step in management is pain assessment, which should include data collection and analysis, as well as a determination of the need for intervention. These processes should be followed by appropriate documentation. Structures can be created to support the processes of pain assessment and documentation.

Routines for pain assessment should be established by practice groups and nursing units. Information regarding these routines should be included in staff orientation classes to increase staff awareness of the importance of and institutional standards for pain assessment. To facilitate communication among disciplines, all care providers should use a common pain measurement method. Assessment standards should include information obtained about the pain at its best and its worst, while the patient is at rest, and during activities of daily living.

To remind staff to ask patients about their pain, spaces for entering information concerning pain intensity and relief should be included on bedside flow charts, patient assessment forms, and critical pathway forms. Separate pain flow charts for documentation of pain assessment, management therapies, and occurrence of side effects may also be useful (Figure 8-5). Use of these forms would also make it easier to record and find pain information on the chart.

Standards for pain relief should be established and clearly stated on nursing care plans and critical pathways. In this way patient status can be compared with the expected course of recovery, variances readily detected, and the need for

UNIVERSITY OF MARYLAND MEDICAL SYSTEM
PAIN MANAGEMENT FLOW SHEET

Pain Assessment Tool (circle one): Verbal Numerical Rating Scale / Visual Analogue Scale / Faces Scale / Poker Chip Tool / CHEOPS / Other ______________

Concentration screen must always be set at 0.0 mg. / ml

Patient's / Family's Acceptable Pain Score ______

ADDRESSOGRAPH

DATE	TIME	DRUG	ROUTE	*PUMP SETTINGS* vol. LIMIT (ml)	vol. GIVEN (ml)	conc.	DOSE (ml)	DELAY (min.)	BASAL RATE (ml/hr)	1 HOUR LIMIT (ml/hr)	BOLUS (ml)	# INJ	## ATT	**ASSESSMENT** PAIN SCORE	RR	† SED SCORE	‡ S / E	CAN RAISE HEELS	INT.	COMMENTS Alternative Therapies, Other Observations, and Plans
						0.0														
						0.0														
						0.0														
						0.0														
						0.0														
						0.0														

ROUTE
- p.o. = By mouth
- IM = Intramuscular
- IV = Intravenous
- SubQ = Subcutaneous
- CLE = Continuous lumbar epidural
- CTE = Continuous thoracic epidural
- IPL = Intrapleural
- IT = Intrathecal
- TD = Transdermal

‡S / E = SIDE EFFECTS
- N = Nausea
- V = Vomiting
- I = Itching
- R = Urinary Retention
- CS = Constipation
- CNF = Confusion
- OH = Orthostatic Hypotension
- MB = Motor Block
- HB = High block
- RD = Respiratory depression

† SEDATION (SED) SCORE
- 0 = None = Alert; easy to arouse
- 1 = Mild = Occasionally drowsy; easy to arouse
- 2 = Moderate = Frequently drowsy; easy to arouse
- 3 = Somnolent = Difficult to arouse
- S = Sleep = Normal sleep; would be easy to arouse

ADJUNCTIVE THERAPIES
- TENS = Tens unit
- H = Heat
- CD = Cold
- RLT = Relaxation therapy
- GuI = Guided Imagery
- D = Distraction
- MuT = Music Therapy
- M = Massage
- L = Linament

Adapted and reprinted from: **Oncology Nursing Forum** with permission from the Oncology Nursing Press, Inc. McMillan, Susan C.,; Williams, Faye A. et al. "A Validity and Reliability Study of Two Tools for Assessing and Managing Cancer Pain. "**Oncology Nursing Forum** 15(6):738, 1988 and Mosby Publishing Co., Pasero, C.L. "Role of the Clinical Nurse Coordinator." (In) Sinatra, R.S.; Hord; A.H.; Ginsberg, B.; Preble, L.M. (eds): **Acute Pain Mechanisms & Management**. 555, 1992.

Infusion system securely taped, tubings patent, pump has volume and is infusing as ordered. If PCA^: "Patient button within reach and functions properly. Tubing / bag / battery changed every 72 hours."

DATE	TIME	SIGNATURE / INITIAL ( )	DATE	TIME	SIGNATURE / INITIAL ( )
DATE	TIME	SIGNATURE / INITIAL ( )	DATE	TIME	SIGNATURE / INITIAL ( )
DATE	TIME	SIGNATURE / INITIAL ( )	DATE	TIME	SIGNATURE / INITIAL ( )
DATE	TIME	SIGNATURE / INITIAL ( )	DATE	TIME	SIGNATURE / INITIAL ( )
DATE	TIME	SIGNATURE / INITIAL ( )	DATE	TIME	SIGNATURE / INITIAL ( )

ASSESSMENTS

ASSESSMENT FOR PATIENT CONTROLLED ANALGESIA (PCA^):

A. Chart pain score, respiratory rate, sedation score and presence of side effects q 1/2 hour x 2 times, q 2 hours x 8 times, then q 4 hours. **

B. Heart rate & BP per routine.

ASSESSMENT FOR OTHER ANALGESICS:

A. Chart pain score, respiratory rate, sedation score, and presence of side effects
q ________ hours x ______ hours, then
q ________ hours x ______ hours, then
q ________ hours **

B. Chart patient response to analgesic therapy (pain score, sedation score, and respiratory rate) and side effect management:
__________ mins. / hours (circle one) after administration of primary analgesic and __________ min. / hours (circle one) after administration of rescue analgesic.

ASSESSMENT FOR EPIDURAL / CAUDAL / INTRATHECAL ANALGESIA VIA SINGLE / INTERMITTENT BOLUS OR CONTINUOUS INFUSION
(Maintain 4 hours post D/C epidural infusion or 18 hours post single / intermittent bolus dose of morphine w/o infusion):

A. For patients < 18 years: Respiratory rate q 1 hour **
Sedation score q 1 hour **

B. For patients > 18 years:
Respiratory rate q 1 hour x 24 hours, then q 2 hours **
Sedation score q 1 hour x 24 hours, then q 2 hours **

C. Pain score and presence of side effects q 2 hours X 24 hours, then q 4 hours.

D. BP and HR per routine

E. Assess ability to raise heels off bed q 4 hours and before weight bearing.

F. Head of bed ≥ 30 degrees (except for 15 minute intervals for physical care) while epidural / caudal in place or 12 hours post last morphine dose.

G. Maintain IV access for 18 hours post infusion / single bolus with morphine.

H. Ambu bag, mask, suction and Yankauer, O_2 flow meter available at all times.

I. All epidural catheter dressing changes by APMS* physician only.

FOR RESPIRATORY RATE
< 20 if < 6 mo. < 16 if < 2 yr. < 14 if < 8 yr.
< 12 if < 16 yr. < 10 if ≥ 16 yr.

A. STOP pump by pushing pump STOP BUTTON twice (2) within 1 second.

B. REMOVE the patient control button from the patient's reach (if applicable).

C. GIVE NALOXONE as ordered.

D. PAGE RESIDENT / APPROPRIATE CONSULTING PAIN SERVICE

* **CHART PUMP SETTINGS UPON:** initiation, bag change, D/C, transfer, prescription change and q 8 hours.

** Increase frequency as needed.

INJ = Injections ## ATT = Attempts
PCA ^ = Patient Controlled Analgesia
APMS ^^= Acute Pain Management Service

NOTIFY APMS ^^/ PCA ^SERVICE FOR:

A. Respiratory rate
< 20 if < 6 mo. < 16 if < 2 yr. <14 if < 8 yr.
< 12 if < 16 yr. < 10 if ≥ 16 yr.

B. Sedation score of 3.

C. Pain uncontrolled by prescribed therapy.

D. No spontaneous void x 6 hours

E. Agitation / confusion / inconsolability

F. N/V, itching, or urinary retention unrelieved by adjunctive therapies.

G. O_2 sat < 95% on oxygen (for pt. in ICU / IMC setting).

H. Catheter disconnects / dressing integrity disruption.

I. pt. c/o numbness higher than nipple line.

J. Decreased ability to move leg(s) or deep breathe.

50424 (REV. 1/95)

Figure 8-5 Pain management flow sheet. (Used by permission of University of Maryland Medical System.)

corrective action identified. Unit quality improvement committees should be charged with the responsibility to monitor and regularly report on pain-related outcomes. This monitoring should include variance reports and patient surveys regarding satisfaction with the pain therapies used and the level of pain relief obtained.

Pharmacologic Interventions

Analgesic medications are the first line of defense against acute pain (American Pain Society, 1992). Nonpharmacologic therapies may be used in conjunction with, but not instead of, pharmacologic agents. Two major types of analgesic medications are used in managing acute pain: opioids and nonsteroidal antiinflammatory drugs (NSAIDs). These two types of medication are also used in combination, usually in compounds composed of a small dose of an NSAID plus a relatively weak opioid. Together they provide better relief than when either is used alone.

Severe pain usually requires the use of a potent opioid analgesic such as fentanyl or morphine. Combination compounds, such as percocet, can be effective for moderate pain. A very large number of analgesic medications and combinations are available with a variety of dosages and routes of administration. For optimal pain management with a reasonable degree of safety, a general practitioner should be familiar with the most commonly used NSAID and opioid analgesic medications. (See Chapter 4 for more complete information on analgesic medications.)

Local anesthetic medications are also used in the treatment of acute pain. They can be administered by local tissue infiltration, in topical creams, and in sprays for very localized, relatively mild pain (e.g., minor lacerations). They are also administered in nerve blocks and via epidural and intrathecal injections. Opioid analgesics are sometimes used in combination with local anesthetic medications for intraspinal analgesia. (See Chapter 14 for a description of these techniques.)

Opioids

Decades of experience in the use of opioid drugs to treat acute pain in experimental and clinical situations have taught practitioners that these drugs are both safe and effective (Portenoy, 1992). Contrary to common belief, the incidence of addiction is low in drug-naive patients treated with opioids for postoperative pain (Porter & Jick, 1980).

The use of opioids involves characteristic side effects, including sedation and drowsiness. These effects are thought to be mediated by neurotransmitters in the brain. Respiratory depression is characterized by decreased respiratory rate and volume accompanied by lowered response to hypercarbia. These respiratory effects are preceded by sedation and are mediated by the pontine and medullary respiratory centers (Jaffe & Martin, 1985).

Peripheral vascular dilation, inhibition of baroreceptor reflexes, and histamine release after opioid administration can cause hypotension, particularly with postural changes and in patients who are hypovolemic. Pruritus is also caused by opioid-mediated histamine release by some opioids. Opioids can also cause nausea and vomiting, particularly when the patient is in upright positions or is moving. Urinary retention can be caused by the increased tone in the detrusor muscle and vesical sphincter resulting from opioid use.

NSAIDs

Nonsteroidal antiinflammatory drugs (NSAIDs) are non opioid drugs thatvinterfere with the production of prostaglandins. Prostaglandins lower the normally high threshold of nociceptors at the site of an injury. They are one of the chemical mediators in a wound that directly stimulate nociceptors and elicit pain. Since prostaglandins directly and indirectly cause pain, any medication that interferes with prostaglandin production will reduce pain.

NSAIDs are generally effective for mild pain, especially that associated with inflammation. In addition to their analgesic effects, these drugs have antipyretic and antiinflammatory properties. Aspirin, ibuprofen, and naproxen are examples of commonly used NSAIDs. Acetominophen is sometimes categorized as an NSAID even though it has no antiinflammatory effects.

The relative safety of NSAIDs has led to their widespread use in over-the-counter forms. NSAIDs are relatively inexpensive and are available in tablet, capsule, and liquid forms for oral administration. Many can also be administered in suppositories. Ketorolac (Toradol) is the only NSAID available for parenteral use. Doses, duration of action, and side effects vary among compounds. (See Chapter 4 for an in-depth review of NSAIDs and dosage guidelines.)

Gastrointestinal upset and fluid retention are common side effects with NSAID agents. An increased tendency to bleed because of altered platelet aggregation is also associated with their use. Choline magnesium trisalicylate is the only NSAID that does not produce this problem (Stuart & Pisko, 1981). In general, most NSAIDs should not be used by people with viral illnesses, hypersensitivity to aspirin, history of asthma, or liver or renal impairment.

Routes of Administration

Medications cannot have an effect until they are absorbed into the bloodstream. The status of the patient's peripheral and gastrointestinal tissue perfusion needs to be considered in selecting an administration route. Absorption of medications from muscle, fat, and the gastrointestinal tract may be impaired in patients with significant acute alterations in cardiac output or tissue perfusion. Patients who are shunting blood flow away from the peripheral and gastrointestinal tissues may not obtain adequate relief from oral, transdermal, or parenteral administration. Intravenous (IV) injection is the most reliable route for medication administration for these patients. It is also used for patients who cannot accept oral administration.

If the pain is severe or the patient is unable to take medications orally, parenteral administration is suggested. Intravenous administration is the preferred parenteral route because it provides the fastest and most efficient route for analgesic medication administration. Delays in drug absorption are avoided, making essentially 100% of the medication available immediately. The rapid onset and peak effect allows the practitioner, over a short period of time, to titrate analgesic doses and gain control over the pain. For most IV medications, smaller doses are used and the duration of effect is shorter, which may reduce the risk of side or toxic effects compared with other routes (Table 8-1).

In titrating, sequential doses of medication are administered IV while the patient is closely monitored for pain relief and occurrence of side effects. Adequate time is allowed between doses for the medication to reach peak effect. Additional doses are administered until adequate relief is achieved or side effects occur.

Continuous and patient-controlled IV infusions provide the smoothest analgesia, using the "kinetic-dynamic relationships" of opioids and avoiding the peaks and valleys of serum concentration encountered with other administration methods. Infusions should always be preceded by a loading dose to gain initial control over the pain. After the patient's pain has been brought under control, the practitioner must provide maintenance doses, on a regular schedule, of continuous or patient-controlled infusions. Edwards and Breed (1990) recommend using the following formula to estimate hourly analgesic dose:

$$\text{Estimated hourly analgesic dose} = \frac{\text{Loading dose}}{\text{Elimination half-life in hours} \times 2}$$

As this maintenance dose is administered, patient monitoring should be continued and dose adjustments made for at least 2 hours.

Opioid agents can also be administered through epidural and intrathecal injections or infusions. When an opioid is mixed with a local anesthetic, smaller doses of both medications can be used to attain the same or better levels of analgesia with fewer side effects. Both techniques require the services of a physician or nurse anesthetist. (See Chapter 14.)

Table 8-1 Intravenous Opioids

Drug	Dose (mg)	Infusion (mg/hr)	Onset (min)	Peak (min)	Duration (hr)	Excretion (first pass/ second pass)
Agonists						
Morphine	2–10	2–8	2–3	20	4–5	Urine/bile
Meperedine (Demerol)	10–30	15–35	1	5–7	2–4	Urine
Hydromorphone (Dilaudid)	0.5–1.0	0.2–1.0	10–15	15–30	2–3	Urine
Methadone (Dolophine)	2.5–10.0	NR*	2–3	15–30	3–4†	Urine/bile
Oxymorphone (Numorphan)	1.0–1.5	NR	5–10	15–30	3–4	Urine
Fentanyl (Sublimaze)	50–100 μg	50–100 μg	1–2	3–5	0.5–1.0	Urine
Sufentanyl (Sufenta)	25–50 μg	NR	Immediate	1.3–3.0	5 min	Urine/bile
Mixed agonists-antagonists						
Buprenorphine (Buprenex)	0.3–0.6	NR	2–5	15–30	6–8	Bile
Butorphanol (Stadol)	0.5–2.0	NR	1	4–5	3–4	Urine/bile
Nalbuphine (Nubain)	10	NR	2–3	30	3–4	Urine
Pentazocine (Talwin)	30–60	NR	2–3	15–30	2–3	Urine/bile

From Wild, L. (1991). Intravenous methods of analgesia for pain in the critically ill. In K. Puntillo (Ed.), *Pain in the critically ill: Assessment and management* (pp. 79-94). Gaithersburg, MD: Aspen. Reprinted with permission.

**NR,* Not reported for analgesic doses.

†Duration lengthens with subsequent doses.

Patient-Controlled Analgesia

The concept of patient-controlled analgesia (PCA) is based on the idea that the patient is in the best position to evaluate pain and pain relief and consequently to determine the need for further analgesic doses. The idea of self-service underlies another principle of PCA—that analgesia is more effective when the patient, rather than the nurse or physician, is in control.

Opioids exhibit a hierarchy of response in that analgesia occurs at a plasma level below that associated with side effects. With PCA the overall plasma concentration of a drug is kept within a narrow range, eliminating the dramatic peaks and valleys common with large bolus injections. By keeping plasma levels within a narrow range around the minimum effective analgesic concentration for the individual, the incidence of side effects is significantly reduced and pain relief is enhanced (Figure 8-6).

A variety of routes of medication administration—including oral, subcutaneous, intramuscular, intravenous, and epidural—can be used in the patient-controlled mode. However, PCA traditionally refers to "the patient's self-administration of intravenous bolus doses of narcotics using a special infusion pump" (McCaffery, 1987, p. 62).

To be a candidate for PCA a patient must be alert, mentally intact, and able to follow simple directions. Many patients with acute pain related to a medical condition—for example, myocardial ischemia, dissecting aortic aneurysm, or sickle cell crisis—should be evaluated for PCA use. Patients admitted to inpatient settings after a major injury or surgical procedure should also be evaluated for therapy. Burn and trauma patients require adequate fluid resuscitation before PCA can be safely initiated. PCA may not be cost effective for patients who will require parenteral therapy with potent opioids for less than 24 hours.

Elderly patients and those with respiratory compromise or hypovolemia may be at high risk for respiratory complications with IV opioids of any type. Patients with significant impairment of renal or hepatic function probably should not use PCA (Table 8-2).

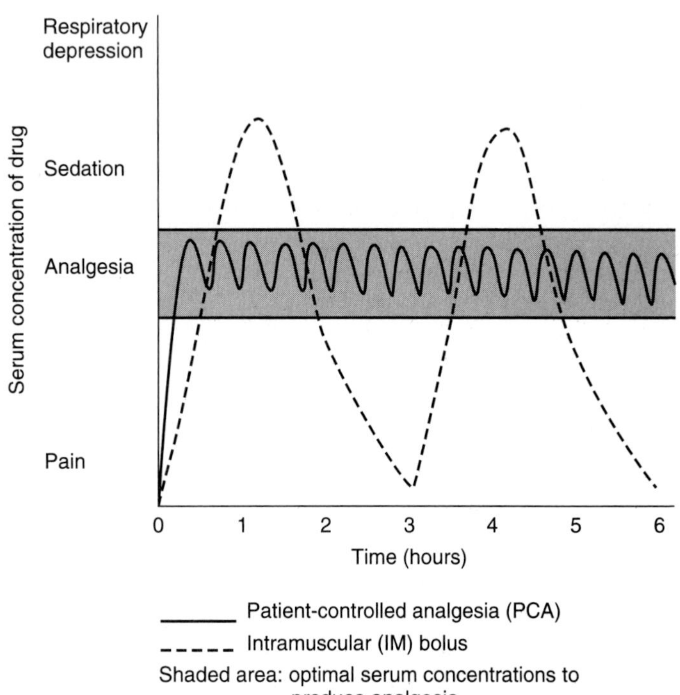

Figure 8-6 Dose-effect relationships for IM and PCA analgesia. (From Wild, L. (1991). Intravenous methods of analgesia for pain in the critically ill. In K. Puntillo (Ed.), *Pain in the critically ill: Assessment and management* (pp. 79-94). Gaithersburg, MD: Aspen.)

To establish PCA, dosing control limits are programmed into the pump memory. The program includes loading dose, PCA dose, lockout interval, and background infusion (Table 8-3).

The loading dose is a one-time analgesic dose administered at the beginning of PCA therapy. It is designed to establish an initial plasma concentration of drug and gain immediate control of the pain. Use of a loading dose reduces the need for the patient to make frequent early demands to establish a

Table 8-2 Patient Selection Criteria for PCA

Indications	Contraindications
Alert and oriented	Altered level of consciousness
Adequate circulating volume	Shock or other significant hemodynamic instability
Able to follow commands	Sepsis
Normal renal and hepatic function	Renal or hepatic failure
Neurologically intact	
Normal respiratory function (or mechanically ventilated)	

From Stanik-Hutt, J. (1991). Use of patient-controlled analgesia with critically ill patients. *AACN Clinical Issues in Critical Care Nursing, 2*(4), 741-747. Reprinted by permission.

Table 8-3 Suggested PCA Settings for Commonly Used Opioids*

	Morphine	Fentanyl	Hydromorphone
Loading dose	2–30 mg	25–250 μg	0.25–5 mg
Basal infusion	0–2 mg	10–25 μg	0–0.5 mg
PCA dose	0.5–2.5 mg	15–75 μg	0.1–0.5 mg
Lockout interval	6–12 min	3–10 min	5–15 min
4-hour limit	35 mg	300 μg	20 mg

From Sevarino, F., & Preble, L. (1992). *A manual for acute postoperative pain management.* New York: Raven Press.

*These recommended doses do not apply to children, adults weighing less than 50 kg, or those with renal or hepatic dysfunction. Clinical therapy should be titrated to patient responses.

baseline plasma concentration of analgesic. The loading dose can be programmed to be delivered by the pump or can be manually administered by the nurse or physician. Patients who have not received opioids previously may be administered a loading dose in small doses (for example, 1 to 5 mg morphine) every 10 minutes until the pain is relieved.

The PCA dose (demand dose) is the amount of analgesic infused in a single bolus dose in response to each patient demand. The PCA dose must be large enough to produce an analgesic effect but not large enough to lead to toxic plasma concentrations.

The lockout interval is the minimum time between successive PCA doses. For most potent opioids this interval is 6 to 10 minutes. The lockout interval should allow adequate time for the onset of analgesic effects from one PCA dose before a subsequent PCA dose is administered. This forced waiting period is intended to prevent overdosage.

The background or basal infusion is a constant-rate infusion of the analgesic that is supplemented by the intermittent PCA doses. The purpose of the background infusion is to prevent subtherapeutic plasma concentrations; however, like the loading dose, the background infusion frequently is omitted in practice and is no longer considered essential to PCA.

Physician orders for PCA should include the following information: (a) name of the medication, concentration, and route of administration; loading dose, basal infusion rate, and bolus dose in milligrams and cubic centimeters; lockout period and 4-hour dose limit; (b) frequency of monitoring respiratory rate and sedation; (c) naloxone administration conditions and dosages; (d) how to reach the physician if necessary; (e) adjunct medications, such as antiemetics and laxatives; and (f) instructions to discontinue all CNS depressant and controlled substance medications. All orders for opioids, sedatives, and anxiolytics are to be written by the PCA physician.

Nursing expertise is a key factor in the successful implementation of PCA. The nurse is involved in patient selection, pain assessment, patient teaching, monitoring the effects of therapy, and designing a treatment plan based on the individual patient's responses. The patient should be observed closely, every 15 to 30 minutes, for the first 2 hours of therapy or after prescription changes. Effectiveness of therapy should be evaluated at least every 4 hours. Patients should be asked to rate their pain and the adequacy of pain relief. Pump recordings of the patient's self-administered doses, attempted doses, and the amount delivered can also be used to evaluate analgesic needs.

If a patient's pain is not significantly reduced after 3 to 4 hours of therapy, a full patient assessment is in order. Areas to be checked include patency of the IV site, patient operation of the equipment, proper equipment functioning, presence of abdominal or bladder distension, functioning of drainage tubes, and status of wounds. If the source of continuing pain is not found, the PCA dose should be increased as opposed to reducing the lockout interval.

Regular assessment of bowel and bladder function, hydration status, respiratory function, and mentation are essential to preventing complications. If the patient is having undesirable side effects with no other apparent cause, the PCA dose can be reduced, the lockout interval lengthened, or another drug used.

Naloxone should always be readily available in the nursing unit where potent opioids are administered parenterally. If the patient becomes severely sedated and the respiratory rate falls below 10 per minute, life-threatening respiratory depression may be imminent. The PCA infusion should be immediately discontinued and the physician notified. Naloxone should be prepared for IV administration in increments of 0.1 mg while level of consciousness and respiratory rate are monitored. Doses can be administered every few minutes until the patient is easily arousable. It is important to remember that the duration of action for naloxone is significantly shorter than that of most opioids. Additional doses may need to be administered every 20 minutes.

Clinical Decision Making

Practitioners need to use patient assessment data to guide their decisions regarding medication therapy for pain. Several core questions need to be answered. First, is pain already present? If so, an effort should be made to provide relief as quickly as possible. If the pain is moderate to severe, a parenteral route should be used to administer the analgesic of choice. Intravenous injection provides 100% absorption, the fastest onset of action, and shortest time to peak effect. For example, the time to peak effect is as short as 1 to 5 minutes for IV fentanyl and 10 minutes for IV morphine. If the pain is mild and the patient can take oral medications, oral administration may be used; however, it is important to remember that onset of action and time to peak effect are prolonged, by at least 30 and 60 minutes, respectively, because of the increased drug absorption time.

How severe is the pain, or what is its anticipated severity? If moderate to severe pain is present (or imminent), potent opioid analgesics should be used. If mild pain is present (or anticipated), pharmacologic therapy may begin with NSAIDs or the combinations of an NSAID with a low-potency opioid.

Which route should be used? As stated earlier, if pain already exists, relief should be provided as quickly as possible. In this situation the use of parenteral routes is preferred, with intravenous injection being the quickest. If the pain is expected but not yet present, or has already been controlled by a previous dose of analgesic, oral, transdermal, and parenteral routes can be used.

Nonpharmacologic Interventions

The AHCPR guidelines (Carr et al., 1992) group nonpharmacologic interventions to relieve acute pain into two broad categories: physical and cognitive-behavioral. Physical interventions are externally applied, noninvasive devices, substances, or procedures that are meant to support the injured area, reduce nociceptor stimulation, or interfere with spinal cord transmission of nociceptor impulses. Cognitive-behavioral therapies are actually psychologic interventions that utilize mental and emotional processes to influence the pain experience.

Physical Interventions

Physical interventions include supportive measures to arrest further pathophysiologic pain-producing changes within the injured area, and stimulation to "close the gate" against nociceptive impulses in the dorsal horn.

Supportive measures are used to prevent further stimulation of nociceptors in the injured area. External support can be applied to the painful area. For example, an elastic bandage can be wrapped around a strained ankle, or a folded blanket can be used against an abdominal incision during turning.

Immobilization can be used to minimize tissue and muscle movement in the painful area. Splinting a fracture and the use of bed rest with logrolling for back pain are examples of immobilization to treat pain. Elevating an injured arm on soft pillows and applying ice packs reduces edema formation and prevents further nociceptor stimulation.

Surface stimulation is used to activate large afferent sensory fibers and block dorsal horn transmission of impulses from nociceptors to ascending spinal cord pathways. These interventions are believed to promote pain relief by activation of the gating mechanism described in the gate control theory of pain. Applications of heat and cold, TENS, and massage are examples of surface stimulation techniques (Carr et al., 1992).

TENS

Transcutaneous electrical nerve stimulation (TENS) consists of the selective stimulation of cutaneous mechanoreceptors with low-intensity electrical current applied via skin electrodes. Its origins can be traced to the ancient Egyptians and Romans, who used electric fish to stimulate the skin and relieve pain. Interest in the technique is based on descriptions of the gate control theory of pain (Melzack & Wall, 1965). Dorsal horn input from A-beta afferent fibers has been demonstrated to interfere with afferent transmission of A-delta and C fiber impulses (Wall & Sweet, 1967).

TENS has been used to relieve acute pain associated with surgery and traumatic injuries. In these settings TENS use has been associated with pain relief 60% to 77% of the time (Brown, 1992; Cooperman & Hall, 1977). It can reduce pulmonary complications (Ali, Yaffee, & Serretti, 1982; Hymes, Raab, Yonehiro, Nelson, & Printy, 1973; Sloan, Muwanga, & Waters, 1986); nausea, vomiting, and ileus (Stubbing & Jellico, 1988; Vulpio, 1988); and analgesic use (Cooperman & Hall, 1977; Merrill, 1989). TENS has also been advocated during the early stages of labor with the use of thoracolumbar electrodes (Bundsen, Ericson, Petersen, & Thiringer, 1982) and during painful procedures (Hargreaves & Lander, 1989).

TENS has been shown to provide good though variable relief from acute pain and is very safe (Carr et al., 1992; McCaffery & Beebe, 1989). However, its use during initial periods of acute pain may be limited because at least 30 to 60 minutes is required for initiation of therapy and onset of effect. TENS can be used in conjunction with pharmacologic analgesic therapies (Carr et al.; Solomon, Viernstein, & Long, 1980). Consultation with an expert practitioner knowledgeable in TENS, its mechanism of action, and neuroanatomy is essential to achieving optimal effects (Sjolund & Eriksson, 1985).

To use TENS, three pieces of equipment are needed: a pulse generator or stimulator box, skin electrodes, and cable wires to connect the stimulator box to the electrodes. The stimulator box is small, about the size of a transistor radio, and portable. Reusable carbonized silicone rubber or disposable electrodes can be used and are available in many sizes and shapes.

Several modes of TENS are used: conventional, acupuncture-like, burst, and brief intense (Brown, 1992). The conventional mode of TENS therapy will be the focus of this discussion. The therapy can be used continuously, intermittently, or in a patient-controlled mode (Christoph, 1985).

Before TENS is begun, it should be verified that the patient meets selection criteria and does not have any condition that would contraindicate its use (McCaffery & Beebe, 1989; Sjolund & Eriksson, 1985). In addition to restrictions on electrode placement—they should not be used on the neck or on the abdomen of a pregnant woman (FDA, 1976)—TENS should not be used on patients with implanted cardiac devices (Eriksson, Schuller, & Sjolund, 1978), over open wounds or skin lesions, or for patients with allergies to conductive gels or adhesives (Table 8-4). TENS has been found to interfere with electronic physiologic monitors. Once the patient has been given an explanation of the procedure and agreed to its use, he or she should be instructed on how to use the device.

Electrodes can be placed in the painful area, for example, the site of injury. Incisional electrodes should be placed

Table 8-4 TENS Patient Selection Criteria

TENS Indicated	TENS Contraindicated
Cooperative patient	Cardiac pacemaker
Intact skin	Automatic implantable cardioverter defibrillator
Localized, relatively limited painful area	Skin lesion, rash, or open wound at electrode sites
	Allergy to conductive gel or electrodes
	Use on neck or pregnant woman's abdomen
	Use with electronic physiologic monitors

0.5 to 2 inches away from and on either side of the wound (Brown, 1992; McCaffery & Beebe, 1989). They may also be positioned around invasive device sites (Christoph, 1985). Alternative placements include areas proximal or distal to the painful area, or contralateral over the dermatome that corresponds to the painful area (McCaffery & Beebe).

Electrodes should be applied only over intact skin. The skin should be gently washed with mild soap, rinsed with water, and dried with a nonabrasive towel (Brown, 1992). Reusable electrodes should be evenly covered with a thin layer of conductive gel and secured with hypoallergenic tape. Sterile, self-adhesive, pregelled disposable electrodes are also available for use. Whatever type of electrode is used, the gel must be moist and there must be good contact between the skin and electrode.

Once the electrodes are in place, they are connected to the stimulator by cable wires. Before the stimulator is turned on a number of parameters, such as pulse frequency (rate), pulse duration (width), and current intensity (amplitude), are set. Pulse frequency, measured in hertz, is the number of stimulation cycles delivered per second. The low-frequency range is from 1 to 50 Hz; 50 to 100 Hz is considered high frequency. The lowest effective frequency should be used. Frequencies above 100 Hz have not been found to increase the effectiveness of TENS. Pulse duration, measured in milliseconds, is the length of time each pulse cycle lasts. TENS duration is set between 0.05 and 0.5 ms (Sjolund & Eriksson, 1985). Current intensity, measured in milliamperes, is the strength of the electric stimulation applied to the electrodes. Current intensity for TENS usually ranges from 10 to 60 mA.

To begin therapy using conventional TENS, the pulse stimulator should be set at 80 Hz, 3 to 10 mA, and 100 μs duration (Brown, 1992; Sjolund & Eriksson, 1985). The patient should initially sense a tingling followed by weak paresthesia just below the electrodes. If the sensation is uncomfortable, the amplitude or frequency settings may need to be adjusted. Once paresthesia is attained, the lowest effective frequency is used, and current is gradually increased until either full paresthesia is attained or the maximal current setting of 75 mA is reached.

The unit is left on for 10 to 30 minutes before further adjustments are made (Brown, 1992; Sjolund & Eriksson, 1985). Pain relief should begin within 2 to 20 minutes. If this does not occur, electrode placement should be checked and possibly modified, and settings should be readjusted. TENS can be used continuously, or, depending on the duration of relief after the stimulator is turned off (aftereffect), the stimulator can be turned on and off by the patient as the pain varies in severity.

The most common side effects of TENS are skin irritation and burns. Fewer than 10% of patients can be expected to demonstrate some degree of skin irritation, and burns are extremely rare. Careful attention to skin preparation and electrode application is essential to avoiding these problems. Use of high current and frequency levels can irritate skin. Proper skin preparation and use of conductive gels minimizes skin impedance, allowing use of lower current levels. Skin irritation is also reduced when current delivery is evenly distributed over the surface of the electrode. Even current distribution is achieved by close contact between skin and electrode. When stimulation is used only intermittently, electrodes should be removed between stimulation sessions. Disposable electrodes should be changed at least every 24 hours. A protocol for routine skin inspection and care should be followed. Electrode placement, and possibly the brand of conductive gel or tape, should be changed at the first sign of irritation.

Psychologic Interventions

Psychologic measures activate the power of the brain to alter the pain experience. These techniques are not effective for all patients, however, and should be used as an adjunct to rather than as a substitute for analgesic medications (Carr et al., 1992). (For in-depth information regarding these interventions, see Chapter 5.)

Some methods distract the individual or influence his or her interpretation of the experience. Others may activate descending CNS mechanisms involving endorphins and thereby alter the afferent transmission of nociceptive impulses within the spinal cord. Preprocedural patient teaching, relaxation, and hypnosis are examples of psychologic interventions that have been shown to alter acute pain experiences. Except perhaps for hypnosis, these interventions do not eliminate the pain but may make the pain less distressing and more bearable (McCaffery & Beebe, 1989).

All psychologic interventions require the cooperation and discipline of the patient, as well as a collaborative relationship between practitioner and patient. The effective application of some methods—deep relaxation and hypnosis, for example—requires the services of a practitioner with special training and experience.

Distraction is a technique in which the patient's attention is focused on stimuli other than the pain sensation (McCaffery & Beebe, 1989). The use of this technique is most appropriate for sudden, short-duration (less than 30 minutes) pain episodes. The box on this page lists types of episodic acute pain that are responsive to distraction.

For mild to moderate pain, playing soothing music of the patient's selection may be a useful adjunct to analgesic medications. It may distract the patient or help him or her to relax. Listening to music has been reported to reduce heart rate and improve peripheral issue perfusion in critically ill patients (Guzzetta, 1989).

TYPES OF EPISODIC ACUTE PAIN RESPONSIVE TO DISTRACTION

Waiting for onset of effect of analgesic medication
Changing position
Transfer from bed to stretcher
Removal/insertion of monitoring device or drainage tube
Internal exam (pelvic, sigmoidoscopy, etc.)
Dressing changes

From Carr, D. B., Jacox, A., Chapman, C. R., Ferrell, B., Fields, H. L., Heidrich, G., Hester, N. K., Hill, C. S., Lipman, A. G., McGarvey, C. L., Miaskowski, C., Mulder, D., Payne, R., Schechter, N., Shapiro, B. S., Smith, R. S., Tsou, C. V., Vecchiarelli, L. (1992). *Acute pain management: Operative or medical procedures and trauma. Clinical practice guideline.* AHCPR Pub. No. 92-0032. Rockville, MD: Agency for Health Care Policy and Research, PHS, USDHHS.

TEAM APPROACH

Acute pain is a complex problem whose effective management requires interdisciplinary collaboration by committed professionals. Recently published clinical practice guidelines for acute pain management stress the importance of establishing formal procedures for ensuring adequate pain management (Carr et al., 1992). Interested professionals from all health care disciplines must work together to develop, implement, and evaluate pain management plans. It is best if one provider is given primary responsibility for effective pain relief, but clearly delineated lines of responsibility and communication must be established so that each individual understands his or her role in pain management.

Presentations on pain, its consequences, and its management should be added to professional education programs. Copies of the acute pain management clinical practice guidelines should be made available and used to form the basis of discussions aimed at improving pain management methods. Individuals with special expertise in pain management by virtue of knowledge, experience, or interest should be identified and made available to practitioners around the clock (Carr et al., 1992). Provisions for pain management should be a routine component of admission and discharge procedures. Finally, clinical practice or quality improvement committees should be charged with the responsibility of monitoring pain management, available programs, and their outcomes.

Patients and their family members should be informed that the patient's pain and its effective management is an important part of the treatment plan. They should be informed of available pain relief methods and have their questions concerning them answered. The roles of patients and family members relative to pain management should be explained. Patients should be allowed to indicate their preferences regarding available pain assessment and management methods. Whenever possible, those preferences should be supported by health care providers.

Family members can be particularly helpful in alerting health care providers to problems with the patient's pain management. They can also assist the patient in accepting and making full use of pain management methods such as distraction. In addition to enhancing pain management, involving family members can give them a feeling of purpose and usefulness in an otherwise frustrating situation.

SUMMARY

Acute pain is a problem that patients and nurses will continue to face. A relationship is known to exist between pain and morbidity, and sometimes mortality, in acutely ill and injured patients. Nurses are in a critical position to plan for, preempt, assess, and manage pain. They must use this position to advocate for patients who are experiencing or at risk for acute pain. Figures 8-7 and 8-8 summarize pain management techniques that nurses should use to advocate for patients.

Keeping in mind that not all therapies work for all patients, nurses must be familiar with the wide variety of available pain management techniques and be prepared to recommend and implement them. They must educate patients and their families regarding their role in pain management.

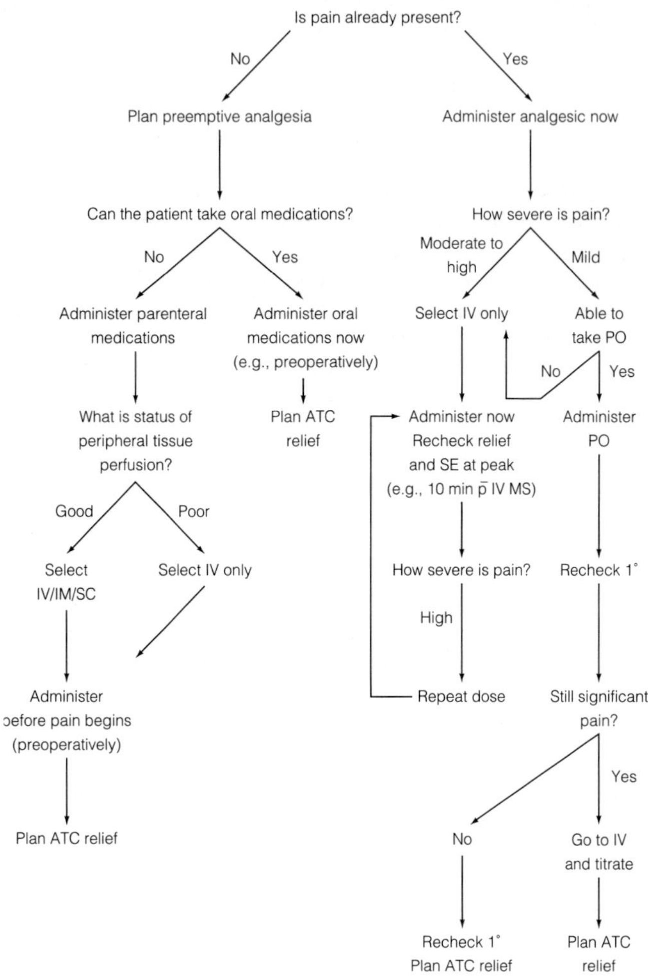

Figure 8-7 Acute pain decision tree. (*ATC,* Around the clock; *IM,* intramuscular; *IV,* intravenous; *MS,* morphine sulfate; *PO,* by mouth; *SC,* subcutaneous; *SE,* side effects.)

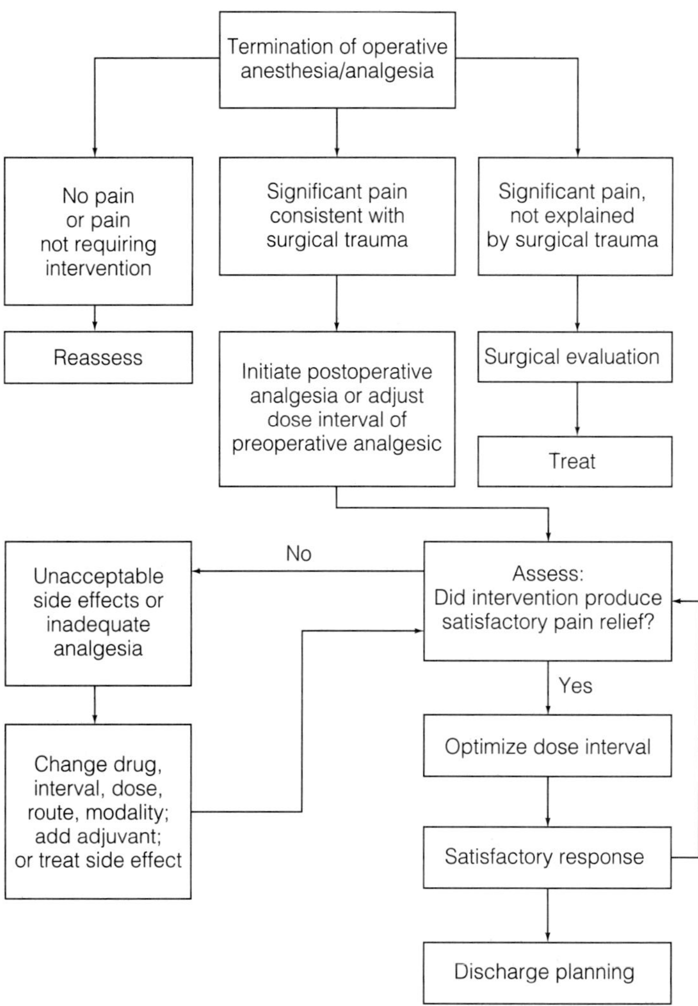

Figure 8-8 Pain treatment flow chart: postoperative phase. (From Carr, D. B., Jacox, A., Chapman, C. R., Ferrell, B., Fields, H. L., Heidrich, G., Hester, N. K., Hill, C. S., Lipman, A. G., McGarvey, C. L., Miaskowski, C., Mulder, D., Payne, R., Schechter, N., Shapiro, B. S., Smith, R. S., Tsou, C. V., Vecchiarelli, L. (1992). *Acute pain management: Operative or medical procedures and trauma. Clinical practice guideline.* AHCPR Pub. No. 92-0032. Rockville, MD: Agency for Health Care Policy and Research, PHS, USDHHS.)

Nurses must also be prepared to work with multidisciplinary groups to develop, implement, and monitor formal programs to improve acute pain management for all patients.

References

Ackerman, M., & Stevens, M. (1989). Acute and chronic pain: Pain dimensions and psychological status. *Journal of Clinical Psychology, 45*(2), 223-228.

Aimone, L. (1992). Neurochemistry and modulation of pain. In R. Sinatra, A. Hord, B. Ginsberg, & L. Preble (Eds.), *Acute pain: Mechanisms and management* (pp. 29-44). St. Louis: Mosby.

Ali, J., Yaffee, C., & Serretti, C. (1981). The effect of transcutaneous electrical nerve stimulation on postoperative pain and pulmonary function. *Surgery, 89,* 507-512.

American Pain Society. (1992). *Principles of analgesic use in the treatment of acute pain and cancer pain* (3rd ed.). Skokie, IL: American Pain Society.

Andrews, I. (1983). Management of postoperative pain. *International Anesthesia Clinics, 21*(1), 31-41.

Armstrong, D., Jepson, J., Keele, C., & Stewart, J. (1957). Pain producing substance in human inflammatory sexudates and plasma. *Journal of Physiology, 135,* 350-370.

Brown, R. (1992). Transcutaneous electrical nerve stimulation for acute and postoperative pain. In R. Sinatra, A. Hord, B. Ginsberg, & L. Preble (Eds.), *Acute pain: Mechanisms and management* (pp. 379-390). St. Louis: Mosby.

Bullit, E. (1989). Induction of c-fos-like protein within the lumbar spinal cord and thalamus of the rat following peripheral stimulation. *Brain Research, 493,* 391-397.

Bundsen, P., Ericson, K., Petersen, L., & Thiringer, K. (1982). Pain relief in labor by transcutaneous electrical nerve stimulation. *Acta Obstetricia et Gynecologica Scandinavica, 62,* 129-136.

Carr, D. B., Jacox, A., Chapman, C. R., Ferrell, B., Fields, H. L., Heidrich, G., Hester, N. K., Hill, C. S., Lipman, A. G., McGarvey, C. L., Miaskowski, C., Mulder, D., Payne, R., Schechter, N., Shapiro, B. S., Smith, R. S., Tsou, C. V., & Vecchiarelli, L. (1992). *Acute pain management: Operative or medical procedures and trauma. Clinical practice guideline.* AHCPR Pub. No. 92-0032. Rockville, MD: Agency for Health Care Policy and Research, PHS, USDHHS.

Chapman, R. (1985). Psychological factors in postoperative pain and their treatment. In G. Smith & B. Covino (Eds.), *Acute pain* (pp. 22-41). London: Butterworths.

Christoph, S. (1985). A comparison of patient-controlled transcutaneous electrical stimulation with traditional analgesics for postoperative pain relief. Unpublished doctoral dissertation, Catholic University of America, Washington, DC.

Collins, J. (1992). Historical overview of pain management: From undermedication to state of the art. In R. Sinatra, A. Hord, B. Ginsberg, & L. Preble (Eds.), *Acute pain: Mechanisms and management* (pp. 1-8). St. Louis: Mosby.

Cooper, D., & Schumann, D. (1979). Postsurgical nursing intervention as an adjunct to wound healing. *Nursing Clinics of North America, 14,* 713-723.

Cooperman, S., & Hall, B. (1977). Use of transcutaneous electrical nerve stimulation in control of postoperative pain: Result of a prospective randomized controlled study. *American Journal of Surgery, 133,* 157-185.

Cousins, M. (1989). Acute and postoperative pain. In P. Wall & R. Melzack (Eds.), *Textbook of pain* (2nd ed., pp. 284-305). Edinburgh: Churchill Livingstone.

Curro, F. (1987). Assessing the physiologic and clinical characteristics of acute versus chronic pain. *Dental Clinics of North America, 31*(4), xiii-xxiii.

Davis, G. (1989a). Measurement of the chronic pain experience: Development of an instrument. *Research in Nursing and Health, 12*(4), 221-227.

Davis, G. (1989b). The clinical assessment of chronic pain in rheumatic disease: Evaluating the use of two instruments. *Journal of Advanced Nursing, 14,* 397-402.

Drain, C., & Cain, R. (1981). The nursing implications of postoperative pain. *Military Medicine, 146,* 127-130.

Edwards, W., & Breed, R. (1990). Treatment of postoperative pain in the post anesthesia care unit. *Anesthesiology Clinics of North America, 8,* 235-265.

Eriksson, M., Schuller, H., & Sjolund, B. (1978). Hazard from transcutaneous nerve stimulation in patients with pacemakers. *Lancet, 1,* 1319.

FDA Advisory Panel on Review of Neurological Devices (1976). *Report on transcutaneous electrical stimulation for pain relief.* Washington, DC: Food and Drug Administration.

Fitzgerald, M. (1990). C-fos and changing the face of pain. *Trends in Neuroscience, 13,* 439-440.

Fordham, M. (1982). The recovery of physical fitness. *International Journal of Nursing Studies, 19,* 205-212.

Fought, S. (1988). Critical care for the multiply injured patient. *Critical Care Nursing Quarterly, 11*(2), 63-69.

Graves, D. A., Foster, R. L., Batenhorst, R. L., Bennett, R., & Baumann, T. (1983). Patient-controlled analgesia. *Annals of Internal Medicine, 99,* 360-366. American College of Physicians.)

Guzzetta, C. (1989). Effects of relaxation and music therapy on patients in a coronary care unit with presumptive acute myocardial infarction. *Heart and Lung, 18*(6), 609-616.

Hargreaves, A., & Lander, J. (1989). Use of transcutaneous nerve stimulation for postoperative pain. *Nursing Research, 38*(3), 159-161.

Harrison, M., & Cotanch, P. (1987). Pain: Advances and issues in critical care. *Nursing Clinics of North America, 22*(3), 691-697.

Hirota, N., Kuraishi, Y., Hino, Y., Sato, Y., Sato, H. M., Takagi, H. (1985). Met-enkephalin and morphine but not dynorphin inhibit the noxious stimuli-induced release of substance P from rabbit dorsal horn in situ. *Neuropharmacology, 24,* 567-570.

Hughes, J. (1983). Postoperative pulmonary care: Past, present and future. *Critical Care Quarterly, 6*(2), 67-71.

Hymes, A., Raab, E., Yonehiro, E., Nelson, G., & Printy, A. (1973). Electrical surface stimulation for control of acute postoperative pain and prevention of ileus. *Surgery Forum, 24,* 447-448.

International Association for the Study of Pain (IASP). (1979). Pain terms: A list with definitions and notes on usage. *Pain, 6,* 249-251.

Jaffe, J., & Martin, W. (1985). Opioid analgesics and antagonists. In A. Gilman & L. Goodman (Eds.), *Goodman and Gilman's pharmacologic basis of therapeutics* (7th ed., pp. 491-531). New York: Macmillan.

Levine, J. (1984). Pain and analgesia: The outlook for more rational treatment. *Annals of Internal Medicine, 100*(1), 269-276.

Masson, A. (1971). The role of analgesic drugs in the treatment of postoperative pain. *British Journal of Anaesthesia, 39,* 713-719.

McCaffery, M. (1987). Patient controlled analgesia: More than a machine. *Nursing 1987, 17,* 62-64.

McCaffery, M., & Beebe, A. (1989). *Pain: Clinical manual for nursing practice.* St Louis: Mosby.

Melzack, R. (1975). The McGill Questionnaire: Major properties and scoring methods. *Pain, 1,* 277-299.

Melzack, R. (1987). The short-form McGill Pain Questionnaire. *Pain, 30,* 191-197.

Melzack, R., & Wall, P. (1965). Pain mechanism: A new theory. *Science, 150,* 971-978.

Mense, S., & Meyer, H. (1981). Bradykinin-induced sensitization of high threshold muscle receptors with slowly conducting afferent fibers. *Pain Supplement, 1,* S204.

Murry, R. (1975). Assessment of psychologic status in the surgical ICU patient. *Nursing Clinics of North America, 10,* 69-81.

Parkhouse, J., Lambrechts, W., & Simpson, B. (1961). The incidence of postoperative pain. *British Journal of Anaesthesia, 33,* 345-352.

Pflugg, A., & Bonica, J. (1977). Physiopathology and control of postoperative pain. *Archives of Surgery, 112,* 773-781.

Portenoy, R. (1992). Clinical application of opioid analgesics. In R. Sinatra, A. Hord, B. Ginsberg, & L. Preble (Eds.), *Acute pain: Mechanisms and management* (pp. 93-101). St. Louis: Mosby.

Porter, J., Jick, H. (1980). Addiction rare in patients treated with narcotics. *New England Journal of Medicine, 302*(2), 123.

Puntillo, K. (1988). The phenomenon of pain and critical care nursing. *Heart and Lung, 17*(3), 262-273.

Puntillo, K. (1991). *Pain in the critically ill: Assessment and management.* Gaithersburg, MD: Aspen.

Rosenthal, S. (1977). Histamine as the chemical mediator for cutaneous pain. *Journal of Investigative Dermatology, 69,* 98-105.

Sabbe, M., & Yaksh, T. (1990). Pharmacology of spinal opioids. *Journal of Pain and Symptom Management, 5,* 191-203.

Schmitt, M. (1977). The nature of pain. *Nursing Clinics of North America, 12,* 621-629.

Sevarino, F., & Preble, L. (1992). *A manual for acute postoperative pain management.* New York: Raven Press.

Sjolund, B., & Eriksson, M. (1985). *Relief of Pain by TENS.* Chichester, England: John Wiley & Sons.

Sloan, J., Muwanga, C., & Waters, E. (1986). Multiple rib fractures: Transcutaneous nerve stimulation versus conventional analgesia. *Journal of Trauma, 26*(12), 1120-1122.

Solomon, R., Viernstein, M., & Long, D. (1980). Reduction of postoperative pain and narcotic use by transcutaneous electrical stimulation. *Surgery, 87,* 142-146.

Stanik-Hutt, J. (1991). Use of patient-controlled analgesia with critically ill patients. *AACN Clinical Issues in Critical Care Nursing, 2*(4), 741-747.

Stanik-Hutt, J. (1993). Strategies for pain management in traumatic thoracic injuries. *Critical Care Nursing Clinics of North America, 5*(4), 713-722.

Stanik-Hutt, J. (1994). Pain experiences of traumatically injured individuals in critical care settings. Unpublished doctoral dissertation, University of Maryland at Baltimore.

Stuart, J., & Pisko, E. (1981). Choline magnesium trisalicylate does not impair platelet aggregation. *Pharmatherapeutica, 2,* 547-551.

Stubbing, J., & Jellico, J. (1988). Transcutaneous electrical nerve stimulation after thoracotomy. *Anesthesia, 43,* 296-298.

Torda, T. (1983). Management of acute and postoperative pain. *International Anesthesia Clinics, 21*(4), 27-41.

Ulmer, J. (1991). Pain, coping, and depression following burn injury. Unpublished doctoral dissertation, University of Maryland at Baltimore.

Vulpio, C. (1988). Transcutaneous electrical stimulation in the prevention of postoperative ileus and pain. *Chirurgia e Patalogia Sperimentale, 36*(1), 3-13.

Wall, P. (1988). The prevention of postoperative pain. *Pain, 33,* 289-290.

Wall, P., & Sweet, W. (1967). Temporary ablation of pain in man. *Science, 55,* 108-109.

Wells, N. (1984). Responses to acute pain and the nursing implications. *Journal of Advanced Nursing, 9,* 51-58.

Wild, L. (1991). Intravenous methods of analgesia for pain in the critically ill. In K. Puntillo (Ed.), *Pain in the critically ill: Assessment and management* (pp. 79-94). Gaithersburg, MD: Aspen.

Woolf, C., & Wall, P. (1986). Morphine sensitive and morphine insensitive actions of C-fibre input on the rat spinal cord. *Neuroscience Letters, 64,* 221-225.

9

Chronic Nonmalignant Pain Management

Mary E. Nossel

Key Points

- Mastery of pain management techniques takes time and practice.
- Untreated pain can lead to anxiety and depression.
- When using adjunct medications start low, go slow.
- Chronic pain has an impact on every aspect of a patient's life and on the family.
- It is imperative that the patient's report of pain be accepted.
- Patients with chronic nonmalignant pain can and do live useful, productive, and fulfilling lives.

This chapter is designed to assist the nurse in caring for patients with chronic nonmalignant pain, who can be some of the most challenging patients that the nurse will ever encounter. Discussed in this chapter are a variety of treatment modalities, both pharmacologic and nonpharmacologic, that the nurse can employ to help these patients. The discussion is not intended to make anyone an expert in chronic pain management. It is meant to help the nurse who is confronted in any clinical situation with a patient with chronic nonmalignant pain by providing guidelines, some structure, and an awareness that this patient can be helped.

In working with a patient with chronic nonmalignant pain (CNMP) it is most important to always believe what the patient says about the pain. Pain is entirely a subjective experience; no one can ever feel exactly what another person is feeling. Any time a nurse, physician, or other caregiver doubts a patient's report of pain or tries to establish that the patient is in less pain than reported, he or she has destroyed any hope of a treatment alliance with the patient and has set up an antagonistic situation that is doomed to failure.

A basic assumption throughout this chapter is that the patient has been thoroughly evaluated by experts in neurology, neurosurgery, regional anesthesia, or other pertinent medical specialty and that there is no direct curative procedure that is likely to help the patient.

DESCRIPTION

A variety of conditions can produce CNMP. A patient may suffer from chronic low back pain, chronic neck pain, peripheral neuropathy, postherpetic neuralgia, reflex sympathetic dystrophy, or headaches.

By far the most common type of CNMP is low back pain. (The Agency for Health Care Policy and Research has published a clinical practice guideline on acute low back problems in adults [Bigos et al., 1994].) This usually is the result of some work-related mishap or automobile accident, but it can occur under other circumstances. In many cases the patient undergoes two, three, or many more surgical procedures with no reduction in the pain. The injury or surgery may have led to arachnoiditis (scarring of the arachnoid layer of the meninges with matting and clumping of nerves) or other forms of scarring in the spine, and additional surgery may only create further scarring.

Patients with low back pain often develop very unusual body postures and gaits and have markedly deconditioned paravertebral muscles that are prone to spasm and pain. Any of these problems can produce CNMP.

Neck pain related to cervical spine disease is probably the next most common CNMP problem. As with low back pain, the problem usually begins with a job-related injury or motor vehicle accident. The underlying pathology can be disk disease, arthritis, or paracervical muscle strain. Like those with low back pain, most of these patients have undergone more than one unsuccessful surgical procedure, and further surgery is not indicated.

Peripheral or polyneuropathy can also lead to CNMP. Disorders such as alcoholism or diabetes are the most frequent cause, but other causes, such as neoplasm medications, should also be considered. The pain is often symmetrical and distal, affecting the feet and hands. It is described as a constant burning or aching sensation with superimposed paroxysmal jabs of pain. Allodynia and hyperalgesia may also be present (Maciewicz, Bouckoms, & Martin, 1985).

Another source of CNMP is postherpetic neuralgia (PHN). This condition occurs in some people after an episode of herpes zoster. These people develop severe pain in the area affected by the zoster virus. About 10% of people affected with herpes zoster develop PHN. The pain is characterized by a constant burning and aching with superimposed shooting, lancinating pain, and yet the skin may be hypesthetic and hypoalgesic and may even be analgesic. Dysesthesias and paresthesias may also accompany the pain (Loesser, 1990).

What has recently become a very controversial type of CNMP and a focus for much research and debate is a condition called reflex sympathetic dystrophy (RSD). Classically patients with RSD experience burning pain and tenderness, allodynia and hyperpathia, swelling with or without pitting edema, dystrophic skin and nail changes, hyperhidrosis, and vasomotor changes of color and temperature. Typically patients complain of pain in a distal extremity that may develop suddenly and insidiously and does not follow a dermatomal or myotomal distribution. (See Chapter 15 for further information.)

Headache is another condition that can present as CNMP. Although most people experience an occasional headache that is either self-limiting or relieved by mild analgesics, some patients suffer from a form of constant daily headache or severe, debilitating, recurrent headaches. Headaches have been classified into 13 types. This classification includes migraines, tension-type headaches, temperomandibular headaches and chronic substance abuse headaches. These headaches most likely result from a complex interplay of neurobiologic and behavioral processes, and thus treatment must be directed toward both the mind and the body (Schoenen & Maertens de Noordhaut, 1994).

ASSESSMENT

The components of a thorough pain assessment were discussed in Chapter 1. This section will focus on parts of the assessment process that are most important for patients with

CNMP. As with other kinds of pain, the location, pattern of radiation, character or quality (what it feels like), and duration are very important, but there are other aspects of assessment that need special attention for CNMP.

The most obvious aspects are aggravating and alleviating factors. Asking a patient with CNMP what makes the pain better or worse can be both part of the assessment and part of the intervention. Sometimes the process of asking about what reduces the pain helps the patient to remember and clarify comfort measures that have not been utilized for some time. For the nurse, knowing what the patient already considers helpful is the best place to begin in planning care. This information can provide a firm foundation for other pain management strategies.

The Holistic Approach

In caring for a patient with CNMP, in addition to acquiring data about the pain itself, it is very important to find out how the pain has affected the patient's life. The nurse should ask the patient about work, family, and leisure activities. For most patients the nurse will discover that the pain has had a profound impact on all areas. Most patients who seek treatment for CNMP are either no longer able to work because of their pain, work part-time only, or have had to change jobs. This change in employment almost always results in a long-term loss of income, a major change in lifestyle, and a subsequent decrease in self-esteem and feelings of diminished self-worth (Sullivan, Turner, & Romano, 1991).

Patients who request treatment for CNMP also frequently experience difficulties in their family situations. They may have marital difficulties and problems managing the children. Some single patients move back in with their parents, and this situation can generate many other problems, including a major financial drain on aging parents with a fixed income.

Patients with CNMP often find that they no longer enjoy activities that previously brought pleasure in their leisure time. They may have trouble sitting long enough to see a movie or play or even to go out to dinner. Their behavior and their pain-focused conversations can be difficult for friends and acquaintances to understand. These friends may begin to call less and less, leaving patients isolated. Those whose leisure activities once involved a good deal of activity, such as hunting, hiking, or sports, have a very difficult time once they are no longer able to engage in these activities. The nurse must examine all of these aspects of a person's life when working with a patient with CNMP.

After completing this part of the assessment, the nurse should try to identify the patient's interests and strengths, as well as coping strategies and problem-solving abilities. Identifying these attributes is essential for planning care. In many clinical settings, the nurse will not have the time or the resources to address these difficulties directly. What the nurse can do is help the patient sort out some of these problems and begin to work on those that are less complex. The nurse can also make appropriate referrals to resources such as vocational rehabilitation, family counseling, or individual counseling. Merely identifying the problem and reassuring the patient that his or her problems are very similar to those of many others with chronic pain can help to normalize the experience and make it less stressful.

The Role of Depression

Depression is often associated with CNMP, and many patients with major depression report multiple pain complaints (Romano & Turner, 1985). Blumer and Heilbronn (1981) posited that pain in the absence of organic pathology should be considered a depressive disorder (Romano & Turner). On the other hand, Pilowsky, Chapman, and Bonica (1977) reported that depression occurred in only a small subset of pain patients (Romano & Turner). A more recent study by Doan and Wadden (1989) showed that 66% of the patients were classified as mildly to severely depressed based on scores on the Beck Depression Inventory. The researchers noted that patients with CNMP who were also depressed were more functionally impaired, were more preoccupied with physical problems, were more irritable, used more sensory descriptors, and were more negative about their ability to cope. In addition, they noted that depression left untreated was strongly associated with poor results from other treatment modalities, including opiates (Doan & Wadden; Bouckoms et al., 1991). Treatment of depression in CNMP patients with antidepressants and psychotherapy improved not only mood, but sleep and pain frequency and severity (Sullivan, Ressor, Mikail, & Fisher, 1992). The nursing assessment of patients with CNMP must therefore include an assessment of mood and mood-related symptoms (see the box below).

SYMPTOMS OF DEPRESSION

1. Depressed mood most of the day, nearly every day as indicated by subjective report (e.g., feels sad or empty) or observation made by others (e.g., appears tearful).
2. Markedly diminished interest or pleasure in all or almost all activities most of the day nearly every day (as indicated by either subjective account or observations made by others).
3. Significant weight loss when not dieting, or weight gain, or decrease or increase in appetite nearly every day.
4. Insomnia or hypersomnia nearly every day.
5. Psychomotor retardation or agitation nearly every day (observable by others, not just subjective feelings of restlessness or being slowed down).
6. Fatigue or loss of energy nearly every day.
7. Feelings of worthlessness or excessive or inappropriate guilt nearly every day.
8. Diminished ability to think or concentrate, or indecisiveness nearly every day.
9. Recurrent thoughts of death, recurrent suicidal ideation without a specific plan, or a suicide attempt or a specific plan for committing suicide.

From American Psychiatric Association. (1994). *Diagnostic and statistical manual of mental disorders* (4th ed.). Washington, DC: APA.

Patients with CNMP may be very reluctant to accept the diagnosis of depression and tend to attribute all of their distress to the pain. In interactions with patients, approaching the depression as an effect of the pain can often facilitate the assessment process and the therapeutic relationship (Sullivan et al., 1991). After a thorough holistic assessment, interventions are planned.

INTERVENTIONS

Pharmacologic

This section will discuss some of the medications available to help patients with CNMP. Included in the discussion are tricyclic antidepressants (TCAs), selective serotonin reuptake inhibitors (SSRIs), anticonvulsants, and opiates. All of these medications can be used safely by elderly patients but require special caution. Elderly patients usually require a very low initial dose compared with younger patients, and medications must be advanced in smaller increments at a slower rate. Doses of nortriptyline, for example, of 5 mg at bedtime are not uncommon.

Tricyclic Antidepressants

First-line medications for patients with CNMP are the TCAs. These drugs are ideal because they have properties that address the depressive aspect of the problem and they also have a direct effect on the pain (Max et al., 1991). Nortriptyline, the active metabolite of amitriptyline, has limited side effects and is usually preferred. Imipramine and desipramine are also available and used frequently. Failure of one TCA does not imply failure of another. In addition to treating both the pain and the depression, TCAs are to varying degrees sedating and most helpful in promoting restful sleep.

The side effects that most patients find annoying are a dry mouth, constipation, and a "hung over" feeling in the morning. The "hung over" feeling appears to be dose related and dissipates as the patient reaches a steady-state blood level. The dry mouth and constipation usually improve a little but can remain as a minor annoyance. Patients should also be observed for postural hypotension when being started on a TCA and for dysrhythmias, although the latter effect is uncommon (AHFS, 1994).

When starting a patient on a TCA, the initial dose should be very low. Patients usually experience side effects before any therapeutic effect of the drug is noted. Therefore it is important to minimize the side effects as much as possible. Using small initial doses and increasing the dose in small, graded increments is a good way to keep side effects to a minimum. It is very unfortunate when a patient refuses a drug because of side effects that could have been prevented by proper dosing; the patient may not be willing to take a medication that might have been very helpful. One other factor that makes TCAs excellent first-line medications is that effective therapeutic blood levels can be determined (*AMA Drug Evaluations*, 1991).

Anticonvulsants

Next to be considered are the anticonvulsants phenytoin, carbamazepine, and valproic acid. The anticonvulsant drugs are especially helpful for patients suffering from the sharp, lancinating pain that occurs in conditions such as trigeminal neuralgia and postherpetic neuralgia, and the paresthetic pain that may occur in peripheral neuropathies (Maciewicz et al., 1985). As with the TCAs, the initial dose should be quite low, and the titration process should go very slowly. A starting dose of carbamazepine can be as low as 50 mg qhs for an elderly person or 100 mg qhs for younger patients. Also as with the TCAs, patients may experience side effects before they experience any therapeutic effect. The nurse must maintain a positive attitude and provide encouragement, support, and thorough medication teaching when therapy is begun. Blood levels should be checked periodically, and the goal should be either pain relief or a level within the therapeutic range.

SSRIs

A new group of excellent antidepressants are the selective serotonin reuptake inhibitors (SSRIs). This group includes fluoxetine, sertraline, and paroxetine. If a patient is unresponsive to a TCA or has intolerable side effects, the SSRIs should be utilized, especially if the patient is depressed. As noted earlier, treating the depression is a vital component of chronic pain treatment. When using a TCA in combination with an SSRI, the dose of the TCA should be lowered and the level checked frequently until steady state is achieved. SSRIs will raise the serum level of TCAs, sometimes quite dramatically (AHFS, 1994).

There is a new antidepressant available called venlafaxine. This drug has properties of both SSRIs and TCAs. Insufficient data are available to determine whether this drug will provide pain relief for patients with CNMP, but clinical use has shown it to be quite effective as an antidepressant (PDR, 1995).

Opiates

In the recent past the use of opiates for CNMP was rejected because of the fear of iatrogenic addiction and perceived risks of opioid-induced toxicity, physical dependence, and tolerance (Portnoy, 1990). Evidence (Portnoy) suggests that some patients with CNMP can be maintained on opiates long term without developing significant toxicity or abuse. Use of these medications must be carefully considered, however, on a patient-by-patient basis. Factors to consider are listed in the box on p. 283. Only after careful consideration of all of these factors can a responsible decision be made.

Nonpharmacologic

Distraction

Many patients with CNMP become socially isolated, give up hobbies, lose interest in formerly pleasurable activities, and become almost completely inactive. They become

FACTORS TO CONSIDER IN USING OPIATES

1. Has the patient been adequately treated with and failed to respond to other pharmacologic interventions?
2. Does the patient suffer from a depression that has not been adequately treated?
3. Does the patient have a past history of alcohol or drug abuse?
4. Does the patient have a strong family history of alcohol or drug abuse?
5. How reliable and compliant has the patient been throughout the treatment process?
6. What kind of monitoring and follow-up care is available?
7. Is the patient willing to be placed on a medicine long term, knowing the potential of physical dependence?

preoccupied with ways to diminish discomfort and invest most of their energy each day in avoiding pain and monitoring their pain level. They believe that this is necessary to achieve an acceptable level of comfort. In fact, the more the patient focuses on pain, the more intrusive and impairing it becomes. At many pain treatment centers patients are required to be up and dressed in the morning, and to participate in a full schedule each day. Throughout their hospital stay patients are encouraged to develop concrete plans for structuring their time at home and to continue diversional activity after discharge.

As old interests are renewed or new interests developed, patients often find it difficult to concentrate on the interest and the pain at the same time. They find that while engaged in an activity, they weren't noticing their pain to the same degree as when not engaged in that activity. Distraction can provide sensory input that promotes inhibition of the pain from the brainstem (McCaffery & Beebe, 1989). The nurse can point out to patients that while they were involved in a certain activity, they may have moved with less guarding or their facial expression was more relaxed, and they were interacting in a more relaxed and spontaneous manner. The nurse can then ask about the pain level during this activity to help patients make the connection between involvement in some distracting activity and diminished pain level.

It is also important for the nurse to help patients identify activities they enjoy and to encourage them to try new things. Many patients will be reluctant to try something new or will resist an old activity out of fear of exacerbating the pain. Helping patients to talk about their fears and then helping them find ways to mitigate the real difficulties and to dispel the groundless fears is another important contribution to patients with CNMP. Simply encouraging someone to go to the movies is clearly not enough. It is important to help the patient determine how to get there, the timing (i.e., don't make yourself rush), where to sit, who goes along, who gets the popcorn, and perhaps even what to see. These plans can be quite daunting to a patient who is preoccupied with the immediate pain perception and frightened about anything that may possibly increase the pain. Going through these planning steps with the nurse is a good way for the patient to realize that an outing may really be possible.

It is important to remember and remind others that even though the distraction is helpful, it does not mean that the patient's pain is not severe. Distraction temporarily raises the pain threshold, enabling the patient to turn attention to something other than the pain.

Exercise

Mention exercise to a patient with CNMP and you are likely to receive a barrage of negative retorts. Be persistent! Exercise provides a variety of benefits to a patient with CNMP. An exercise program that includes general conditioning provides patients with a general feeling of improving health as they see their stamina and endurance increase and as they realize that they actually can be active. In addition, general aerobic conditioning exercises promote the production of endorphins, the body's own pain relievers. Along with general conditioning, an exercise program also should include strengthening and stretching. Muscles that are strong and flexible are less likely to be sore or to develop painful spasms. As patients see their ability to participate in an exercise program improve, they begin to regain the confidence in their body and its functioning that they had lost because of their persistent pain.

When a patient begins a new exercise program, consideration of other underlying medical problems such as cardiovascular disease is essential. This is especially true for elderly patients. Many of these patients have been sedentary for a long time and may believe that because they are older exercise is no longer needed or that it might even be dangerous. After careful assessment of a patient's general medical condition has confirmed that it is safe for the elderly patient to begin an exercise program, encouragement should be provided.

Heat and Cold

Heat and cold are often used along with other therapies in the treatment of CNMP involving the musculoskeletal system. Either one may be used to reduce painful muscle spasms or provide a counterirritant effect (Lehman & de Lateur, 1994). The muscle relaxation effect is especially helpful in interrupting the vicious cycle of muscle spasm, ischemia, pain, and more muscle spasm (Lehman & de Lateur). Unfortunately, the effect of heat or cold on spasticity is not permanent; however, even temporary relief is welcome to the patient with CNMP. Chapter 5 discusses the physiologic effects of heat and cold.

Relaxation

Relaxation exercises are utilized by a wide variety of practitioners to treat an even wider variety of difficulties. Relaxation techniques have been shown to be helpful in the treatment of anxiety disorder, headache, insomnia, baruxism, Raynaud's disease, and the management of acute and chronic pain regardless of its etiology (Schwartz et al., 1987). Most patients with CNMP find very early that their pain is worse when they are in a stressful situation. Learning relaxation exercises is one way to abort the exacerbation of CNMP caused by an increase in stress. Chapter 5 discusses relaxation in depth.

Learning to achieve this relaxed state can be very difficult. Biofeedback equipment can provide very useful data to a patient who is just beginning to learn relaxation techniques. The external signals provide tangible cues that can be used until internal cues and feeling states can be recognized. After a person has mastered the relaxation technique using biofeedback, the equipment can be left behind and the technique can be used any time, anywhere.

TENS

Transcutaneous electrical nerve stimulation (TENS) is a process in which a low-voltage electrical pulse is directed through the skin via electrodes placed on the skin. This electrical pulse is believed to stimulate nerve fibers in the peripheral nervous systems in a nonpainful way and thus interfere with the conduction of painful stimuli to the brain (Mannheimer & Lampe, 1988). The degree to which TENS can be helpful is often dependent on how much professional supervision and encouragement can be provided to the patient in the use of the TENS unit. Chapter 8 contains an in-depth discussion of the indications, placement, and patient teaching required with TENS.

Medication Misuse

Another issue that may face nurses caring for patients with CNMP is medication misuse. These patients may be taking extraordinary amounts of opiates or benzodiazepines. They may be intoxicated from these medications, cognitively impaired, physically deactivated, and complaining of severe, debilitating pain. Cognitive difficulties related to the overuse of the medications may cause difficulty in remembering when or how much of the medicine was taken, so that the condition continues to reinforce itself and worsen. Before an accurate assessment of the pain and its impact on the patient's life can be performed, it is essential that the patient be free of these medicines.

An attempt should be made to determine an accurate estimation of the patient's daily dose of opiate or benzodiazepine. The patient should be stabilized on this dose, and then the dose should be gradually tapered to zero. Only after the patient has been detoxified can an adequate assessment of pain be made, and only then should trials of other medications begin.

Clinical experiences in this regard have provided some interesting outcomes. Frequently the patient will report much less pain after the detoxification process is complete and will feel much more able to manage the remaining pain. Outpatient detoxification is very difficult to accomplish, especially with patients who suffer with CNMP. Regular detoxification centers commonly fail to consider the patient's pain as a factor, and the detoxification is frequently abrupt. Therefore an inpatient chronic pain treatment center is the best place to accomplish detoxification for patients with CNMP. This setting can provide the needed support during the detoxification process. In addition, the patient can learn new ways to manage pain and see others who have been in treatment and are improving. This helps the patient persevere and increase the chances for success.

Team Approach

The treatment of patients with CNMP requires a number of different professions working in concert. Physicians in regional anesthesia and neurosurgery are most helpful in the early stages of diagnosis and treatment. Psychiatrists are very helpful in the diagnosis and management of depression and in the use of antidepressant medication. Psychologists, social workers, and psychiatric nurse clinical specialists are invaluable in providing individual and family psychotherapy to help patients and their families cope with chronic pain. Physical therapists are needed to develop and supervise appropriate exercise programs, and occupational therapists are important in helping patients learn appropriate body mechanics,

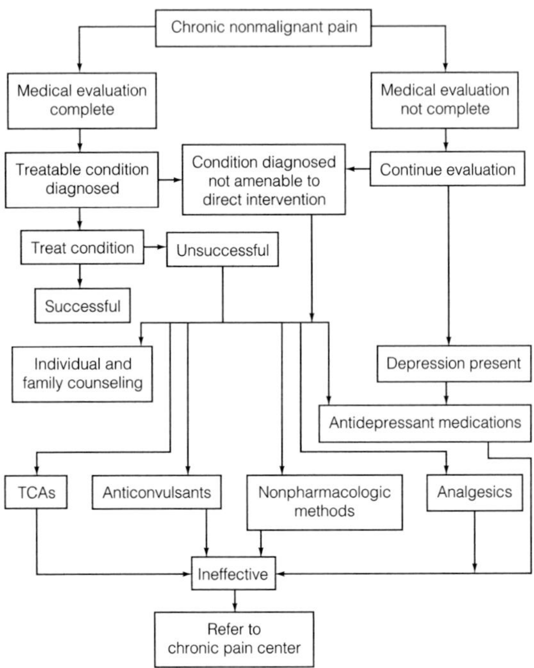

Figure 9-1 Chronic nonmalignant pain algorithm.

learn how to structure time, develop goals, and identify ways to accomplish these goals. Crucial in this team approach, the nurse coordinates and assists team members. The nurse identifies the patient's needs, makes the appropriate referrals, and supports and encourages the patient during treatment. It is the nurse who improves communication among the other team members and with the patient. It is the nurse who reinforces teaching and ensures patient understanding of the treatment plan and who evaluates the effectiveness of each component of the plan. CNMP requires a team approach, and the nurse is an integral part of that team (see Figure 9-1).

OUTCOME

In working with a patient with CNMP, the decision of how to define a successful outcome is very individualized. For some patients it may mean a return to work; for others it may mean the ability to be up and about for more hours than are spent in bed. The nurse must remain aware of this range of what is considered successful. It is important to include the patient in this process and not arbitrarily set goals for the patient. The nurse must also keep in mind that the patient may need help in establishing goals that are realistic and attainable. Very often the patient will identify the primary goal as being pain free. Except for rare instances the achievement of a pain-free state is not possible for patients with CNMP. Patients need help in adjusting to the reality that this is not an achievable goal and help in modifying this goal to one that is realistic. On the other hand, a patient may have been suffering for so long that he or she sets goals that are clearly less than can be achieved, and it is up to the nurse to help the patient see that things can be better than the patient can presently imagine.

Goals and outcome measures can be subjective—for example, "My mood will be better" or "I will feel like my old self." These goals can be somewhat objectified through the use of rating scales, such as visual analog scales, and patients can state that they want to achieve a pain level of 5 or less on a 0 to 10 scale. These measures are still subjective but are an attempt at objectivity. More objective goals are also possible. Patients can state that they want to be able to sit for 1 hour or walk 100 feet without resting. Objective goals such as these can be included in establishing outcome criteria for each patient.

General outcome goals focus more on the patient's developing a working knowledge of the variety of techniques available for the management of pain. Most of these methods take practice, and their helpfulness to the patient should improve over time. Nurses in inpatient settings are likely to have an opportunity only to introduce a patient to these methods, whereas nurses in home care or other outpatient situations will have an opportunity to help patients master these techniques.

SUMMARY

This chapter has presented an armamentarium of both pharmacologic and nonpharmacologic methods to help the patient with CNMP. Although CNMP can be very challenging, perhaps daunting, it is not hopeless. Many patients use some or all of these treatment modalities and live full and active lives. The nurse caring for these patients should always try to convey an attitude of hope and a conviction that the pain can be effectively managed. Using the tools described here, the nurse can be very effective in helping patients with CNMP.

References

AHFS. (1994). *American Hospital Formulary Service drug information '94,* Bethesda, MD: American Society of Hospital Pharmacists.

AMA drug evaluations. (1991). Milwaukee: American Medical Association.

American Psychiatric Association. (1994). *Diagnostic and statistical manual of mental disorders* (4th ed.). Washington, DC: APA.

Bigos, S. T., Bowyer, O. R., Braen, G. R., Brown, K. C., Deyo, R. A., Haldeman, S., Hart, J. L., Johnson, E. W., Keller, R. B., Kido, D. K., Liang, M. H., Nelson, R. M., Nordin, M., Owen, B. D., Pope, M. H., Schwartz, R. K., Stewart, D. H., Susman, J. L., Triano, J. J., Tripp, L., Turk, D., Watts, C., & Weinstein, J. (1994). *Acute low back problems in adults. Clinical practice guideline no. 14.* AHCPR Pub. No. 95-0642. Rockville, MD: Agency for Health Care Policy and Research, PHS, USDHHS.

Blumer, D., & Heibronm, M. (1981). The pain-prone disorder: A clinical and psychological profile. *Psychosomatics, 22,* 395-402.

Bouckoms, A. J., Prakash, M., Murray, G. B., Cassem, E. H., Stern, T. A., & Tesar, G. E. (1992). Chronic nonmalignant pain treated with long-term oral narcotic analgesics. *Annals of Clinical Psychiatry, 4*(3), 185-191.

Doan, B. D., & Wadden, N. P. (1989). Relationships between depressive symptoms and descriptions of chronic pain. *Pain, 36,* 75-84.

Lehman, J. F., & de Lateur, B. J. (1994). The application of heat and cold. In P. D. Wall & R. Melzack (Eds.), *Textbook of pain* (3rd ed.). New York: Churchill Livingstone.

Loesser, J. D. (1990). *Management of pain* (2nd ed.). New York: Raven Press.

Maciewicz, R., Bouckoms, A., & Martin, J. B. (1985). Drug therapy of neuropathic pain. *Clinical Journal of Pain, 1,* 39-49.

Mannheimer, J. S., & Lampe, N. (1988). *Clinical transcutaneous electrical nerve stimulation.* Philadelphia: Davis.

Max, M. B., Kishare-Kumar, R., Schafer, S. C., Meister, B., Gracely, R. H., Smoller, B., & Dubner, R. (1991). A randomized controlled trial of desipramine in painful diabetic neuropathy. *Pain, 1,* 3-10.

McCaffery, M., & Beebe, A. (1989). *Pain: Clinical manual for nursing practice.* St. Louis: Mosby.

PDR. (1995). *Physician's Desk Reference* (49th ed.). Montvale NJ: Medical Economics, pp. 2264-2667.

Pilowsky, I., Chapman, C. R., & Bonica, J. J. (1977). Pain, depression and illness behavior in a pain clinic population. *Pain, 4,* 183-192.

Portnoy, R. S. (1990). Chronic opioid therapy in nonmalignant pain. *Journal of Pain Management, 5,* 546-562.

Romano, J. M., & Turner, J. A. (1985). Chronic pain and depression: Does the evidence support a relationship? *Psychological Bulletin, 97,* 18-34.

Schoenen, J., & Maertens de Noordhout, S. (1994). Headaches. In P. Wall & R. Melzack (Eds.), *Textbook of pain.* New York: Churchill Livingstone.

Schwartz, M., et al. (1987). *Biofeedback.* New York: Guilford Press.

Sullivan, M. J. L., Ressor, K., Mikail, S., & Fisher, R. (1992). Treatment of depression in chronic low back pain: Review and recommendations. *Pain, 50,* 5-13.

Sullivan, M. D., Turner, J. A., & Romano, J. (1991). Chronic pain in primary care: Identification and management of psychosocial factors. *Journal of Family Practice, 32*(2), 193-199.

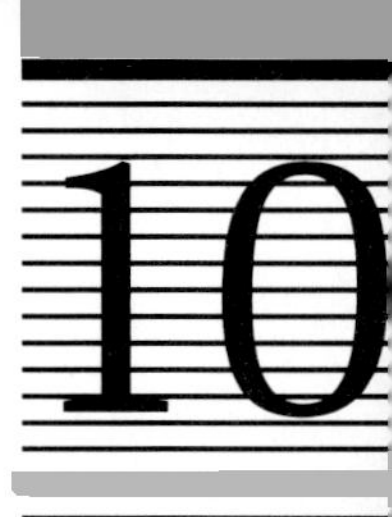

Cancer Pain Management

Barry Kinzbrunner

Janet Pate McGough

- Administer Analgesics on a Regular Basis after Initial Titration
- Use Drug Combinations Appropriately
  - Treatment of Specific Pains
    - Bone Pain
    - Neuropathic Pain
    - Depression and Mood
    - Gastrointestinal Pain Syndromes
- Watch for the Development of Tolerance
- Prevent Acute Withdrawal
- Do Not Use Placebos to Assess the Nature of Pain
- Anticipate and Treat Complications and Side Effects

Nonpharmacologic Interventions

- Physical Medicine
- Behavior Modification
- Anesthetic and Neurosurgical Techniques
- Radiotherapy
- Chemotherapy and Hormonal Therapy

Summary

Key Points

- Pain is the most common and most feared symptom of patients with cancer.
- Identification of the cause(s) of the pain is necessary to maximize patient comfort.
- Expertise in agonist-antagonist as well as adjunctive medications is required of health care providers caring for individuals with cancer.
- The expectation must exist that pain can be controlled.

Pain is the most common and most feared symptom of patients with cancer. It has been shown that 30% to 50% of patients receiving active cancer treatment and 60% to 80% of patients with advanced cancer will suffer from significant pain (Elliott & Elliott, 1991). Despite evidence that for 90% or more of the patients with cancer the pain should be controllable (Teoh & Stjernsward, 1992), recent studies suggest that between 50% and 75% of these patients will not receive adequate treatment of their pain (Bonica, 1990; Cleeland et al., 1994; Von Roenn, Cleeland, Gonin, Hatfield, & Pandya, 1993).

During the early 1990s the inadequate treatment of cancer pain became a major public health issue. In a recent malpractice action a health care provider was held liable for failing to provide adequate pain relief for a patient (Shapiro, 1994). It is the physician's responsibility to order adequate pain medication, and the nurse caring for the patient has the responsibility of assessing the pain experienced and being knowledgeable of available drugs, their side effects, and the administration of pain medication. The results of a survey (Hamilton & Edgar, 1992) of 318 nurses concerning their knowledge of pain control indicated that nurses tended to be most knowledgeable in identification of drugs. Their knowledge regarding addiction, ceiling effect, respiratory depression, and other factors was generally weak. The debate over the legalization of physician-assisted suicide appears to be motivated by the fear of patients and loved ones of the prospect of dying in uncontrolled pain. This fear underlines the need for expertise in pain management for the terminally ill patient. This chapter will discuss principles underlying the pain management techniques required for the care of the cancer patient population.

CAUSES OF CANCER PAIN

As illustrated in Table 10-1, pain that occurs in cancer patients may be secondary to the cancer (70%), may be related to the cancer treatment (15% to 20%), or may be unrelated to

Table 10-1 Causes of Cancer Pain

Source	Cause of Pain
Tumor (70%)	Release of pain-causing substances produced by the tumor or by the immune system in response to the presence of tumor Invasion of tumor into bone, nerves, viscera, blood vessels, mucous membranes, soft tissue
Treatment (15%-20%)	Surgery: acute postoperative pain, chronic pain syndromes (postthoracotomy, postmastectomy, phantom limb) Chemotherapy: extravasation, phlebitis, mucositis, neuropathy, diarrhea, constipation, aseptic bone necrosis Radiation therapy: skin desquamation, mucositis, diarrhea, implants, gastric ulcer, fat necrosis, fibrosis, myelopathy, nerve plexopathy, osteoradionecrosis Biotherapy: myalgia/arthralgia, neuropathy Miscellaneous: insertion of central lines, infection
Diagnostic tests	Biopsies Invasive radiologic procedures Venipuncture Positioning on hard table
Nursing care	Injections Venipuncture Dressing changes Movement of painful body parts
Comorbid conditions (10%-15%)	Diabetic neuropathy Low back pain Headache Arthritis Decubitus Muscle spasm/cramps Peripheral vascular disease Postherpetic neuralgia Prolonged immobility

From Gross, J., Johnson, B.: *Handbook of Oncology Nursing,* second edition. ©1994. Boston: Jones and Bartlett Publishers. Reprinted with permission.

the cancer or its treatment (10% to 15%) (Foley, 1985; Gross & Johnson, 1994; Supportive Care, 1994).

One must attempt to determine the causes of pain—whether related to the malignancy, secondary to treatment, or unrelated to the illness—based on subjective and objective data. In some instances no physiologic cause can be offered to explain the patient's pain; nonetheless it does not mean there is no physiologic basis for the pain. Following is a discussion of the more common etiologies of pain seen in cancer patients based on the predominant location of the symptoms.

Bone Metastasis and Other Causes of Bone Pain

Bone metastases are most typically observed in cancers of the breast, prostate, and lung and in multiple myeloma. Involvement of the bone may be seen in other malignancies as well. Pain is the most common symptom, occurring in about 75% of patients with bone metastasis, and because bone invasion is usually multifocal, patients will often complain of pain in multiple sites. The pain is predominantly somatic in nature, caused by direct invasion of bone, and is described as dull and aching. Pain caused by bone metastasis is often exacerbated by movement or weight bearing (Jacox et al., 1994).

A serious complication of bone metastasis is spinal cord compression, usually occurring secondary to extension of metastasis from vertebral bodies into the spinal canal. Back pain is the most common symptom and may occur weeks before any frank neurologic deficits are found. Often patients complain of a shooting pain in a radicular distribution caused by compression of nerve roots exiting the affected vertebral body. Signs of frank spinal cord compression may include motor and sensory deficits, as well as bladder and bowel dysfunction. Failure to diagnose and treat spinal cord compression can result in complete loss of neurologic function below the level of the lesion. This finding must be approached as a medical emergency. Treatment consists of analgesics, steroids, radiotherapy, and occasionally surgery (Jacox et al., 1994).

Special attention must be paid to patients who complain of pain in weight-bearing bones. Early diagnosis and treatment of metastatic lesions of these bones will reduce the risk of pathologic fracture.

It is important to remember that nonmalignant causes of bone and joint pain, such as arthritis and bursitis, must be considered in evaluating patients with metastatic cancer. These conditions may be present along with documented bone metastasis.

Headache

Patients with metastatic cancer may develop headache, which may be secondary to skull metastasis or brain metastasis. Metastasis to the skull should be considered whenever a patient has headache associated with changes in ocular movement and vision, painful head and neck movement, and difficulty with chewing or tongue movement. Symptoms associated with increased intracranial pressure from brain metastasis include emesis with minimal or no nausea, change in mental status, and neurological symptoms (motor or sensory) typical of a lesion in the central nervous system (Jacox et al., 1994).

Neuropathies and Plexopathies

Neuropathies and plexopathies are exceedingly important pain syndromes because they are extremely difficult to treat. They represent some of the greatest therapeutic challenges to health care personnel treating cancer pain. These syndromes may be caused by direct tumor invasion of nervous system structures; damage to nerves and plexi caused by surgery, radiation, or chemotherapy; and conditions not directly related to the malignant process.

Direct Tumor Invasion

Tumor invasion of peripheral nerves generally causes pain described as constant or burning in nature and that is often unilateral. In patients with bone metastasis, neuropathic pain due to invasion of nerves surrounding bony structures may accompany somatic bone pain. Failure to recognize the neuropathic component of the pain and to incorporate the appropriate adjunctive analgesics into the patient's pain regime probably accounts for a significant percentage of patients whose pain is inadequately controlled (Jacox et al., 1994).

Cervical plexopathy is generally characterized by an aching in the neck area, usually either secondary to local extension of primary head and neck cancers or due to cervical lymph node metastasis from a variety of tumors. Pain in the shoulder with shooting or electric sensations in the thumb and index finger are generally associated with involvement of the upper brachial plexus. Invasion of the lower portion of the brachial plexus is characterized by shoulder pain combined with pain in the elbow, arm, medial forearm, and the fourth and fifth digits.

Cancers of the breast and lung and lymphoproliferative disorders involving the lower neck and chest are the most common causes of brachial plexopathy. Malignant involvement of the lumbosacral plexus is usually marked by pain in the lower abdomen, buttock, and leg or, if sacral nerves are predominantly involved, perineal and perirectal pain. Neurologic symptoms, including weakness, sensory loss, and urinary incontinence, will follow in weeks to months. Intraabdominal and pelvic neoplasms—including colorectal, renal, and endometrial cancers; sarcomas; and lymphomas—are the most common causes of lumbosacral plexopathy (Elliot & Foley, 1989; Jacox et al., 1994). Tumor involvement of the spinal cord, leading to the syndrome of spinal cord compression, was discussed previously.

Pain Associated with Treatment of Cancer

A number of neuropathic pain syndromes are associated with the treatment and management of malignant disease. Patients who have undergone radical neck dissection may experience tightness, burning, dysesthesias, and shocklike sensations in and around the surgical site. Pain associated with drooping of the shoulder on the same side as the neck dissection has also been described. Postmastectomy patients may complain of tightness, constriction, or burning in the arm, axilla, and anterior chest wall of the affected side. The pain may be exacerbated by movement. Patients who have had a thoracotomy may experience pain and tenderness at the incision site and possible sensory loss in the area. Nephrectomy is another surgical procedure associated with neuropathic pain. In the patient who has undergone an amputation, phantom limb pain will be present if the patient had pain in the limb prior to its removal. Pain at the stump site is characterized as burning dysesthesias sometimes exacerbated by movement. It may be present years after surgery (Jacox et al., 1994; Kelly & Payne, 1991).

Some commonly used chemotherapeutic agents may cause neuropathic syndromes. Drugs such as vincristine and newer agents such as vinorelbine tartrate may produce both sensory and motor symptoms including parasthesias, dysesthesias, hyporeflexia, and weakness in the distal muscles of the hands and feet. An unusual neuropathic syndrome associated with vincristine and vinorelbine is severe jaw pain. Cisplatinum neurotoxicity is primarily sensory (Campa & Payne, 1993). Another new chemotherapeutic agent, paclitaxel, may also cause sensory and motor neuropathies and has been reported to cause painful myalgias starting 2 to 3 days posttreatment and lasting for about 5 days (Donehower & Rowinsky, 1994).

Radiation therapy may cause constriction of nerves or plexi secondary to fibrosis from surrounding tissues. This may result in pain that is less severe than the neuropathic symptoms caused by direct tumor involvement of the affected nerve or plexus. Possible long-term effects of radiotherapy include direct injury of larger nerve trunks and the spinal cord. Neurogenic tumors, such as fibrosarcomas, are long-term risks associated with radiotherapy (Campa & Payne, 1993; Jacox et al., 1994).

Pain Unrelated to the Malignant Process

Neuropathic pain not directly related to the malignant process is most commonly related to infection or chronic disease. The most common infectious agent associated with neuropathy is the herpes zoster virus commonly known as shingles. Acute shingles may be accompanied by a burning, aching pain, and the pain may occur several days prior to the development of the characteristic vesicular lesions. Postherpetic pain is persistent pain following healing of the skin lesions, is characterized by shocklike paroxysmal pain, and is extremely challenging to treat (Jacox et al., 1994).

Abdominal Pain

Common causes of abdominal pain related to the malignant disease include painful tumor masses, bowel obstruction, abdominal distension secondary to ascites, and abdominal carcinomatosis. Medications used to treat pain and symptoms may result in painful constipation or diarrhea. Patients generally complain of pain that is "colicky" in nature. It may be worse after eating and is often associated with nausea. When there is abdominal obstruction, vomiting may also occur. Pain due to hepatic metastasis may be pleuritic and referred to the right shoulder. Intraabdominal malignancies may cause neuropathy and plexopathy due to infiltration of nervous system structures such as the celiac plexus in pancreatic carcinoma or the lumbosacral plexus in colorectal carcinoma (Jacox et al., 1994).

Radiation therapy and chemotherapy may cause mucositis. Mucositis related to chemotherapy usually begins 3 to 5 days after the agents are administered and resolves in about 2 weeks. Radiation-induced mucositis occurs in the radiated area, usually beginning about the end of the second week of treatment. The symptoms may persist 2 to 3 weeks after treatment is completed. Affected patients generally complain of pain described as a burning sensation, especially on oral intake. Therefore recognition and treatment of this troublesome symptom is important to help maintain the patient's nutritional status (Campa & Payne, 1993; Jacox et al., 1994).

Although it usually affects the oral cavity and esophagus, mucositis may also affect any portion of the gastrointestinal tract. Patients with this condition, usually referred to as radiation- or chemotherapy-induced enteritis, typically have nausea, emesis, and diarrhea (sometimes bloody) in addition to abdominal pain (Campa & Payne, 1993).

Medications used to treat pain and other symptoms may contribute to abdominal pain. Corticosteroids and nonsteroidal antiinflammatory drugs (NSAIDs) may cause gastritis or the development of peptic ulcers. Steroids may also cause candidiasis, contributing to oral mucositis and esophagitis (Ettinger & Portenoy, 1988; Watanabe & Bruera, 1994). Morphine and other opioid analgesics will cause constipation. If this symptom is not adequately treated, it can contribute to abdominal symptoms. When a patient complains of suprapubic abdominal pain, the possibility of urinary retention must be considered. Patients with cancer may also develop abdominal conditions unrelated to their malignancy. Intestinal obstruction secondary to adhesions or cholecystitis is one such condition. Cancer-associated dyspepsia syndrome (CADS) is another cause of pain that has been reported. Believed to be related to delayed gastric emptying without evidence of obstruction, CADS symptoms include stomach pain, early satiety, bloating, and anorexia. This syndrome may be treated effectively with metoclopramide (Nelson & Walsh, 1993).

PAIN ASSESSMENT

In a recent study (Von Roenn et al., 1993) oncologists stated that an inadequate pain assessment was the single most important cause of failure to satisfactorily treat cancer pain. Nurses dealing with cancer patients must recognize the importance of adequately assessing the severity and cause of the pain. Pain relief goals should be based on the assessment findings. One way to assist in the nursing assessment is to utilize an organized method of data collection. An example of one such method is shown in Figure 10-1.

For assessing pain, Kinzbrunner and Salerno (1994) suggest the following:

1. *In patients with cancer pain, the operative definition of pain is: "Pain is whatever the experiencing person says it is, existing whenever the experiencing person says it does"* (McCaffery & Beebe, 1989, p. 7). Pain is subjective and real to the patient. The goal of a pain assessment is to determine the cause of the pain. It may be physical, psychosocial, or a combination of the two. The prescribed treatment must encompass all components.
2. *Avoid personal biases in responding to a patient's requests for pain relief.* Patients' behavior varies with their personal belief system and background. In addition, the severity and duration of pain are factors. In concert with the patient, the family, and other members of the health care delivery team, a pain management plan that is specific to the patient's needs may be developed. Professionals often become frustrated with patients when they have difficulty controlling pain. The patient sometimes feels responsible, resulting in a sense of failure and humiliation. This sense of responsibility may further increase the patient's perception of pain.
3. *Recognition of pain in a patient who is not willing to communicate openly is critical to achieving good pain control.* Many patients will not readily admit that they have pain or in some circumstances may be unable to say that they hurt. Others with pain may deny it or refuse medication. Nonverbal behavior can be a major clue to unexpressed or uncontrolled pain and includes such signals as crying, restlessness, rigid posture, lack of concentration, grimaces, a gasp or scream upon being touched or when the bed

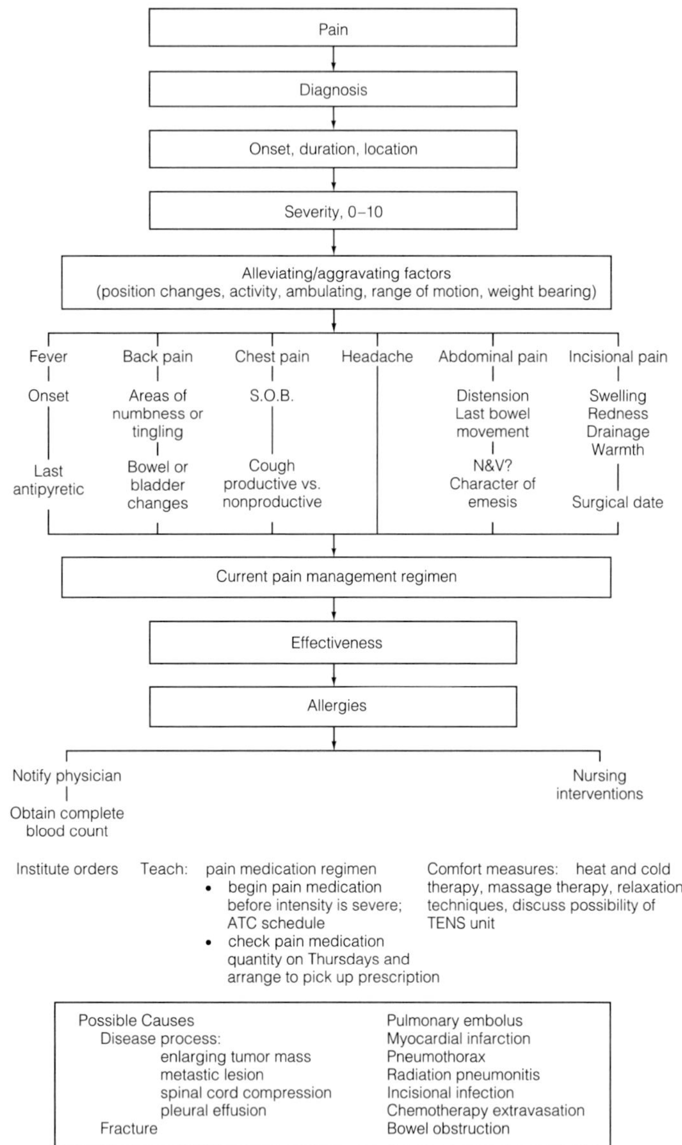

Figure 10-1 Data collection guide for assessing the severity and cause of pain. (From Texas Oncology, Dallas.)

is accidentally bumped, increased immobility, and alterations in sleep patterns.

4. *Professionals need to be aware that the typical sympathetic system response to pain is often not a valid measure for the patient with chronic cancer pain.* Acute pain is characterized by physiologic responses including increases in pulse rate, blood pressure, respiratory rate, and perspiration. Patients with acute pain will focus on their pain, cry, moan, frown, grimace, report the pain, rub a specific painful area, or have increased muscle tension. Patients with chronic pain, because of adaptation, may display few if any of the physiologic changes that typify acute pain. Terminally ill patients may not report pain unless asked. They may appear quiet, sleep for long intervals, or turn their attention to other things. Physical inactivity, immobility, or a flat affect characterized by a blank facial expression may be the only sign present. It is important that the nurse be aware of any physiologic and behavioral changes in caring for their patients.

Health care professionals should keep in mind that unrelieved pain or a lack of response to analgesics is nearly always due to inadequate pain assessment resulting in inadequate drug dosing, improper drug dosing intervals, or inadequate use of coanalgesics and other adjunctive treatments.

Jacox and co-workers (1994) recommend four major steps for a proper pain assessment: a detailed history, a physical examination with emphasis on the neurologic examination, a thorough psychosocial assessment, and, when indicated, appropriate diagnostic studies to definitively determine the cause of the pain.

Pain History

Always obtain a thorough history, preferably from the patient. This should include a full description of the characteristics of each type of pain. A patient may have more than

PQRST PAIN ASSESSMENT PROCESS

P:	Palliative	What *palliates* the pain? (What makes it better?)
	Provocative	What *provokes* the pain? (What makes it worse?)
Q:	Quality	What is the *quality* of the pain? (What is it like?)
R:	Radiation	Where does the pain *radiate?* (Does the pain spread anywhere else?)
S:	Severity	How *severe* is the pain? (Rate the pain on a 0-10 scale.)
T:	Temporal	Is the pain *acute* or *chronic?* (Is it there all the time or does it come and go?)

one pain or more than one cause for the pain experienced. A mnemonic that is useful in obtaining a thorough pain history and in assessing the characteristics of the pain is *PQRST*, described in the following discussion and summarized in the box above.

Palliative or *Provocative:* Determining that a complaint of chest pain is "palliated" when the patient sits and is "provoked" when the patient lies down or takes a deep breath suggests a pleuritic type of pain, which could be secondary to pleural involvement with cancer, inflammatory pleurisy, pathology in the rib cage, or, if on the right side, possible liver metastasis. Increased pain with weight bearing may indicate an impending pathologic fracture, and relief of abdominal pain with milk products or antacids suggests gastritis or peptic ulcer disease.

Quality: Determining the quality of the pain is important to differentiate somatic from neuropathic pain, so that appropriate analgesic and adjuvant therapy can be prescribed. When the pain is described as sharp, dull, or aching, it is usually somatic in nature. This type of pain usually responds well to opioid analgesics or NSAIDs. When the patient complains of pain of a burning, shooting, or tingling quality, associated with paresthesia or dysesthesia (electric shock sensations), the pain is most likely neuropathic. This individual may respond to a tricyclic antidepressant or anticonvulsant.

Radiation: Because of the distribution of sensory nerves, pain often radiates or is perceived at a site somewhat distant from the actual location of the pain stimulus. This is called referred pain. It is important to determine the pattern of radiation of pain. For example, pain or dysesthesia radiating in a girding fashion around the abdomen in the area of the umbilicus suggests pathology involving the T10 sensory nerve roots. Depending on other findings, this could indicate early herpes zoster infection, or it could be a sign of impending spinal cord compression due to a metastatic lesion.

Severity: The measurement of severity is one of the more critical aspects of pain assessment. Some common ways of measuring severity are discussed in Chapter 1.

Temporal: Determining the temporal aspects of pain is also important. Recognizing the differences between the signs of acute and chronic pain is vital, as is understanding that patients may develop acute pain superimposed on chronic pain. For example, pain that increases suddenly, such as after a fall, in a patient with known bone pain secondary to metastatic bone disease might suggest a new pathological fracture in an already involved site of bone metastasis. Temporal information may also be helpful in planning treatment. Pain that occurs in association with a specific planned activity might be managed by using a small additional dose of an analgesic prior to the activity rather than by increasing the patient's regular medication dose.

In addition to obtaining as much information as possible about the pain itself, a complete history of the patient's malignant illness—including prior diagnostic tests, surgical procedures, radiation and chemotherapy treatments, and a history of any concurrent illnesses—should be obtained. A careful medication history, including both over-the-counter (OTC) and prescription drugs and any past or current recreational drug use, is also important.

Physical Exam

A neurologic assessment of the painful areas is crucial. Assessment of pain in the neck or back requires a full motor, sensory, and reflex examination to rule out plexopathy and spinal cord lesions. Patients with headache or skull pain should be examined for possible cranial nerve defects.

Psychosocial Assessment

It is important to include a full psychosocial assessment as part of a comprehensive pain evaluation. Studies (Portenoy, 1988; Welk, 1991) have clearly shown that the associated social, cultural, spiritual, emotional, bureaucratic, and financial challenges have a significant impact on the patient's perception of physical pain. Uncontrolled physical pain will adversely affect many of these factors, creating a vicious cycle (Ferrell, Grant, Rhiner, & Padilla, 1992). It is critical that the psychosocial factors influencing the patient be fully assessed and treated. These factors are considered along with the pharmacologic and nonpharmacologic interventions that address the physical pain stimulus.

Diagnostic Evaluation

A complete nursing assessment is important in the evaluation and treatment of cancer pain. When a patient who has been in remission or has been responding to antineoplastic therapy develops new pain, one of the major concerns is recurrent or progressive cancer. The nurse assists in obtaining the appropriate laboratory studies, such as tumor markers and liver function tests. Nuclear medicine studies, CT scans, or MRI scans may also be required to determine the origin of the pain.

For patients with more advanced cancer, where true palliative care is the most appropriate therapy, diagnostic studies should be performed only when the results clearly dictate an alternative treatment option. For example, in a patient with increasing bone pain and known bone metastasis who has a malignancy that is not amenable to chemotherapy, routine bone scanning to evaluate how much the bone metastases have progressed is not indicated. On the other hand, if the increasing pain is confined to one bone and the possibility of palliative radiation therapy to that site is being considered, an x-ray of that site might be appropriate. The nurse caring for such a patient may play an integral role in gathering the initial information from the individual and communicating those findings to the physician.

Completion of the Pain Assessment

Patients should be informed of the findings and recommendations resulting from the pain assessment. Assure the patient that the pain can be controlled while establishing a realistic time frame to achieve relief goals. For example, because somatic pain responds more rapidly to intervention than neuropathic pain, the patient and family need to be made aware that it might take longer for neuropathic pain to be controlled.

Reassess the patient's status frequently. The AHCPR clinical practice guidelines on the management of cancer pain (Jacox et al., 1994) recommend that pain be assessed and documented:

a. At regular intervals after starting the treatment plan
b. With each new report of pain
c. At a suitable interval after each pharmacologic or nonpharmacologic intervention, such as 15 to 30 minutes after parenteral drug therapy and 1 hour after oral administration

By following these simple guidelines and paying attention to the patient's verbal and nonverbal communication, the health care team can improve their ability to manage the patient with cancer pain (Jacox et al.). See the following box for strategies to implement the cancer pain guidelines.

STRATEGIES TO IMPLEMENT CANCER PAIN GUIDELINES

Teach staff regarding pain management and the AHCPR guidelines.

Identify problems of inadequate pain management through chart audits.

Communicate to staff, physicians, and administration the status of pain management and the need for improvement (be specific).

Assign an expert pain management nurse on each shift or in each department (outpatient), and give that individual the responsibility to direct staff and address untreated pain issues.

Provide education to physicians and other health care professionals through seminars, articles, audiotapes, and other methods.

Institute a uniform pain assessment instrument to be used by all health care professionals.

Establish standards of care for pain control.

Encourage other specialized professionals (pharmacist, social worker, chaplain, etc.) to participate on the pain management team.

Involve and educate the patient and the family in the treatment and prevention of pain. Include pain management discussion in patient support groups.

Develop nonpharmacologic interventions of pain management as adjuvants to drug therapy (music therapy, heat and cold therapy, etc.).

STRATEGIES TO IMPLEMENT CANCER PAIN GUIDELINES—cont'd

Post equinanalgesic charts on the wall. Develop and distribute assessment scales and equinanalgesic charts for the staff.

Teach the nursing staff about basic principles of pain management. Regularly update the staff on new and additional information in this area. Teach staff to expect to control pain in their patients.

Include pain management philosophy, approaches, and strategies in the new employee orientation program.

Coordinate inpatient, outpatient, and home care. Document and communicate pain assessments and outcomes.

Regularly evaluate the program and be prepared to change as needed. Actively include the patient in pain management assessments and decisions and consider patient and family satisfaction when evaluating the pain program.

Identify regulatory barriers to pain control and work with professional organizations to overcome those barriers.

Treat patients with the same pain management you would seek for your own family.

Modified from Ferrell, B. R., Jacox, A., Miaskowski, C., Paice, J., & Hester, N. (1994). Cancer pain guidelines: Now that we have them, what must we do? *Oncology Nursing Forum, 21,* 1230.

TREATMENT OF CANCER PAIN

Various modalities are available to treat pain. The best approach to therapy depends largely on the results of a thorough pain assessment. Based on currently available data, 75% to 85% of patients with cancer pain are successfully managed with oral, rectal, or transdermal analgesia (Jacox et al., 1994; Supportive Care, 1994). The remaining 15% to 25% of individuals can be treated successfully with intravenous or subcutaneous analgesia. Only a small percentage of patients require intraspinal analgesia, nerve blocks, palliative surgery, or ablative surgery to achieve pain control

GUIDELINES FOR THE PHARMACOLOGIC TREATMENT OF CANCER PAIN

1. Use a specific type of drug for a specific type of pain.
2. Know the pharmacology of the drug prescribed.
3. Adjust the route of administration to the patient's needs.
4. Administer analgesics on a regular basis after initial titration.
5. Use drug combinations to provide additive analgesia and reduce side effects.
6. Avoid drug combinations that increase sedation without enhancing analgesia.
7. Watch for the development of tolerance.
8. Prevent acute withdrawal.
9. Do not use placebos to assess the nature of pain.
10. Anticipate and treat complications and side effects.

Modified from Foley, K. (1985). The treatment of cancer pain. *New England Journal of Medicine, 313,* 84–95, 1985.

(Jacox et al., 1994). Often these various forms of primary pain management can be combined with other therapies. These interventions may include adjuvant medications, palliative radiotherapy and chemohormonal therapy, physical therapy, and psychosocial care to achieve optimal pain control.

Pharmacologic Therapy

The primary treatment of cancer pain is pharmacologic therapy. It is critical to know how to properly utilize the agents described in detail in Chapter 4. By carefully following the guidelines listed in the box above and explained in the following discussion (Foley, 1985), success in controlling cancer pain may be achieved.

Use a Specific Type of Drug for a Specific Type of Pain

The World Health Organization (WHO) recommends a ladder approach to pain management that provides for incremental analgesic increases based on the severity of a patient's pain, as illustrated in Figure 10-2 (WHO, 1986). This approach has been accepted by most experts as the standard for pain management and has been included in the AHCPR clinical practice guidelines on the management of cancer pain

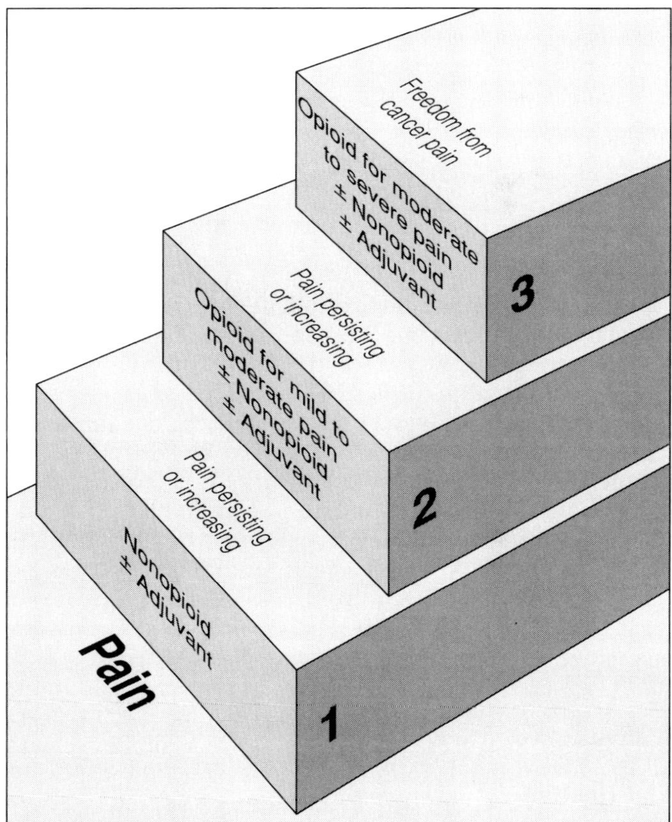

Figure 10-2 The WHO three-step analgesic ladder. (From World Health Organization. (1990). *Cancer pain relief and palliative care: Report of a WHO expert committee.* Geneva: World Health Organization. Used with permission.)

(Jacox et al., 1994). Ferrell, Jacox, Miaskowski, Paice, and Hester (1994) challenge nurses caring for oncology patients to treat the clinical practice guidelines as strategies. Following a thorough pain assessment, patients rate their pain as either mild (severity scale 1-3), moderate (severity scale 4-6), or severe (severity scale 7-10). Appropriate analgesic medication is then selected based on this determination. Adjuvant medications and nonpharmacologic modalities are added as needed based on the pain assessment.

Step 1: Mild pain (severity scale 1-3) The nonopioid analgesics, recommended for the treatment of mild pain, include acetaminophen and the NSAIDs, of which aspirin is the prototype. Acetaminophen is one of the most popular analgesics available today for the treatment of mild pain. In step 2 and, to a lesser degree, step 3 of the WHO ladder, acetaminophen is often used in combination with other analgesics, such as codeine and oxycodone. It has both analgesic and antipyretic effects but is not an antiinflammatory agent. Acetaminophen is generally well tolerated and has minimal toxicity provided that the dose is limited to less than 4 grams per day (Kinzbrunner & Salerno, 1994). Patients who exceed this dose, especially those with impaired liver function, face significant risk of developing progressive hepatic failure, which may be irreversible. Because acetaminophen is found in many over-the-counter preparations, it is important to have full knowledge of all medications taken by the patient.

The other major class of agents used to treat mild pain are the NSAIDs. These drugs have, in addition to the antipyretic and analgesic properties of acetaminophen, significant antiinflammatory properties. They are specifically useful in the treatment of bone pain (to be discussed later).

Aspirin, like acetaminophen, is often combined with codeine or oxycodone to treat moderate pain. Unfortunately, the utilization of aspirin to treat cancer pain is severely limited because of the associated high incidence of gastrointestinal toxicity and its irreversible interference with platelet function, which contribute to the potential for bleeding complications. The nonacetylated salicylates, which include salsalate, choline Mg trisalicylate, and diflusinal, are better tolerated than aspirin by the stomach and have a lesser effect on platelets.

Other commonly used NSAIDs are ibuprofen, naproxen, and indomethacin. Both ibuprofen and naproxen are better tolerated than aspirin and are now available OTC. Indomethacin, despite its fairly high risk of gastrointestinal toxicity, has been useful in treating fever secondary to malignancy and pleuritic pain. Piroxicam is an NSAID in capsule form that is long acting and may be given in one dose daily. Ketorolac has been extremely efficacious in the management of acute inflammatory painful conditions and is especially effective when given parenterally. Because ketorolac has an extremely high risk of toxicity, it should be administered for no more than 5 consecutive days or in no more than 20 doses.

It generally takes about 2 hours for the patient to note any significant effect of an NSAID, and the maximal effect occurs after 2 hours as drug levels rise. In managing a patient with an NSAID, dosing should continue for 1 to 2 weeks before the maximal effects of the drug are assessed. If pain continues after that time, an alternative NSAID or another type of analgesic should be initiated, if careful reassessment so indicates.

Unlike most of the opioid analgesics, NSAIDs have ceiling effects and dose-limiting toxicities, including gastrointestinal irritation and renal toxicity. Since acetaminophen and the NSAIDs relieve pain primarily through peripheral mechanisms, and the opioid analgesics work centrally, the two groups of medications may be combined in a synergistic fashion (Jacox et al., 1994).

Step 2: Moderate pain (severity scale 4-6) Most agents used to treat moderate pain, step 2 on the WHO ladder, are combinations containing either acetaminophen or aspirin. Acetaminophen with codeine is one of the more common available combinations and comes in the following strengths: 300 mg of acetaminophen and either 7.5 mg, 15 mg, 30 mg, or 60 mg of codeine (Kinzbrunner & Salerno, 1992). Individuals should take no more than two tablets every 4 hours due to the potential for acetaminophen toxicity at higher doses. Also, codeine has a ceiling effect and, when administered in doses beyond 65 mg every 4 hours, has been reported to produce increased side effects without a concomitant increase in analgesia (Jacox et al., 1994).

Another popular combination is oxycodone with acetaminophen. Each tablet contains 5 mg of the opioid oxycodone and 325 mg of acetaminophen. The usefulness of this combination is also limited by potential acetaminophen toxicity. Unlike codeine, oxycodone does not appear to have a ceiling effect. It is available without acetaminophen for treatment of severe pain. Another popular combination is hydrocodone with acetaminophen.

Both codeine and oxycodone with aspirin are available, but because of the side effects of aspirin, the use of this combination is severely limited in the treatment of cancer pain.

Step 3: Severe pain (severity scale 7-10) For the treatment of severe pain, opioid agonists such as morphine are the medications of choice. Morphine is available in the following formulations: oral liquids with concentrations of 2 mg/ml and 20 mg/ml, short-acting tablets (insoluble: 15 mg and 30 mg; soluble: 10 mg, 15 mg, and 30 mg), long-acting tablets (15 mg, 30 mg, 60 mg, 100 mg, and 200 mg strengths), rectal suppositories, and intraspinal and parental preparations. This variety allows for flexibility in treating patients with severe cancer pain.

For patients with severe pain, a typical morphine starting dose is 10 to 20 mg orally every 4 hours around the clock (ATC) of a short-acting preparation, with incremental increases as necessary to achieve pain control. In patients being switched from a step 2 opioid, such as an oxycodone-acetaminophen combination, an equianalgesic dose of morphine should be determined and implemented as the starting dose. (See Chapter 4.) Dosage adjustments are based on the patient's response, and the dose should be increased as necessary. Although there is no set formula for dosage titration, the following guidelines may be helpful:

1. If the pain is almost controlled with the present regimen but the patient has some discomfort, the drug dose may be increased by approximately 10%.
2. If the pain is only partially controlled, increase the dosage by 25% to 50%.
3. If the pain is severe and little or no pain relief has been noted with the current dose of analgesic, a dose increase of up to 100% may be appropriate (Kinzbrunner & Salerno, 1994; McCaffery & Beebe, 1989).

After the patient's pain has been controlled with a relatively stable dose of short-acting morphine, conversion to a long-acting morphine may be accomplished for patient convenience. Whether the patient is maintained on a short-acting morphine preparation or is converted to a long-acting morphine, the availability of short-acting morphine for the treatment of breakthrough pain on a prn basis is mandatory. Recommended doses of short-acting morphine for breakthrough pain are calculated at either 5% to 10% of the 24-hour total dose, given every 2 to 3 hours as needed (Portenoy & Hagen, 1990), or 25% of the 12-hour dose, given at intervals of 3 to 4 hours (Ferrell, 1991).

There are a number of other commonly used opioid agonist analgesics. Hydromorphone is generally started at a dose of 2 mg every 3 to 4 hours and is available in oral (2 and 4 mg tablets), suppository (1 mg and 3 mg), and parenteral forms. For patients who require subcutaneous injection, hydromorphone is advantageous because it is more potent than morphine milligram for milligram. Because of this higher concentration, a smaller amount of subcutaneous hydromorphone is required to achieve a similar analgesic effect (Storey, Hill, St. Louis, & Tarver, 1990). Oxycodone, traditionally considered a step 2 agent in combination with acetaminophen or aspirin, is now available uncombined. Oxycodone does not have a ceiling effect and therefore is used as a step 3 opioid analgesic (Glare & Walsh, 1993).

Fentanyl, an opioid agonist traditionally used as an anesthetic, is now available in a transdermal formulation. A full discussion of the pharmacology of the fentanyl transdermal system is presented in Chapter 4, and a discussion of the advantages and disadvantages of the transdermal route of administration appears later in this chapter.

Other agonist analgesics are methadone and levorphanol. These analgesics have long half-lives, leading to drug accumulation and potential toxicity, which limits their use in geriatric patients and those with advanced malignancy (Kinzbrunner & Salerno, 1994).

Certain opioid analgesics should be avoided. Meperidine, an opioid agonist that is fairly popular in the acute postoperative setting, should not be prescribed for the treatment of chronic cancer pain (Jacox et al., 1994). This medication has a very short half-life, must be dosed every 2 to 4 hours, and has poor oral bioavailability. Most important, meperidine is metabolized in the body to normeperidine, which will accumulate with prolonged administration, with high doses, or in patients with impaired renal or liver function. Normeperidine is responsible for serious toxic effects associated with meperidine, including significant mood changes, CNS stimulation, tremors, and multifocal myoclonus and seizures (Kaiko et al., 1983).

Prescribing a partial agonist or agonist-antagonist opioid drug such as pentazocine, butorphanol, nalbuphine, dezocine, or buprenorphine is also discouraged. These agents have a ceiling dose effect. Agonist-antagonist drugs bind to opioid receptors to produce analgesia, but because they also have antagonist effects, they could reverse opioid analgesia and precipitate opioid withdrawal (Jacox et al., 1994).

Know the Pharmacology of the Drug Prescribed

There are a large number of opioid analgesics and NSAIDs to choose from. It is important to develop significant expertise with at least two or three agents in each class of drugs.

Not all patients react in the same fashion to the same medication. A medication that works well for one patient may be toxic for another. Therefore familiarity with more than one medication in each class will allow flexibility in tailoring the drug regime to each patient's needs. Many patients with chronic pain are being treated with medications such as meperidine or the agonist-antagonist agents; therefore it is important for health care professionals to safely convert patients to more appropriate analgesics.

Adjust the Route of Administration to the Patient's Needs

Oral administration of analgesics is the preferred route, and other routes should be reserved for patients who cannot be managed with oral analgesics. Orally administered analgesics are safe, simple, cost effective, and, with long-acting morphine preparations now available in higher dosage forms, very convenient for the patient.

A small percentage of patients cannot tolerate oral agents at some time during their illness. It is difficult to manage patients with oral analgesics who are experiencing intractable nausea and vomiting because of the analgesic, other medication, cancer treatment, or the disease; who are having difficulty swallowing secondary to an oral or esophageal cancer; or who are nearing the end of life (Jacox et al., 1994). Although it is all too commonplace in these circumstances to consider invasive methods of drug delivery, a number of noninvasive alternatives are available, including buccal, sublingual, rectal, and transdermal routes of analgesic administration (Whedon & Ferrell, 1991).

There are currently no approved buccal or sublingual analgesic medications available in the United States. Buprenorphine, a partial agonist, is available in Europe in sublingual form, but it has a ceiling dose and a risk of precipitating analgesic withdrawal when given with an opioid agonist. Treatment of terminally ill cancer patients with high-concentration oral morphine solution held in the patient's mouth, on either the buccal or the sublingual surface, is thought to be effective in controlling pain. Theoretically, a higher amount of drug should reach the morphine receptors because the portal circulation and any first-pass metabolic effects from the liver are avoided when the drug is absorbed buccally or sublingually. Questions as to whether the drug is actually absorbed directly from the mucosal surface or trickles down the throat have not been answered. Whether the higher drug concentration actually reaches the receptor is also unknown (Payne, 1987).

Administration of opioids by rectal suppository is an effective means of treating the patient who can no longer take medication by mouth. Although the degree of rectal absorption is actually less than that of absorption through the small intestine, because rectal blood flow avoids the liver, the blood levels are about the same (Cole & Hanning, 1990). The efficacy of rectal morphine administration in terminally ill patients makes this a viable alternative to administering analgesics invasively in the last several days of life (Kinzbrunner, Policzer, Miller, & Neiber, 1990). With the use of gelatin capsules and hydrophilic morphine tablets, one can now provide virtually any dosage level of morphine via the rectal route (Kinzbrunner & Salerno, 1994). Also, long-acting morphine may be placed in a gelatin capsule and may provide prolonged effects. This method reduces the number of times a patient requires suppository insertion and is especially important in patients with thrombocytopenia (Maloney, Kesner, Klein, & Bockenstette, 1989; Wilkinson et al., 1992). Acetaminophen and several of the NSAIDs, including aspirin and indomethacin, may also be administered via the rectal route (Kinzbrunner & Salerno).

Transdermal fentanyl provides another noninvasive treatment option for patients who are unable to take opioids by mouth. Because fentanyl is 20 times more potent than morphine milligram for milligram and is readily absorbed through the skin and mucous membranes, it is well suited to a transdermal delivery system (Plezia, Kramer, Linford, & Hameroff, 1989; Miser et al., 1989). Treatment is generally initiated at a dose of 25 μg every 3 days. If the patient is already taking an opioid analgesic, the appropriate bioequivalent dose is used. There are challenges involved with the use of the fentanyl transdermal system, including irregular drug absorption in patients who are febrile, the long half-life, and practical concerns regarding patch placement, that have limited the effectiveness of transdermal analgesia. A detailed discussion of how to use the fentanyl transdermal system effectively and safely is presented in Chapter 4.

There are several alternative parenteral routes of administration available for patients who are unable to have pain effectively controlled by a noninvasive route of analgesia administration. These include intravenous, intramuscular, and subcutaneous injections and subcutaneous and intravenous infusions.

For patients with severe, uncontrolled acute pain the use of injectable opioids on an interim basis will allow for more rapid analgesic blood levels and short-term control of pain. At the same time, appropriate long-term pain control measures may be initiated. The intravenous route would be the route of choice, with subcutaneous injections reserved for patients without venous access. Intramuscular injections should be avoided because of pain at the injection site and unreliable absorption of the medication (Jacox et al., 1994).

The preferred method for long-term intravenous (IV) administration of analgesics is by continuous infusion. Continuous infusion of analgesics provides patients with consistent blood levels and can be easily titrated to effect. Indications for providing analgesia by continuous IV infusion include persistent nausea and vomiting, severe dysphagia and swallowing disorders, and severe alterations in mental status (Jacox et al.,1994).

Continuous infusion of opioid analgesics may be accomplished either intravenously or, when patients do not have reliable venous access, subcutaneously (Storey et al., 1990). Some form of infusion control device, either mechanical (for example, a syringe driver pump) or computerized, is employed to ensure proper drug delivery. Some computerized delivery systems include the ability to provide patient-controlled analgesia (PCA) (Bruera & Ripamonti, 1993b). With these systems patients have the option of self-administering predetermined bolus doses of extra analgesia while also receiving a continuous dose. This is especially effective in ambulatory patients who might need breakthrough medication prior to activity (Graves, Foster, Batenhorst, Bennett, & Baumann, 1983). (For an in-depth discussion on the administration of PCA, refer to Chapter 8.)

Intraspinal infusion of analgesic medication should be reserved for patients with pain that cannot be adequately controlled by either noninvasive routes of administration, continuous IV infusion, or subcutaneous infusion. (Treatment of pain by intraspinal techniques is discussed in Chapter 14.)

Administer Analgesics on a Regular Basis after Initial Titration

Around-the-clock therapy for effective chronic pain management is critical to achieving good pain control. Fig-

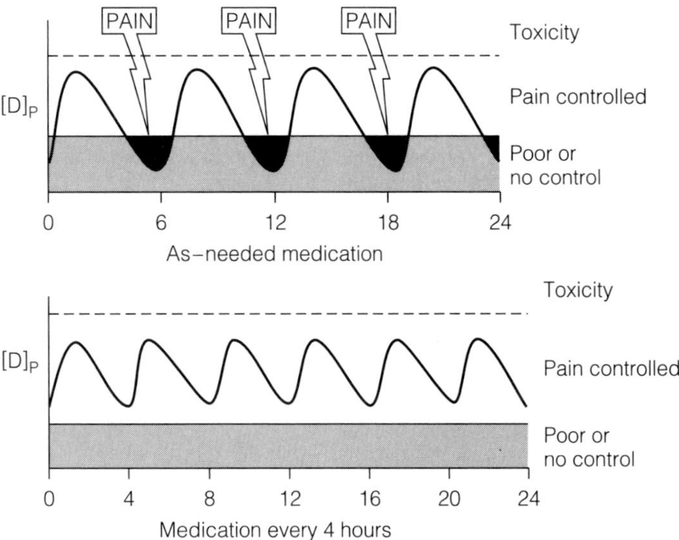

Figure 10-3 Illustration of the results of pain medication given on an as-needed basis versus regular 4-hour administration of morphine sulphate. $[D]p$, Plasma concentration of drug. (From Twycross, R. G. (1994). *Pain relief in advanced cancer.* Edinburgh: Churchill Livingstone.)

ure 10-3 illustrates the pharmacokinetics associated with ATC treatment versus "as needed" or prn dosing of analgesia. Patients on a prn schedule will receive medication only when they complain of and are experiencing pain. In contrast, when analgesia is provided on a regular basis, in anticipation of recurring pain, the establishment and maintenance of drug levels within a therapeutic range will effectively prevent the recurrence of pain. The knowledge that the pain does not have to recur prior to the next dosing of analgesia can be of great importance in reducing patient anxiety. This reduction of anxiety may itself have significant therapeutic benefit (Portenoy, 1988; Ferrell et al., 1992).

For patients with intermittent pain, prn dosing is appropriate. When patients with chronic pain that is generally well controlled experience increased pain on an irregular basis (such as related to activity), supplemental "as needed" medication should be provided (Portenoy & Coyle, 1990).

Use Drug Combinations Appropriately

The purposes of using drug combinations are to provide additive analgesia and to reduce side effects. A number of adjuvant medications are indicated for the treatment of specific types of pain, and these are often used in conjunction with the opioid analgesics. Table 10-2 presents a list of some of the more common pain syndromes and the associated adjuvant medications. To identify patients with cancer pain who will benefit from these adjuvant medications, a thorough pain assessment is mandatory. Failure to use adjuvant medications, especially when patients have pain that is difficult to control with opioid analgesics alone, is one of the major reasons many patients do not have their cancer pain adequately controlled.

Treatment of specific types of pain

Bone pain Bone pain is mediated by prostaglandins produced as a result of the enzyme cyclooxygenase (prostaglandin synthetase), which converts arachidonic acid to cylic endoperoxidases to prostaglandins. The NSAIDs inhibit cyclooxygenase, reducing prostaglandin production. Because

Table 10-2 Adjuvant Pharmacologic Treatment of Pain

Type of Pain	Recommended Adjuvant Medications
Bone pain	NSAIDs
	Biphosphonates
	Calcitonin
Neuropathic pain	Tricyclic antidepressants (amitryptyline)
	Oral antiarrythmics (mexilitene)
	Anticonvulsants (phenytoin, carbamazepine, corticosteroids)
	Clonidine
Headache from increased intracranial pressure	Corticosteroids
Muscle spasm	Baclofen
	Diazepam
Abdominal pain	Carafate
	Antacids
	H_2-blockers (cimetidine)
	Metoclopramide
Bladder spasms	Belladonna and opium
	Urispas
Mucositis	Capsaicin cream
	Topical lidocaine
	Kaopectate and Benadryl
	Topical antifungal agents
	Acyclovir cream
Anxiety	Lorazepam
Depression	Methylphenidate
	Antidepressants

prostaglandins are responsible for causing much of the pain and inflammation associated with bone pain, NSAIDs can be very effective in treating it. They may be used either alone or in conjunction with an opioid analgesic (Stambaugh, 1993). (See the previous discussion of step 1 pain and Chapter 4 for additional information on NSAIDs.)

Another class of agents that may be effective in controlling bone pain are the biphosphonates (etidronate, pamidronate), which are currently indicated for the treatment of hypercalcemia. These medications inhibit bone resorption in vivo, and studies (Jacox et al., 1994) have suggested that some patients have experienced decreased bone pain and required less analgesia when receiving these agents. Calcitonin, another agent used to treat hypercalcemia, has also been shown to be beneficial in reducing analgesic requirements in some patients with bone pain (Jacox et al.).

Neuropathic pain Although not totally resistant to opioids, neuropathic pains are clearly less sensitive to opioids than nociceptive pains, and they frequently require the addition of adjuvant analgesics to achieve pain control. Tricyclic antidepressants, steroids, and anticonvulsant medications are used to treat neuropathic pain.

The tricyclic antidepressants have been shown to treat neuropathic pain by three different mechanisms: mood elevation, potentiation or enhancement of opioid analgesics, and direct analgesic effects (France, 1987; Max et al., 1988; Ventafridda et al., 1990). Amitriptyline is the medication that has been most extensively studied. Although some patients achieve analgesia with lower doses of the medication than are typical for achieving antidepressant effects, doses as high as 150 mg per day may be required for pain relief. Because it often takes 1 to 2 weeks to obtain serum levels and 4 to 6 weeks to achieve peak effect, patients need to be aware that it will take time to perceive any significant pain relief from the medication (Kehoe, 1993; Watson, 1994a). Side effects include sedation, dry mouth, constipation, and urinary retention limit. To minimize toxicity, it is recommended that treatment be initiated with a small dose (10 to 25 mg) at bedtime, with increases at similar increments every 3 to 4 days (Jacox et al., 1994). (See Chapter 9 for an in-depth discussion on the management of pain with antidepressants.)

Corticosteroids are especially effective in treating neuropathic symptoms accompanied by inflammation and edema. Headaches due to increased intracranial pressure and the pain and neurologic deficits of spinal cord compressions are examples of neuropathic symptoms. Dexamethasone in high doses is generally the steroid medication of choice.

Corticosteroids may also be helpful in treating other forms of neuropathic pain and plexopathy. They are especially effective when there is a significant component of inflammation and soft tissue swelling (Ettinger & Portenoy, 1988; Watanabe & Bruera, 1994).

Anticonvulsants such as phenytoin and carbamazepine may be effective in treating neuropathic pain that is lancinating or burning in nature, as may be caused by nerve injury (Bruera & Ripamonti, 1993a; Jacox et al., 1994). (Chapters 4 and 9 discuss the use of these agents.)

Other agents with anecdotal success in the treatment of neuropathic pain are the antihypertensive clonidine (Bruera & Ripamonti, 1993a), systemically administered local anesthetics such as IV lidocaine, and oral mexiletine and tocainide (Bruera & Ripamonti; Edmondson, Simpson, Stubler, & Beric, 1993; Tanelian & Brose, 1991). Muscle spasms often accompany neurologic injury and can be quite painful. In cases of spinal cord compression or other central nervous system impairment associated with spastic paresis, baclofen in gradually escalating doses from 10 mg daily to 10 mg tid may be very effective. Other muscle relaxants, such as diazepam or cyclobenzaprine, may be used as well (Bruera & Ripamonti; Kinzbrunner & Salerno, 1994).

Depression and mood As has been well documented, pain perception is often exacerbated by depression and anxiety (Ferrell et al., 1992; Portenoy, 1988). Antidepressants in full therapeutic doses may be useful (Kehoe, 1993). It may take several weeks for antidepressant effects to be felt; therefore for patients with short life expectancy who require antidepressant therapy, the psychostimulant methylphenidate has been found to be an effective agent due to its rapid onset of action (Gurian & Rosowsky, 1990; Woods, Tesar, Murray, & Cassem, 1986).

Anxiety may be another symptom complicating uncontrolled pain. In treating anxiety along with pain, avoid medications that will cause additive toxicity without necessarily achieving the desired effects. Benzodiazepines, such as lorazepam, may be useful. Some of the older medications, such as diazepam, have significant depressant effects and additive sedative potential when used with opioid analgesics, and their use should be avoided. With the exception of some limited studies (Patt, Proper, & Reddy, 1994) using the agent methotrimeprazine, neuroleptic drugs, including the phenothiazines and butyrophenones, have not been shown to have any additive analgesic effects and should be avoided unless patients have severe symptoms of agitation.

Gastrointestinal pain syndromes A number of agents are available for the treatment of mucositis. For oral mucositis treatment should be directed at the pain and possible superimposed infection. For the latter topical antifungal agents such as Mycelex troches or Mycostatin cream may be useful. For more stubborn fungal infection oral agents such as Diflucan may be required. Acyclovir tablets or cream may be required if a superimposed infection is viral in origin. Topical lidocaine may be helpful in reducing the pain associated with eating and drinking, although its effects are very short-lived. A recent report (Watson, 1994b) suggested that capsaicin, the spice found in chili peppers, may be an effective analgesic for the treatment of mucositis when applied topically. Some clinicians have found that antacids or Kaopectate combined with diphenhydramine liquid and applied topically to the affected mucosa can be beneficial.

Management of pain associated with inflammation of esophageal and gastric mucosa may include treatment similar to that described for oral mucositis. An H_2 blocker such as cimetidine, antacids, or carafate may be added if gastric inflammation is suspected. In patients with cancer-associated dyspepsia syndrome, metoclopramide may be helpful (Nelson & Walsh, 1993). Pain related to gaseous abdominal distension may be helped by an antiflatulent such as simethicone.

Suprapubic and lower abdominal pain must be carefully evaluated as well. Bladder spasms may respond well to a combination of belladonna and opium or a medication such as Urispas. Patients who complain of suprapubic pain and fullness secondary to bladder outlet obstruction may benefit from a medication such as Urecholine or a Foley catheter. If pain is related to constipation, appropriate measures should be taken to ensure proper bowel function (which is discussed later).

Watch for the Development of Tolerance

Tolerance is defined as the need for escalating doses of a medication to maintain an analgesic effect without an increase in nociception (Portenoy & Coyle, 1990; Weissman, Dahl, & Joranson, 1990). Physicians, nurses, and patients are often concerned that early use of opioid analgesics in the management of cancer pain will result in the development of tolerance to the analgesic effects of the medication. They fear that this will leave the patient in a state of uncontrolled pain near the end of life (Cleeland, 1987; Von Roenn et al., 1993). Although many patients require higher doses of analgesics as their disease progresses, this is not usually because of tolerance but is due to increased pain stimulated by the direct or indirect effects of the progressive illness (Kanner & Foley, 1981; Portenoy & Coyle). If tolerance to a specific opioid analgesic does occur, increase the dose of analgesic to effect (Weissman et al., 1990). When dosage escalation is cumbersome, it is recommended that treatment be switched to an alternative opioid analgesic. Since cross-tolerance of opioids is incomplete, it is recommended that the starting dose of the alternative analgesic be 50% of the equianalgesic dose of the medication to which tolerance has developed (Foley, 1985). Tolerance tends to develop more quickly with parenteral administration of opioids and more slowly when the medication is given orally or rectally (Weissman et al.).

Unlike tolerance to the analgesic effects of opioids, tolerance to opioid side effects such as sedation, nausea, and respiratory depression occurs commonly and rapidly. It is important not to abandon an analgesic after several doses because of side effects, but to manage the patient through the side effects and observe for improvement in symptoms as tolerance to the untoward effects develops (Portenoy & Coyle, 1990).

Prevent Acute Withdrawal

There are a number of situations in which reduction in the opioid dose is appropriate. For example, patients with malignancies that are responsive to chemotherapy, hormonal therapy, or radiation therapy may have significant pain reduction as response to therapy and remission is achieved. In such situations it is important not to abruptly discontinue the opioid analgesic, or else symptoms of physical withdrawal will ensue. The medication should be discontinued in a planned, gradual fashion, such as reducing the dose by either 10% per day for 10 days or 5% per day for 20 days (Kinzbrunner & Salerno, 1992).

In patients who are nearing death and who have been on opioid analgesics for chronic pain, it is important to continue at least a partial dose of medication to prevent withdrawal symptoms. Since many of these patients can no longer take medication by mouth, an alternative route of opioid administration may be required (i.e., oral switched to rectal; transdermal fentanyl would *not* be appropriate, since it takes 24 hours to have an effect). Although many of these patients may be managed on the same bioequivalent dose of analgesic, some health care providers prefer to reduce the dose to ensure that some of the observed changes in the patient's condition are not due to side effects of the opioid. Depending on the level of consciousness of the patient, dosage reductions of 25% to 75% are common. This is an acceptable approach and will avoid acute withdrawal symptoms. It is, however, critical that the individuals caring for the patient remain focused on controlling the patient's pain. Careful use of dose titration is necessary to maintain good patient comfort and pain control (McCracken & Gerdsen, 1991).

Do Not Use Placebos to Assess the Nature of Pain

Although it is very well recognized that there is a placebo response to treatment of pain, the deceptive use of placebos to treat patients who are not believed to have "real" pain is inappropriate (Foley, 1985; Jacox et al., 1994).

Anticipate and Treat Complications and Side Effects

The side effects and potential complications of analgesics can have serious consequences but should not preclude the proper, safe use of these agents. The most important method of controlling side effects and complications is by anticipation and prevention. (A full discussion of the side effects of opioid and nonopioid analgesic medications can be found in Chapter 4, and treatment of many of the symptoms is discussed in Chapter 16.)

Concern over inducing respiratory depression in patients on chronic use of morphine is one of the major reasons many patients with cancer pain have their pain undertreated (Portenoy & Coyle, 1990). The concern over inducing respiratory depression prevents health care professionals from increasing opioid analgesia in patients who are nearing death and experiencing progressive pain. For patients nearing death, opioid medications are commonly withheld in an attempt to avoid aggravating the slowing of the respiratory rate that occurs during the dying process. These concerns are usually unsupported (Santiago & Edelman, 1985). Tolerance to the respiratory depressant effects of opioid analgesics develops early in the course of treatment with these agents (Portenoy & Coyle). Patients with chronic obstructive lung disease have demonstrated improvement in exercise tolerance and decreased sense of breathlessness with oral morphine (Light et al., 1989) and dihydrocodeine (Woodcock et al., 1981). Studies (Bruera, Macmillan, Pither, & MacDonald, 1990; Bruera, MacEachern, Ripamonti, & Hanson, 1993) on the efficacy of morphine in the treatment of dyspnea in terminally ill cancer patients have shown that for patients receiving chronic morphine medication for pain, an increase in morphine will control symptoms of breathlessness without significant physiologic effects on respiratory function (Bruera et al., 1990; Bruera et al., 1993). It has been demonstrated that the use of opioid analgesics in the management of dyspnea in patients with chronic obstructive pulmonary disease and advanced cancer is safe (Cowcher & Hanks, 1990). The dose of analgesic medication necessary to control progressive pain in patients on chronic use of opioid analgesia may be administered without an overriding concern that this will result in the induction of significant respiratory depression.

Constipation is one of the most significant side effects of analgesic agents but is preventable. Patients started on any analgesic therapy should be placed on a program that may include increased fiber and fluid consumption, mild laxatives, and stool softeners. Close attention to maintaining regular bowel movements is necessary to prevent severe constipation. When severe constipation occurs, corrective measures may include oral laxatives, rectal suppositories, hyperosmotic agents, or, in very severe cases, manual disimpaction (Jacox et al., 1994).

Dry mouth is another common side effect. It can be treated by frequent moistening of the mucous membranes, and an explanation should be given to the patient that the dry mouth is secondary to the medication.

A complaint of suprapubic abdominal pain may not be related to constipation or gastrointestinal distress but to the opioid side effect of urinary retention. Since overflow incontinence is often associated with urinary retention, the patient may not realize that he or she is unable to urinate. Treatment may include a trial of an anticholinergic medication such as urecholine or a Foley cathcter.

Side effects of analgesics that occur infrequently are postural hypotension, allergic reactions and anaphylaxis, antidiuresis, autonomic reactions, and adverse interactions with MAO inhibitors.

Nonpharmacologic Interventions

In addition to the many analgesic agents available to treat cancer pain, there are a number of other useful interventions that, when combined with the analgesics, allow for more effective pain management. These interventions include physical medicine techniques, behavior modification, anesthetic and neurosurgical techniques, radiation therapy, and chemotherapy.

Physical Medicine

Physical medicine techniques that are beneficial to many patients with cancer pain include immobilization, range-of-motion exercises, and transcutaneous electrical stimulation. Immobilization methods include use of a corset to help support the vertebral bodies and help control back pain secondary to vertebral metastasis, and a shoulder support to reduce pain secondary to a brachial plexopathy. Range-of-motion exercises might be beneficial for patients who are partially immobilized by reducing spasticity or preventing the development of contractures (Jacox et al., 1994). (A more thorough discussion of the indications for physical approaches to cancer pain management can be found in Chapter 5.)

Behavior Modification

Hypnosis, relaxation techniques, music therapy, and other forms of behavior modification may be useful for selected patients, especially if there are strong psychosocial issues contributing to their perception of pain (Jacox et al., 1994). (Refer to Chapters 5 and 7 for a discussion of these interventions and other appropriate psychologic and spiritual interventions.)

Anesthetic and Neurosurgical Techniques

In cases of pain involving a dermatome (e.g., pain secondary to shingles) or involving a specific nerve or plexus (e.g., the celiac plexus in patients with pancreatic carcinoma) nerve blocks may be an appropriate intervention. Surgical disruption of nerve trunks, such as portions of spinal cords or roots, may be indicated for treating isolated areas where pain cannot be controlled with analgesics. These procedures have limitations because of the deafferentation that results from disruption of the nerve trunk, which may be as distressing to the patient as the pain that previously existed. Anesthetic and neurosurgical techniques, especially those requiring invasive surgery, should be reserved for patients who have persistent pain despite adequate trials of oral and parenteral analgesia (Jacox et al., 1994). (Chapter 14 discusses these techniques in more detail.)

Radiotherapy

Radiotherapy may be a very useful intervention, especially when pain can be localized. Pain caused by bone metastasis from a variety of neoplasms resolves with radiation therapy in 75% or more of patients (Ashby, 1993).

While the patient is being treated, analgesic therapy should continue until pain relief is apparent, and then the analgesic should be tapered. Dose fractionation is somewhat dependent on patient prognosis, with regimens of 10 or more treatments prescribed for patients with prognoses greater than 6 months (Ashby, 1993; Jacox et al., 1994). Patients with shorter life expectancies may be treated with 1 to 5 fractions to achieve equivalent pain relief (Ashby, 1991; Bates, 1992; Price et al., 1986).

Diffuse bone pain may be treated with hemibody radiation. A single fraction of 6 to 8 Gy is administered to one half of the body. Vomiting is common, but with antiemetics and partial shielding to reduce lung toxicity, palliation of pain has been reported in between 50% and 75% of treated patients (Poulter et al., 1992; Jacox et al., 1994).

Radiopharmaceuticals have also been used to treat bone pain secondary to metastatic disease. Iodine-131 has been used to treat bone metastasis secondary to thyroid cancer, and phosphorus-32 has been utilized in the past to treat bone metastasis from breast and prostate carcinoma (Jacox et al., 1994). More recently strontium-89 has been found to be effective in over 60% of patients with bone metastasis from prostate carcinoma (Bolger et al., 1993; Robinson,

Preston, Baxter, Dusing, & Spicer, 1993). Other radiopharmaceutical agents, including rhenium-186 and samarium-153, are currently being studied (Jacox et al.).

Pain secondary to tumor infiltration or compression of nerves or other structures in the body may also be treated with radiation therapy (Ashby, 1993; Jacox et al., 1994). The approaches required for the various lesions are beyond the scope of this discussion.

Chemotherapy and Hormonal Therapy

For patients who have malignancies that are responsive to chemotherapy or hormonal therapy, these modalities will provide relief of pain. As for patients with radiation therapy, it is important that patients receiving systemic antineoplastic therapy not be allowed to remain in pain while the therapy's effectiveness in treating the malignant disease is being assessed (Bonadonna & Molinari, 1979; Brule, 1979; Kurman, 1993).

SUMMARY

As illustrated in Figure 10-4, success in controlling pain in patients with cancer requires skill in pain assessment and expertise in the application of many therapeutic techniques. The ability to recognize the need for adjuvant medication and nonpharmacologic interventions will further help treat patients suffering from cancer pain. If the nurse clinician can combine these skills, the complex challenges presented by patients with uncontrolled cancer pain can be overcome.

References

Ashby, M. (1991). The role of radiotherapy in palliative care. *Journal of Pain and Symptom Management, 6,* 380-388.

Ashby, M. (1993). Radiotherapy in the palliation of cancer. In R. B. Patt (Ed.), *Cancer pain.* Philadelphia: Lippincott.

Bates, T. (1992). A review of local radiotherapy in the treatment of bone metastases and cord compression. *International Journal of Radiation Oncology, Biology, Physics, 23,* 217-221.

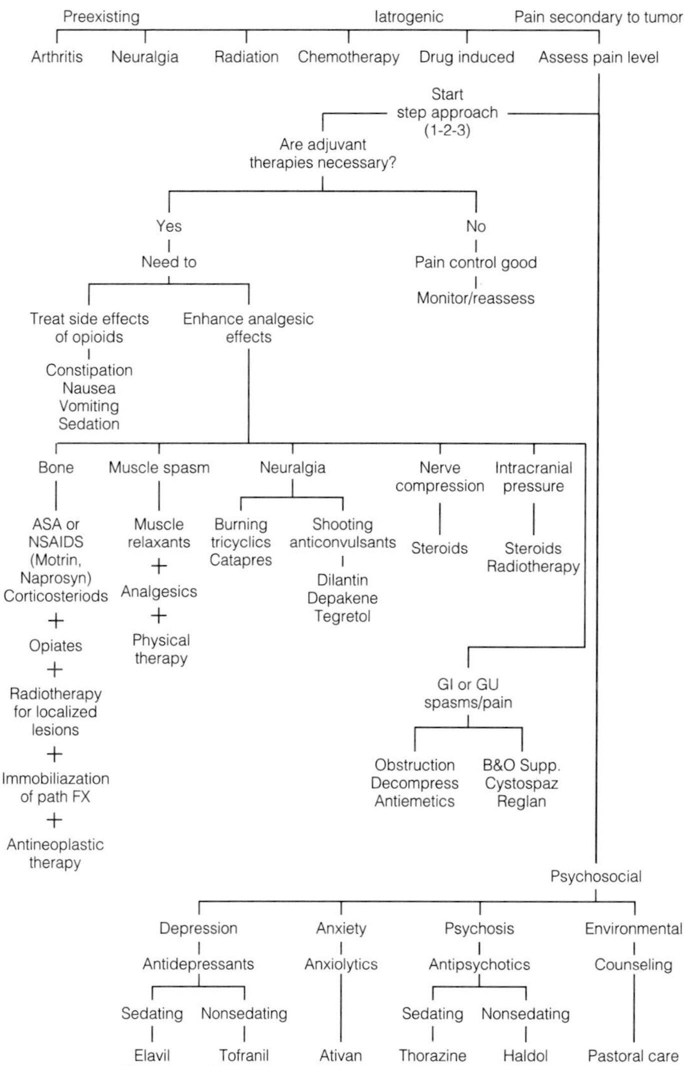

Figure 10-4 Pain management summary chart. (From Kinzbrunner, B. M., & Salerno, E. (1994). *Vitas pain management formulary* (2nd ed.). Miami: Vitas Healthcare Corp.)

Bolger, J. J., Dearnly, D. P., Kirk, D., Lewington, V. J., Mason, M. D., Quilty, P. M., Reed, N. S., Russell, J. M., & Yardley, J. (1993). Strontium-89 (Metastron) versus external beam radiotherapy in patients with painful bone metastases secondary to prostate cancer: Preliminary report of a multicenter trial. *Seminars in Oncology, 20*(3) (suppl. 2), 32-33.

Bonadonna, G., & Molinari, R. (1979). Role and limits of anticancer drugs in the treatment of advanced cancer pain. In J. J. Bonica & V. Ventafridda (Eds.), *Advances in pain research and therapy* (vol. 2, pp. 131-138). New York: Raven Press.

Bonica, J. J. (1990). Cancer pain. In J. J. Bonica (Ed.), *The management of pain* (2nd ed., pp. 400-460). Philadelphia: Lea & Febiger.

Bruera, E., MacEachern, T., Ripamonti, C., & Hanson, J. (1993). Subcutaneous morphine for dyspnea in cancer patients. *Annals of Internal Medicine, 119,* 906-907.

Bruera, E., Macmillan, K., Pither, J., & MacDonald, R. N. (1990). Effects of morphine on the dyspnea of terminal cancer patients. *Journal of Pain and Symptom Management, 5,* 341-344.

Bruera, E., & Ripamonti, C. (1993a). Adjuvants to opioid analgesics. In R. B. Patt (Ed.), *Cancer pain* (pp. 143-159). Philadelphia: Lippincott.

Bruera, E., & Ripamonti, C. (1993b). Alternate routes of administration of opioids for the management of cancer pain. In R. B. Patt (Ed.), *Cancer pain* (pp. 161-184). Philadelphia: Lippincott.

Brule, G. (1979). Role and limits of oncologic chemotherapy in advanced cancer pain. In J. J. Bonica & V. Ventafridda (Eds.), *Advances in pain research and therapy* (vol. 2, pp. 139-144). New York: Raven Press.

Campa, J. A., & Payne, R. (1993). Pain syndromes due to cancer treatment. In R. B. Patt (Ed.), *Cancer pain.* Philadelphia: Lippincott.

Cleeland, C. S. (1987). Barriers to the management of cancer pain. *Oncology, 1*(2), S19-S26.

Cleeland, C. S., Gonin, R., Hatfield, A. K., Edmonson, J. H., Blum, R. H., Stewart, J. A., & Pandya, K. J. (1994). Pain and its treatment in outpatients with metastatic cancer. *New England Journal of Medicine, 330,* 592-596.

Cole, L., & Hanning, C. (1990). Review of the rectal use of opioids. *Journal of Pain and Symptom Management, 5,* 118-126.

Cowcher, K., & Hanks, G. W. (1990). Long-term management of respiratory symptoms in advanced cancer, *Journal of Pain and Symptom Management, 5,* 320-330.

Donehower, R. C., & Rowinsky, E. K. (1994). Paclitaxel. *PPO Updates, 8*(10), 3-16.

Edmondson, E. A, Simpson, R. K., Stubler, D. K., & Beric, A. (1993). Systemic lidocaine for poststroke pain. *Southern Medical Journal, 86,* 1093-1096.

Elliott, K., & Foley, K. (1989). Neurologic pain syndromes in patients with cancer. *Neurology Clinician, 7*(2), 333-360.

Elliott, T. E., & Elliott, B. A. (1991). Physician acquisition of cancer pain management knowledge. *Journal of Pain and Symptom Management, 6*(4), 224-225.

Ettinger, A. B., & Portenoy, R. K. (1988). The use of corticosteroids in the treatment of symptoms associated with cancer. *Journal of Pain and Symptom Management, 3,* 99-103.

Ferrell, B. R. (1991). Managing pain with long-acting morphine. *Nursing '91,* October, 34-39.

Ferrell, B. R., Grant, M. M., Rhiner, M., & Padilla, G. V. (1992). Home care: Maintaining quality of life for patient and family. *Oncology, 6*(suppl.), 136-140.

Ferrell, B. R., Jacox, A., Miaskowski, C., Paice, J., & Hester, N. (1994). Cancer pain guidelines: Now that we have them, what do we do? *Oncology Nursing Forum, 21,* 1229-1230.

Foley, K. (1985). The treatment of cancer pain. *New England Journal of Medicine, 313,* 84-95.

France, R. D. (1987). The future for antidepressants: Treatment of pain. *Psychopathology, 20*(suppl. 1), 99-113.

Glare, P. A., & Walsh, T. D. (1993). Dose-ranging study of oxycodone for chronic pain in advanced cancer. *Journal of Clinical Oncology, 11,* 973-978.

Graves, D. A., Foster, B., Batenhorst, R., Bennett, R., & Baumann, T. (1983). Patient-controlled analgesia. *Annals of Internal Medicine, 99,* 360-366.

Gross, J., & Johnson, B. (Eds.). (1994). *Handbook of oncology nursing.* London: Jones and Bartlett, p. 286.

Gurian, B., & Rosowsky, E. (1990). Low dose methylphenidate in the very old. *Journal of Geriatric Psychiatry Neurology, 3,* 152-154.

Hamilton, J., & Edgar, L. (1992). A survey examining nurses' knowledge of pain control. *Journal of Pain and Symptom Management, 7,* 22-23.

Jacox, A., Carr, D. B., Payne, R., Berde, C. B., Breitbart, W., Cain, J. M., Chapman, C. R., Cleeland, C. S., Ferrell, B. R., Finley, R. S., Hester, N. O., Hill, C. S., Leak, W. D., Lipman, A. G., Logan, C. L., McGarvey, C. L., Miaskowski, C. A., Mulder, D. S., Paice, J. A., Shapiro, B. S., Silberstein, E. B., Smith, R. S., Stover, J., Tsou, C. V., Vecchiarelli, L., & Weissman, D. E. (1994). *Management of cancer pain. Clinical practice guideline.* AHCPR Pub. No. 94-0592. Rockville, MD: Agency for Health Care Policy and Research, PHS, USDHHS.

Kaiko, R. F., Foley, K. M., Grabinski, P. Y., Heidrich, G., Rogers, A. G., Inturrisi, C. E., & Reidenberg, M. M. (1983). Central nervous system excitatory effects of meperidine in cancer patients. *Annals of Neurology, 13,* 180-185.

Kanner, R. M., & Foley, K. M. (1981). Patterns of narcotic use in a cancer pain clinic. *Annals of the New York Academy of Science, 362,* 161-172.

Kehoe, W. A. (1993). Antidepressants for chronic pain: Selection and dosing considerations. *American Journal of Pain Management, 3,* 161-165.

Kelly, J. B., & Payne, R. (1991). Pain syndromes in the cancer patient. *Neurology Clinician, 9*(4), 937-953.

Kinzbrunner, B. M., Policzer, J., Miller, B., & Neiber, L. (1990). Noninvasive pain control in the terminally ill patient. *American Journal of Hospice and Palliative Care, 7*(4), 26-29.

Kinzbrunner, B. M., & Salerno, E. (1994). *Vitas pain management formulary* (2nd ed.). Miami: Vitas Healthcare Corporation.

Kurman, M. (1993). Systemic therapy (chemotherapy) in the palliative treatment of cancer pain. In R. B. Patt (Ed.), *Cancer pain* (pp. 251–274). Philadelphia: Lippincott.

Light, R. W., Muro, J. R., Sato, R. I., Stansbury, D. W., Fischer, C. E., & Brown, S. E. (1989). Effects of oral morphine on breathlessness and exercise tolerance in patients with chronic obstructive pulmonary disease. *American Review of Respiratory Disease, 139,* 126-133.

Maloney, C. M., Kesner, R. K., Klein, G., & Bockenstette, J. (1989). The rectal administration of MS contin: Clinical implications of use in end stage cancer. *American Journal of Hospice Care, 6*(7), 34-35.

Max, M. B., Schafer, S. C., Culnane, M., Smoller, B., Dubner, R., & Gracely, R. M. (1988). Amitriptyline, but not lorazepam, relieves postherpetic neuralgia. *Neurology, 38,* 1427-1432.

McCaffery, M., & Beebe, A. (1989). *Pain: Clinical manual for nursing practice.* St. Louis: Mosby.

McCracken, A. L., & Gerdsen, L. (1991). Sharing the legacy: Hospice care principles for terminally ill elders. *Journal of Gerentologic Nursing, 17*(12), 4-8.

Miser, A. W., Narang, P. K., Dothage, J. A., Young, R. C., Sindelar, W., & Miser, J. S. (1989). Transdermal fentanyl for pain control in patients with cancer. *Pain, 37,* 15-21.

Nelson, K. A., & Walsh, T. D. (1993). Metoclopromide in anorexia caused by cancer associated dyspepsia syndrome (CADS). *Journal of Palliative Care, 9*(2), 14-18.

Patt, R. B., Proper, G., & Reddy, S. (1994). The neuroleptics as adjuvant analgesics. *Journal of Pain and Symptom Management, 9,* 446-453.

Payne, R. (1987). Novel routes of opioid administration in the management of cancer pain. *Oncology,* April (suppl.), 10-18.

Plezia, P. M., Kramer, T. H., Linford, J., & Hameroff, S. R. (1989). Transdermal fentanyl: Pharmacokinetics and preliminary clinical evaluation. *Pharmacotherapy, 9,* 2-9.

Portenoy, R. K. (1988). Practical aspects of pain control in patients with cancer. *CA: A Cancer Journal for Clinicians, 38,* 327-352.

Portenoy, R. K., & Coyle, N. (1990). Controversies in the long-term management of analgesic therapy in patients with advanced cancer. *Journal of Pain and Symptom Management, 5,* 307-319.

Portenoy, R. K., & Hagan, N. A. (1990). Breakthrough pain: Definition, prevalence, and characteristics. *Pain, 41,* 273-281.

Poulter, C. A., Cosmatos, D., Rubin, P., et al. (1992). A report of RTOG 8206: A phase III study of whether the addition of single dose hemibody irradiation to standard fractionated local field irradiation is more effective than local field irradiation alone in the treatment of symptomatic osseous metastases. *International Journal of Radiation Oncology, Biology, Physics, 23,* 207-214.

Price, P., Hoskin, P. J., Easton, D., Austin, D., Palmer, S. G., & Yarnold, J. R. (1986). Prospective randomised trial of single and multifraction radiotherapy schedules in the treatment of painful bone metastases. *Radiotherapy and Oncology, 6,* 247-255.

Robinson, R. G., Preston, D. F., Baxter, K. G., Dusing, R. W., & Spicer, J. A. (1993). Clinical experience with strontium-89 in prostatic and breast cancer patients. *Seminars in Oncology, 20*(3), 44-48.

Santiago, T. V., & Edelman, N. H. (1985). Opioids and breathing. *Journal of Applied Physiology, 59,* 1675-1685.

Shapiro, R. S. (1994). Liability issues in the management of pain. *Journal of Pain and Symptom Management, 9,* 146-152.

Stambaugh, J. E. (1993). Role of nonsteroidal anti-inflammatory drugs in the management of cancer pain. In R. B. Patt (Ed.), *Cancer pain* (pp. 105-117). Philadelphia: Lippincott.

Storey, P., Hill, H. H., St. Louis, R. H., & Tarver, E. E. (1990). Subcutaneous infusions for control of cancer symptoms. *Journal of Pain and Symptom Management, 5,* 33-41.

Supportive care. (1994). In B. D. Cheson, R. L. Schlisky, F. R. Appelbaum et al. (Eds.), *Medical knowledge self-assessment program in the subspecialty of oncology (MKSAP)* (pp. 231-241). Philadelphia: American College of Physicians.

Tanelian, D. L., & Brose, W. G. (1991). Neuropathic pain can be relieved by drugs that are use-dependent sodium channel blockers: Lidocaine, carbamazepine, and mexiletine. *Anesthesiology, 74,* 949-951.

Teoh, N., & Stjernsward, J. (1992). WHO cancer pain relief program—Ten years on. *IASP Newsletter,* 5-6.

Twycross, R. G. (1988). The management of pain in cancer: A guide to drugs and dosages. *Oncology, 2*(4), 35-44, 47.

Ventafridda, V., Bianchi, M., Ripamonti, C., Sacerdote, P., DeConno, F., Zecca, E., & Panerai, A. E. (1990). Studies on the effects of antidepressant effects on the antinociceptive action of morphine and on plasma morphine in rat and man. *Pain, 43,* 155-162.

Von Roenn, J. H., Cleeland, C. S., Gonin, R., Hatfield, A. K., & Pandya, K. J. (1993). Physician attitudes and practice in cancer pain management: A survey from the Eastern Cooperative Oncology Group. *Annals of Internal Medicine, 119,* 121-126.

Watanabe, S., & Bruera, E. (1994). Corticosteroids as adjuvant analgesics. *Journal of Pain and Symptom Management, 9,* 442-445.

Watson, C. P. N. (1994a). Antidepressant drugs as adjuvant analgesics. *Journal of Pain and Symptom Management, 9,* 392-405.

Watson, C. P. N. (1994b). Topical capsaicin as an adjuvant analgesic. *Journal of Pain and Symptom Management, 9,* 425-433.

Weissman, D. E., Dahl, J. L., & Joranson, D. E. (1990). Oral morphine for the treatment of cancer pain. *PPO Updates, 4*(6), 1-8.

Welk, T. (1991). An educational model for explaining hospice services. *American Journal of Hospice and Palliative Care, 8*(5), 14-17.

Whedon, M., & Ferrell, B. (1991). Professional and ethical considerations in the use of high-tech pain management. *Oncology Nursing Forum, 18*(7), 1135-1143.

Wilkinson, T. J., Robinson, B. A., Begg, E. J., Duffull, S. B., Ravenscroft, P. J., & Schneider, J. J. (1992). Pharmacokinetics and efficacy of rectal versus oral sustained-release morphine in cancer patients. *Cancer Chemotherapy and Pharmacology, 31,* 251-254.

Woodcock, A. A., Gross, E. R., Gellert, A., Shah, S., Johnson, M., & Geddes, D. M. (1981). Effects of dihydrocodeine, alcohol, and caffeine on breathlessness and exercise tolerance in patients with chronic obstructive lung disease and normal blood gases. *New England Journal of Medicine, 305,* 1611-1616.

Woods, S. W., Tesar, G. E., Murray, G. B., & Cassem, N. H. (1986). Psychostimulant treatment of depressive disorders secondary to medical illness. *Journal of Clinical Psychiatry, 47,* 12-15.

World Health Organization (WHO). (1986). Comprehensive cancer pain management. In *Cancer pain relief* (pp. 7-8). Geneva: World Health Organization.

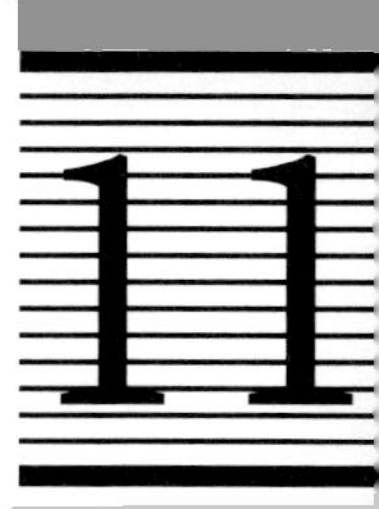

Pediatric Pain Management

Jackie Ochsenreither

Maria L. Cubina

Key Points

- Assessment of pain in pediatric patients may include approaches such as self-report, report by proxy, observational methods, or examination of physiologic indicators.
- Children may have difficulty describing their pain, and measuring it may be difficult.
- Reliable, valid, and developmentally appropriate pain assessment instruments should be utilized to measure and assess pain in pediatric patients.
- Nonpharmacologic and psychosocial interventions can be used as adjuncts to pharmacologic methods in the overall pain management plan.

- Children experience pain as adults do.
- Children have a larger volume of distribution and may have altered elimination half-lives compared with adults.
- A multidisciplinary pain management service can provide children with a broad-based approach to pain management incorporating pharmacologic and nonpharmacologic interventions.

Pain in the pediatric patient may be caused by acute, chronic, or malignant conditions. Although pediatric pain was underestimated and undertreated in the past, practitioners have recently come to recognize the necessity for research and study on pain management in children. A number of factors have contributed to the lack of research and study in this area. These include difficulties in pain assessment, ethical constraints, and lack of financial incentive for pharmaceutical companies to perform drug research on children. Since the landmark survey from Mather and Mackie (1983), which described the practice of pediatric pain management in two major teaching institutions and their inadequate management of pediatric pain, there has been a renewed interest in the management of pediatric pain. Mather and Mackie showed that analgesic medication was not ordered for 16% of the postoperative pediatric patients. When an opioid medication was ordered, 40% of these patients did not receive this medication in the regular inpatient care area. In addition, the pain medication ordered was the lowest amount possible, and it was ordered as pro re nata (prn). Once the medication was ordered, the nursing staff rarely gave the medication because they felt the children were "acting out" or that they needed to "grin and bear it." By the end of the first postoperative day the number of patients reporting no pain had increased, but the number of patients reporting severe pain had also increased (Mather & Mackie).

Multidisciplinary pediatric pain management services have been instituted in many of the major teaching institutions to combat the mismanagement of pediatric pain. This chapter will discuss the key issues in pediatric pain management.

DESCRIPTION

The study of pain in children has been only recently recognized (Anand, Sippell, & Aynsley-Green, 1987) as an area of clinical practice that requires more examination, discussion, and research. Children's pain can be categorized as acute, chronic (nonmalignant), recurrent, or cancer related. Acute pain can be produced by noxious or tissue-damaging stimuli of short duration. Chronic (nonmalignant) pain is a persistent pain that can be associated with chronic disease progression or with unresolved pain that has not relinquished despite tissue or bone healing. Children often interpret this painful event as a warning sign that something is wrong. Recurrent pain has been defined as the occurrence of more than three painful episodes within a 3-month period (Apley, 1976). Cancer pain is frequently undertreated in children (Miser, Dothage, Welsey, & Miser, 1987). Children with cancer experience pain from a variety of sources including cancer-related, therapy-related, debilitation, procedure-related, and other, unrelated medical conditions.

THERAPEUTIC MANAGEMENT

Assessment

Reliable, valid, and developmentally appropriate pain assessment instruments should be utilized to measure and assess pain in pediatric patients. Utilizing developmentally appropriate pain assessment methods can assist practitioners with identification of pain needs and formation of successful pain management strategies. Successful pain management strategies promote healing and recovery for the pediatric patient and assist the child in returning to a state of optimal health.

Assessment of pain in the pediatric patient may include approaches such as self-report, report by proxy, observational methods, and, as a last resort, examination of physiologic indicators. Self-report is a pain assessment method that can be used to estimate pain intensity and location in children more than 4 years of age (McGrath, 1990a, b). Practitioners utilizing self-report measures to assess pain in pediatric patients should recognize that some children who experience pain may deny or underreport it. This may be a result of the child's fear that admission of pain might stimulate additional painful procedures or tests, the child's lack of understanding regarding pain management and treatment, the desire to "live with the pain" according to religious upbringing or cultural bias, or the child's need to protect family and friends from knowledge of possible disease progression.

A variety of self-report methods for pain assessment and measurement have been reported (Beyer, Villarruel, & Denyes, 1993; Hester, Foster, Kristensen, & Bergstrom, 1989; McGrath, 1990b). The Oucher (Beyer et al.) and the Poker Chip Tool (Hester et al.) are two self-report methods appropriate for use with children more than 4 years of age. The Oucher pain rating scale, shown in Figure 11-1, is reliable, has adequate content validity, and correlates well with other visual analog scales (Mathews, McGrath, & Pigeon, 1993). However, the child must be able to understand proportionality to use the scale effectively. The numerical rating scale (McGrath & Unruh, 1987), the horizontal word graphic scale (Savedra, Tesler, Holzemer, & Ward, 1989), and the visual analog scale (Tesler, Savedra, Holzemer, Wilkie, & Paul, 1991) are additional examples of self-report methods that children more than 7 years of age may use to communicate their pain needs to practitioners (Figure 1-5 shows some of these scales). Although these scales are reliable, valid, and versatile, intervals on the numeric scales may not be equal from a child's perspective (Mathews et al.). In other words, the child may not perceive that the degree of pain measured between each pair of points directly correlates with the amount of escalating or declining pain being experienced.

Interestingly, some practitioners have used pediatric face interval scales as instruments of pain measurement in young children (Bieri, Reeve, Champion, Addicoat, & Ziegler, 1990;

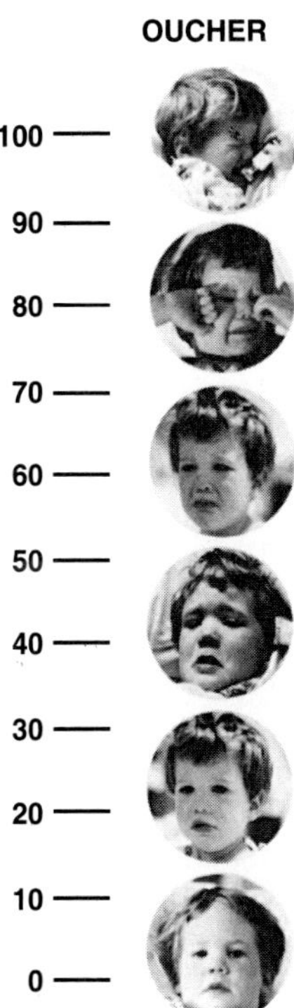

Figure 11-1 The Caucasian version of the Oucher, developed and copyrighted by Judith E. Beyer, RN, PhD, 1983.

McGrath, deVeber, & Hearn, 1985). Another faces scale (Whaley & Wong, 1987) remains popular, but reports of the degree of its reliability and validity are nearly impossible to find. These scales, for younger children (ages 3 to 6 years), may be preferable to more abstract scales. Although much information is available about these scales, there is little information regarding their use in the postoperative period (Maunuksela, Olkkala, & Korpela, 1987; Tyler, Douthit, & Chapman, 1993).

Also available is the Adolescent Pediatric Pain Tool (Savedra, Tesler, Holzemer, Wilkie, & Ward, 1989). Children can use the Adolescent Pediatric Pain Tool, shown in Figure 11-2, to illustrate the location of their discomfort to practitioners via a body map. Children 4 years of age or older can use crayons, chalk, or markers to color in the area(s) where they have pain on the body map. The older the child, the more precise the drawing. Further study is needed to evaluate its efficacy in younger patients.

Not surprisingly, children who are stressed from hospitalization or from demands of coping with an ongoing disease process may regress developmentally. Within this population, pain assessment and measurement may be even more challenging for experienced practitioners. In addition, practitioners may come to rely heavily on parents' perceptions of their child's pain (by proxy) to accurately assess the child's pain. However, this form of reporting is inexact and may be difficult to interpret correctly.

Behavioral observation is another pain assessment method practitioners can employ to assess and measure pain in the pediatric patient. Behavioral observation is the method of choice for pain assessment and measurement in preverbal and nonverbal children. It is also an alternative pain assessment and measurement method for use in verbal children.

Observation of pain behaviors in pediatric patients involves assessment of vocalizations, verbalizations, facial expressions, muscle tension and rigidity, ability to be consoled, guarding of body parts, temperament, activity, and general appearance (Jacox et al., 1994). The Attia (Attia, Ameil-Tison, Mayer, Shnider, & Barrier, 1987) and the Children's Hospital of Eastern Ontario (CHEOPS) pain rating scales (McGrath et al., 1985) are two examples of behavioral rating methods that can be used in preverbal or nonverbal children to assess and measure pain. The CHEOPS scale, in Table 11-1, has accumulated evidence for reliability and validity in the assessment of short, sharp pain. The Attia scale has been reported (Attia et al.) to be a reliable and

Text continues on p. 353.

CODE ____________

DATE ____________

ADOLESCENT PEDIATRIC PAIN TOOL (APPT)

INSTRUCTIONS:

1. Color in the areas on these drawings to show where you have pain. Make the marks as big or small as the place where the pain is.

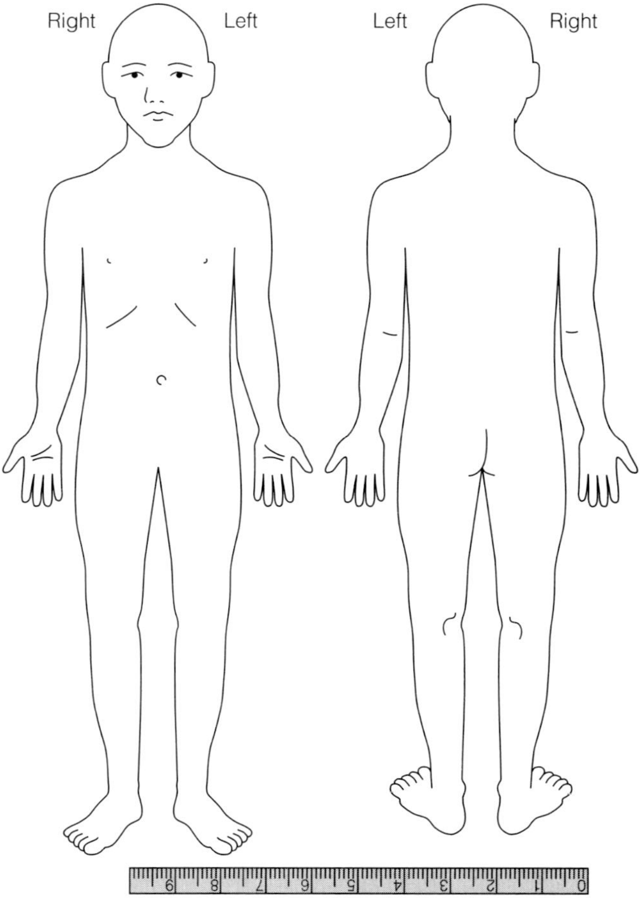

Right Left Left Right

Figure 11-2a Adolescent pediatric pain tool (APPT). (From Savedra, M. C., Tesler, M. D., Holzemer, W. L., & Ward, J. A. (1989). *Adolescent Pediatric Pain Tool (APPT) preliminary user's manual.* San Francisco: University of California School of Nursing.)

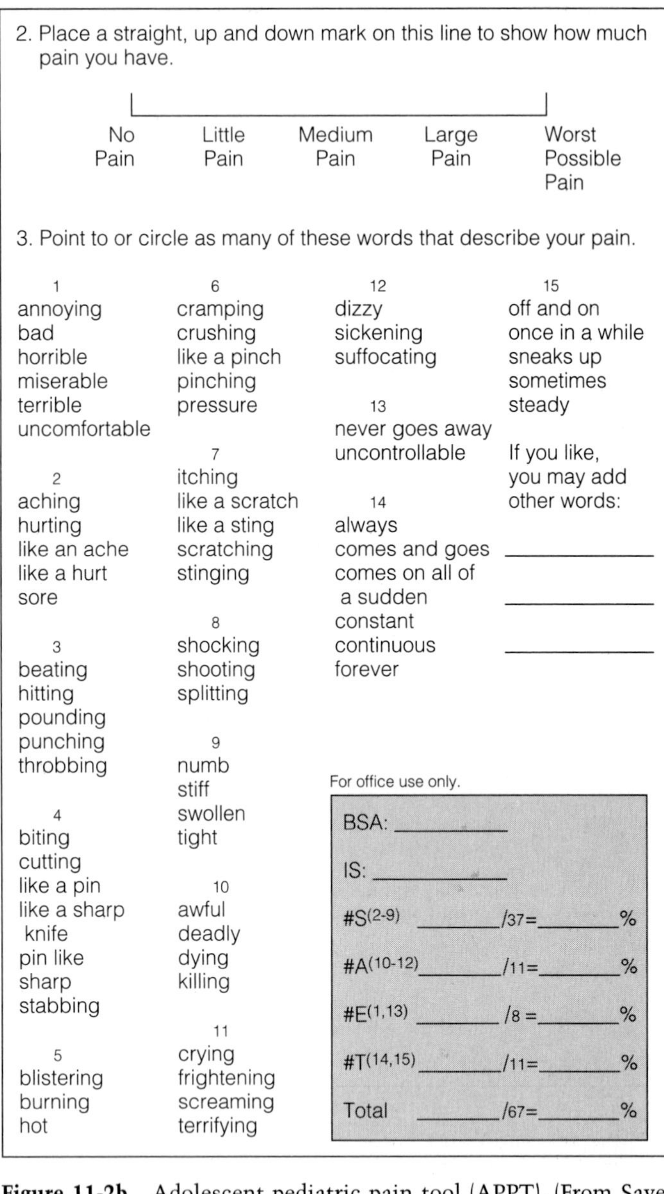

2. Place a straight, up and down mark on this line to show how much pain you have.

No Pain	Little Pain	Medium Pain	Large Pain	Worst Possible Pain

3. Point to or circle as many of these words that describe your pain.

1
annoying
bad
horrible
miserable
terrible
uncomfortable

2
aching
hurting
like an ache
like a hurt
sore

3
beating
hitting
pounding
punching
throbbing

4
biting
cutting
like a pin
like a sharp knife
pin like
sharp
stabbing

5
blistering
burning
hot

6
cramping
crushing
like a pinch
pinching
pressure

7
itching
like a scratch
like a sting
scratching
stinging

8
shocking
shooting
splitting

9
numb
stiff
swollen
tight

10
awful
deadly
dying
killing

11
crying
frightening
screaming
terrifying

12
dizzy
sickening
suffocating

13
never goes away
uncontrollable

14
always
comes and goes
comes on all of a sudden
constant
continuous
forever

15
off and on
once in a while
sneaks up
sometimes
steady

If you like, you may add other words:

____

____

____

For office use only.

BSA: __________

IS: __________

#S(2-9) ______/37=______%

#A(10-12) ______/11=______%

#E(1,13) ______/8 =______%

#T(14,15) ______/11=______%

Total ______/67=______%

Figure 11-2b Adolescent pediatric pain tool (APPT). (From Savedra, M. C., Tesler, M. D., Holzemer, W. L., & Ward, J. A. (1989). *Adolescent Pediatric Pain Tool (APPT) preliminary user's manual.* San Francisco: University of California School of Nursing.)

Table 11-1 CHEOPS

Item	Behavior	Rating	Definition
Cry	No crying	1	Child is not crying
	Moaning	2	Child is moaning or quietly vocalizing silent cry
	Crying	2	Child is crying, but the cry is gentle or whimpering
	Scream	3	Child is in a full-lunged cry; sobbing
			may be scored with complaint or without complaint
Facial	Composed	1	Neutral facial expression
	Grimace	2	Score only if definite negative facial expression
	Smiling	0	Score only if definite positive facial expression
Child verbal	None	1	Child is not talking
	Other complaints	1	Child complains but not about pain (e.g., "I want to see mommy" or "I am thirsty")
	Pain complaints	2	Child complains of pain
	Both complaints	2	Child complains about pain and other things (e.g., "It hurts, I want mommy")
	Positive	0	Child makes any positive statement or talks about other things without complaint

Continued.

Table 11-1 CHEOPS—cont'd

Item	Behavior	Rating	Definition
Torso	Neutral	1	Body (not limbs) is at rest; torso is inactive
	Shifting	2	Body is in motion in a shifting or serpentine fashion
	Tense	2	Body is arched or rigid
	Shivering	2	Body is shuddering or shaking involuntarily
	Upright	2	Child is in a vertical or upright position
	Restrained	2	Body is restrained
Touch	Not touching	1	Child is not touching or grabbing at wound
	Reach	2	Child is reaching for but not touching wound
	Grab	2	Child is grabbing vigorously at wound
	Restrained	2	Child's arms are restrained
Legs	Neutral	1	Legs may be in any position but are relaxed; includes gentle swimming or serpentine movements
	Squirming/kicking	2	Definitive uneasy or restless movements in the legs and/or striking out with foot or feet
	Drawn up/tensed	2	Legs tensed and/or pulled up tightly to body and kept there
	Standing	2	Standing, crouching, or kneeling
	Restrained	2	Child's legs are being held down

From McGrath, P. J., Johnson, G. L., Goodman, J. T., Schillinger, J., Dunn, J., & Chapman, J. (1985). The CHEOPS: A behavioral scale to measure postoperative pain in children. In H. L. Fields, R. Dubner, & F. Cervero (Eds.), *Advances in pain research and therapy* (pp. 395-402). New York: Raven Press.

valid measurement scale for postoperative pain in infants; however, replication studies are needed. In addition, clarification of how this scoring system might account for different coping strategies among infants should be examined.

Also available is the Pain Assessment Inventory for Neonates (Johnson, 1990). This scale incorporates behavioral state, respiratory rate, respiratory quality, heart rate, cry presence and intensity, facial expression, movements, color, and oxygen saturation into its scoring system. This scale was created to provide a multidimensional means of assessing acute pain in infants. Unfortunately, this measurement scale remains largely untested.

The Neonatal Infant Pain Scale (NIPS), designed by Lawrence and colleagues (1993), is a multiitem pain instrument that lends objectivity to the bedside nurse's assessment and documentation of infant behavior. The NIPS scale, in Figure 11-3, is reported to be nonintrusive and objective and provides a global assessment of pain (Lawrence et al., 1993). However, no studies have been done to evaluate its efficacy in the immediate postoperative period.

Observation of pain-related behaviors is not without difficulty. It can be arduous at times to accurately distinguish pain behaviors from behaviors resulting from other types of distress. Pediatric patients who are hungry or anxious may exhibit behaviors similar to those of children experiencing pain. These behaviors may include crying, screaming, or restlessness. Sleeping children are often misinterpreted as being pain free when in fact they may be overcome with pain and are sleeping from being exhausted by it (Jacox et al., 1994). Interestingly, facial expression interpretation has been found to be an alternative observational means of rating subtle behaviors in infants (Grunau & Craig, 1987). However, no work has been done to study this phenomenon in older children.

Additional factors that may inhibit accurate assessment and measurement of a child's pain intensity include intubation, depression, use of paralytic or sedative medications,

ID #: __________ Procedure: __________

Name: __________ Date of Procedure: __________

D.O.B.: __________ Procedure #: __________

Tape #: __________

	Before time		During time					After time		
	1	2	1	2	3	4	5	1	2	3
Facial expression 0 - Relaxed 1 - Grimace	1	2	1	2	3	4	5	1	2	3
Cry 0 - No cry 1 - Whimper 2 - Vigorous	1	2	1	2	3	4	5	1	2	3
Breathing patterns 0 - Relaxed/restrained 1 - Change in breathing	1	2	1	2	3	4	5	1	2	3
Arms 0 - Relaxed/restrained 1 - Flexed/extended	1	2	1	2	3	4	5	1	2	3
Legs 0 - Relaxed/restrained 1 - Flexed/extended	1	2	1	2	3	4	5	1	2	3
State of arousal 0 - Sleeping/awake 1 - Fussy	1	2	1	2	3	4	5	1	2	3
Total										

*Time is measured in one (1) minute intervals.

Figure 11-3 Neonatal infant pain scale (NIPS). (From Lawrence, J., Alcock, D., McGrath, P., Kay, J., MacMurray, S. B., & Dulberg, C. (1993). The development of a tool to assess neonatal pain. *Neonatal Network, 12*(6), 60.)

weakness, and critical illness (Mathews et al., 1993). When these factors exist, observational methods of pain assessment and measurement may become difficult to interpret. Examination of physiologic indicators may be incorporated into the assessment plan to aid the practitioner with estimation of a child's pain intensity. These indicators include heart rate, blood pressure, transcutaneous oxygen saturation, sweating, pupillary dilation, and EEG. Most important, physiologic indicators should not be used as a sole means of pain interpretation in children since indicators such as heart rate, respiratory rate, blood pressure, and saturated oxygen levels alter with a variety of stress arousal events. They should be examined and incorporated into the overall assessment plan in conjunction with other pain assessment methods.

Pharmacologic Interventions

A wide variety of pharmacologic interventions are available for the pediatric population. The most important aspect is to treat pain with the appropriate amount and type of medication. Pediatric pain should be managed by practitioners who have experience in the treatment of the pediatric patient. This does not mean that the person managing the pain must be a pediatrician or a pediatric anesthesiologist, but the practitioner must be sensitive to the issues specific to the pediatric patient. The knowledge of pharmacodynamic and pharmacokinetic properties of analgesics as they relate to the pediatric patient is key. The practitioner must understand that these properties may change in the ongoing developmental process from neonate to adolescent. Neonates must not be considered very tiny adults. Medication may have different pharmacodynamics on patients of different ages. These fundamental concepts must be well understood by the practitioner managing pain in the pediatric population so that proper doses are administered.

The most common nonopioid analgesic used in the pediatric population is acetaminophen or paracetamol. Although drug absorption and half-life may be prolonged in neonates (McGrath, 1990a), infants have pharmacokinetic properties similar to those of adults. Following oral administration acetaminophen blood levels peak in 30 to 60 minutes with a half-life of 2 hours. Actual analgesic levels are unknown since antipyretic levels are the only guide at this point. The most significant variable to be addressed is the route of delivery of the acetaminophen. Rectal suppositories have a wide range of absorption with almost a 50% bioavailability. Therefore larger rectal doses are necessary compared with oral administration. Dosages of 20 to 30 mg/kg rectally will achieve adequate antipyretic levels in the bloodstream. Oral dosing should be 10 to 15 mg/kg every 4 hours.

Nonsteroidal Antiinflammatory Analgesic Drugs

Nonsteroidal antiinflammatory drugs (NSAIDs) are effective in the treatment of a variety of pain syndromes, such as rheumatoid arthritis; bone, joint, and muscle pain; dental pain; menstrual pain; and headaches in the pediatric population. A major indication for their use is the types of pain associated with tissue swelling. It can also be used for closure of a patent ductus arteriosis in newborn and preterm infants. Aspirin, like other NSAIDs, inhibits platelet aggregation. Aspirin produces an irreversible inhibition lasting up to 2 weeks, whereas for the other NSAIDs inhibition lasts 48 to 72 hours. Gastritis is another side effect of all NSAIDs and should be a consideration in choosing these medications, especially for children who have preexisting gastrointestinal disease.

Acetylsalicylic acid (aspirin) continues to be used even though it poses a significant risk of Reye's syndrome in children. Aspirin has nonlinear elimination kinetics, showing slower elimination at higher serum salicylate levels. In neonates the elimination is significantly slower with progression to adult rates by 1 year of age (Levy & Garretson, 1974).

The newest NSAID, ketorolac, has not been approved for use by the Food and Drug Administration in the pediatric population. It is the first parenteral NSAID available in the United States and because of this has gained popularity quickly within the medical community. Ketorolac is also available in oral form. The rationale for using ketorolac is that it is not associated with respiratory depression or nausea and vomiting. Investigation in the adult population has shown that 30 mg given intramuscularly (IM) is equivalent to 12 mg of IM morphine (O'Hara, Fragen, Kinzer, & Pemberton, 1987). Children, although they have a larger volume of distribution and plasma clearance than adults, have a similar elimination half-life to that of adults (Olkkala & Maunuksela, 1991). Studies are still under way in the pediatric population, but a dose of 1 mg/kg is recommended as a loading dose and then 0.5 mg/kg every 6 hours intravenously/intramuscularly (IV/IM) is suggested (Olkkala & Maunuksela). It should be recognized that although the route of delivery is different from that of the other NSAIDs, the side effects are similar. Gastritis and gastrointestinal bleeding have been reported. In addition, there is some degree of platelet dysfunction due to prostaglandin synthesis suppression, making the use of this medication in the perioperative period questionable. In addition, as with other NSAIDS, there is a concern of significant depression of renal function in susceptible patients as well as a potential for hyperkalemia (Rotenberg & Giannini, 1992).

Ibuprofen, another NSAID available for oral dosing in liquid or tablet form, has both antiinflammatory and analgesic effects. The former occur peripherally, and the antipyretic effects occur centrally. The pharmacokinetics are similar to those of other antiinflammatory medications. Dosing for acute pain is 10 mg/kg every 6 hours. Diclofenac, another NSAID, has a plasma clearance in children about twice that of adults, and its elimination is mainly through metabolism in the liver. The maintenance dose must be higher in children to achieve a steady state (Korpela & Olkkala, 1990). Piroxicam is an antiinflammatory agent that has a very prolonged half-life in children. This allows for once-a-day dosing. The elimination half-life is 30 to 35 hours, which is about

20 hours shorter than for adults. This seems to be caused by the higher clearance of piroxicam in children. The volume of distribution is the same as for adults (Mäkelä, Olkkala, & Mattila, 1991).

Opioids

Opioid analgesics are reserved for moderate to severe pain. The respiratory depression associated with all opioids should cause the practitioner to think twice about administering opioids to the pediatric population. However, with careful titration and monitoring in all patients this complication can be quickly recognized and treated. This is especially important in the infant less than 2 months of age because the incidence of respiratory depression is greatest in this age group. Infants less than 2 months of age, especially premature infants, have immature respiratory centers that may be more sensitive to the depressant effects of the opioids. In addition, renal and hepatic function of the neonate may still be immature, and excretion of opioids may be delayed. The opioids discussed in this section include morphine, fentanyl, meperidine, hydromorphone, codeine, and opioid agonist-antagonists. Discussion about these opioids (presented in depth in Chapter 4) centers around the special needs of the pediatric patient.

Morphine, a derivative of the opium plant, is one of the most widely administered analgesics. The intravenous dose for the pediatric patient is 0.1 mg/kg every 3 to 4 hours. The half-life clearance of morphine in children older than 2 months is similar to that for adults. When used in the infant less than 2 months of age it should be administered in a monitored setting such as an intensive care unit (ICU) or intermediate care area (Schechter, Berde, & Yaster, 1993). In patients with severe pain who are less than 8 years of age, a group for which patient-controlled analgesia (PCA) is difficult to use, a continuous infusion of morphine at dosages of 0.02 to 0.03 mg/kg/hr is effective. In the older child (usually more than 8 years of age), PCA has been used with excellent results. (Chapter 8 discusses PCA in depth.) It allows children to have control in a setting where many health care providers are deciding their care. A recommended dose is 0.015 mg/kg with a lockout time of 5 to 8 minutes and a total hourly maximum of 0.1 mg/kg/hr. If pain is not well controlled with this strategy, a background continuous infusion of 0.015 mg/kg/hr may be added with the same total hourly maximum of 0.1 mg/hr.

It should be stressed that these are only guidelines, and each child should be treated as an individual with a possible need of increasing or decreasing the dose. In addition, greater amounts of an opioid are associated with a higher incidence of side effects, and this should be taken into consideration in deciding on a dose of medication.

Morphine may also be administered orally. Only 30% to 40% of the orally administered dose of morphine reaches the systemic circulation (Gourlay, Plummer, Cherry, Foate, & Cousins, 1989; O'Hara, McGrath, D'Astous, & Vair, 1987). A key factor in converting an intravenous dose of morphine to an oral dose is that the oral dose is approximately three times the intravenous dose. The oral dose is available in immediate-release and slow-release preparations. The decision of which to use depends on the intensity and chronicity of pain. For a child with a chronic condition where a constant blood level of opioid is needed, a slow-release preparation given three or four times a day may be better than the immediate-release form given every 2 hours. The immediate-release preparation is available as a liquid or a tablet.

Fentanyl, a highly lipid-soluble opioid, is 100 times more potent than morphine. Its rapid onset and short half-life make it an ideal analgesic for short procedures such as reduction of fractures or suturing of lacerations. It can be used in doses of 1 to 3 μg/kg, titrated slowly IV, and may be repeated or used as an infusion of 1 to 3 μg/kg/hr. Fentanyl's pharmacokinetics differ among infants, children, and adults. The plasma clearance in children from 3 to 12 months of age is greater than in children older than 12 months or adults

(Singleton, Rosen, & Fisher, 1987). Repeated doses of fentanyl (over a 24-hour period) in a child 12 months old or older may cause accumulation of fentanyl, which may lead to respiratory depression. On the other hand, the greater clearance of fentanyl in children 3 to 12 months old may allow them to tolerate more of the opioid and be less sensitive to the respiratory depressant effect of fentanyl (Schechter et al., 1993). Intravenous fentanyl should be titrated slowly, with the appropriate monitoring in place, and emergency airway equipment should be available at the bedside. Sufentanil and alfentanil, derivatives of fentanyl, are rarely used for pain management in the pediatric patient. Sufentanil is 10 times more potent than fentanyl, and alfentanil is 10 times less potent than fentanyl. Equipotent doses, however, would provide similar analgesia.

Meperidine, a synthetic opioid, may be used for children as a postoperative analgesic or as a premedication for anesthesia. It is 10 times less potent than morphine and also differs from morphine in that very large doses may produce slow waves on the EEG. In addition, very high levels of meperidine's primary metabolite, normeperidine, may cause tremors or convulsions. It is therefore suggested that meperidine not be used for prolonged periods of time. The suggested dose of 1 mg/kg every 2 to 3 hours may be used for management of acute pain. Meperidine, as a one-time dose of 0.5 to 1 mg/kg, may also be used to counteract shivering that may occur after anesthesia. Respiratory depression or gastric dysmotility are side effects that occur as with other opioids, with the exception that respiratory depression is seen as a decrease in tidal volume rather than a decrease in respiratory rate. The one opioid side effect that is not shared by merperidine is sphincter of Oddi spasm. For this reason meperidine may be a better opioid choice for the patient with gall bladder disease. In addition, administration of meperidine causes tachycardia and a 20% decrease in cardiac output (Priano & Vatner, 1981).

Hydromorphone, a derivative of morphine, is 6 to 7 times more potent and 2 to 10 times more lipid-soluble than morphine. It has a rapid onset and a duration of 4 to 6 hours.

Used frequently as a substitute for morphine because it is associated with fewer side effects and less sedation, it is effective when administered IV, subcutaneously (SQ), epidurally, and orally. The IV route is the most popular for postoperative pain relief. The loading dose is 0.005 to 0.015 mg/kg. It may be followed by a continuous infusion of 0.003 to 0.005 mg/kg/hr. If bolus doses of hydromorphone are needed, the dose should be 0.003 to 0.005 mg/kg administered every 3 to 4 hours or in the form of PCA by the patient.

Codeine is one of the most popular oral opioids given today. It is an excellent oral analgesic, especially when given in combination with acetaminophen. It can also be used as an antitussive. Intravenous administration of codeine is associated with apnea and hypotension; therefore IV administration is not recommended for the pediatric patient. The usual dose of oral codeine is 0.5 to 1 mg/kg combined with 15 to 20 mg/kg of acetaminophen. The dose as an antitussive is one-half the analgesic dose. Other, similar opioids such as oxycodone are also available. Their advantage may be better gastrointestinal tolerance.

Opioid agonist-antagonists are used in the pediatric population with increasing frequency. These medications are becoming popular not only as first-line analgesics but as adjuvants to help counteract the side effects associated with opioids, such as respiratory depression, nausea, vomiting, and pruritus, without decreasing the analgesic effect of the opioid (Bailey et al., 1987; Moldenhauer et al., 1985; Murphy, 1989). Their primary disadvantage as analgesics is the "ceiling effect" associated with larger doses of medication and the sedation they produce. Nalbuphine is the most commonly used opioid agonist-antagonist in the pediatric population. The most common side effect is sedation, but it has the added advantage that dysphoria is rare. The dosage of nalbuphine to help reverse the side effects of opioids is 0.05 to 0.1 mg/kg given every 4 to 6 hours prn. Nalbuphine can be given orally or parenterally, althought the oral form is not available in the United States. Only 20% to 30% of the oral dose reaches the systemic circulation.

Regional Analgesia

Regional analgesia is widely used in the pediatric population for both therapeutic and diagnostic reasons. The disadvantage of using regional analgesia in the pediatric population is the difficulty of placing a regional technique on a young child. For these reasons, regional analgesia or anesthesia is usually started while the child is asleep with a general anesthetic or under deep sedation. Continuing the regional technique for postoperative analgesia is very popular. An epidural catheter, placed following the induction of anesthesia, is dosed and maintained during the anesthetic. The analgesia of the epidural anesthetic is then carried to the postoperative period for pain relief. Epidural analgesia can be dosed with a variety of medications, the most popular being morphine. Epidural fentanyl at the lumbar area has been found to be as effective as parenteral fentanyl, and fentanyl administered at the thoracic area has been found to provide superior analgesia to parenterally administered fentanyl (Salomaki, Laitinen, & Nuutinen, 1991).

The most popular medications infused via the epidural catheter are combinations of local anesthetic and opioid. The infusion must be made by a pharmacist or a health care provider trained in mixing the infusion. Local anesthetics, such as bupivacaine, are most commonly used. Low doses of bupivacaine block pain fibers well with minimal motor block (see Chapter 14). Dosing of epidural analgesia should be done only by an anesthesiologist well versed in the management of epidural analgesia or by a clinical nurse specialist or nurse practitioner under the direction of an anesthesiologist.

Much has been written about the worrisome complication of central nervous system toxicity associated with epidural analgesia in the pediatric population (Berde, 1992; Rasch, Webster, Polard, & Gurkowski, 1990; Valley & Bailey, 1991; Wood, Goresky, Klassen, Kuwahara, & Neil, 1994). Berde has developed guidelines to assist the practitioner in the management of epidural analgesia in the pediatric population. Children are not more resistant to local anesthetic toxicity, as was previously thought (McIlvaine, Chang,

& Jones, 1988; McIlvaine, Knox, Fennessey, & Goldstein, 1988). It is suggested that the practitioner not exceed recommended local anesthetic infusion rates in the pediatric population. The infusion rate after a loading dose of 2 to 2.5 mg/kg of bupivicaine should probably not exceed 0.4 to 0.5 mg/kg/hr for infants and older children or 0.2 to 0.25 mg/kg/hr for neonates (Agarwal, Gutlove, & Lockhart, 1992). An alternative to increasing the infusion is adding an opioid to the epidural infusion. It is strongly suggested that parenteral opioids not be given in addition to opioids in the epidural infusions since the incidence of respiratory depression is greatly increased in these circumstances (Valley & Bailey). In addition, patients with history of a seizure disorder should probably have lower infusion rates (Berde).

Although postoperative pain relief is the most common use for epidural analgesia, it can also be used for chronic pain syndromes. Reflex sympathetic dystrophy (RSD) is a complicated pain syndrome that can become very debilitating, causing children to miss school, and can have severe psychologic ramifications. Epidural analgesia has been used to help in the diagnosis and treatment of RSD. In addition, epidural analgesia can be used to manage the chronic pain associated with cancer.

Other regional techniques can be used in the pediatric population, including axillary blocks for arm surgery, celiac plexus blocks for abdominal pain, interscalene and cervical plexus blocks for shoulder and arm pain, and intercostal nerve blocks for rib, chest, and upper abdominal pain. These techniques, in the hands of a skilled pediatric anesthesiologist can offer pain relief to both acute and chronic pain patients. (Refer to Chapter 14.)

There are also other medications that can assist the health care provider in relieving pain, especially in the emergency department, where suturing or other painful procedures are common. One is the use of a eutectic mixture of local anesthetic (lidocaine and prilocaine), or EMLA. Placed 1 hour in advance to the area where an IV will be placed or a lumbar punture is to be performed, the procedure will reduce pain. There is a potential to induce methemoglobinemia if an excessively large amount is applied for longer than necessary. A popular medication for use in the suturing of lacerations is a tetracaine, adrenaline, and cocaine mixture known as TAC. This medication can be placed on a pledget or sponge and placed directly on the wound to be sutured. Using a dilute solution (1.0% tetracaine, adrenaline 1:4000, and 4.0% cocaine) at a dose of 1.5 ml/10 kg will deliver 1.5 mg/kg tetracaine and 6.0 mg/kg cocaine. With this concentration there is little potential of achieving toxic systemic levels (Coté, 1994).

Procedural pain and sedation is a topic that has gained much attention recently. There are techniques in addition to the use of pharmacologic interventions that can assist the practitioner. The time of sedation needed for the procedure and the pharmacokinetics of the medications used must be considered. In other words, one should not use a medication that will last 2 or more hours for a 10-minute procedure. Techniques such as distraction can assist the practitioner in making a child comfortable for a procedure. Having the parent present may also be helpful. It should be clearly explained to both parent and child what the procedure will entail. The most important issue to keep in mind is careful monitoring and titration, allowing each dose of medication time to take effect before the next dose is administered. The person who is to perform the procedure should not be the person who is sedating or documenting the vital signs of the patient.

Nonpharmacologic Interventions

Cutaneous stimulation, exercise, immobilization, transcutaneous nerve stimulation (TENS), and acupuncture are examples of nonpharmacologic physical modalities that children can use to manage pain. These modalities assist children with relaxation and distraction from painful stimuli. Most of these methods are noninvasive and can be utilized by children at home or at school. In addition, these measures can be used with other pharmacologic methods to augment the overall pain management plan. (Chapter 5 explains these interventions in detail.) The interventions described here are useful for children.

Cutaneous stimulation can involve massage, vibration, pressure, and cold or heat application to afflicted or non-afflicted body parts. It has been found to be an adjunct therapy for pain relief in children, although an increase in pain may occur briefly before relief is experienced with its use (McCaffery & Beebe, 1989). Cutaneous stimulation provides relief from discomfort and activity-limiting affliction by increasing blood flow to the skin and superficial organs, reducing inflammation and edema to injured areas, and relaxing tightened or knotted musculature. Caution is necessary when placing a heat or cold application on body parts. Young children should be supervised by adults when these modalities are used since thermal or frostbite injuries may occur if temperature levels are inexact or if hot or cold packs are applied directly to skin surfaces without protective barriers.

Some children use exercise as a strategy for pain relief and stress reduction. Exercise enables children to maintain some level of activity by mobilizing joints, stretching muscles, and restoring coordination and balance. An exercise program should be appropriate to the child's developmental level and current conditioning. Proper supervision is necessary for children engaging in a nonformalized exercise program to decrease the incidence of possible injury related to overstraining or improper technique.

Immobilization can be employed to manage acute injuries related to bone fractures or limb or joint disturbances. Immobilization of afflicted body parts may help reduce pain and discomfort for the child and possibly reduce the need for pharmacologic intervention. However, prolonged immobilization can lead to contracture formation, muscle atrophy, and other untoward effects.

Transcutaneous electrical nerve stimulation (TENS) has been reported (Sjolund & Eriksson, 1985) to stimulate endogenous pain-modulating pathways by direct stimulation of peripheral nerves. (Chapter 8 discusses TENS in greater detail.) The TENS unit delivers controlled, low-voltage electric current to peripheral nerve fibers via cutaneous electrodes. The child can wear the device at school, at home, or when playing with friends or family. The child can also modulate the frequency, intensity, and pattern of current delivered to the targeted area. The TENS unit offers children who suffer from muscle strain or injury an alternative, noninvasive means of treatment that allows them to actively participate in their plan of care with some sense of control.

Acupuncture is a neurostimulatory technique that is an alternative therapy for the treatment of pain in adults and children. (Refer to Chapter 7 for more information.) It involves the insertion of fine needles into the skin to varying depths of musculature. There have been few well-controlled studies (Patel, Gutzwiller, Paccaud, & Marrazzi, 1989; ter Riet, Kleijnen, & Knipschild, 1990) documenting acupuncture's role in pain relief. It is not known which type of pain best responds to acupuncture intervention. Adjunctive treatment with pharmacologic methods may be necessary to manage specific pain needs unrelieved by this technique.

Cognitive and behavioral interventions assist children in coping with anxiety and discomfort related to painful procedures or stimuli. Cognitive methods can influence children's perception of events and bodily sensations. Cognitive techniques help children regain a sense of control over their pain and help them return to activities of daily living. Early intervention with these techniques can assist patients and families in coping with acute or chronic pain needs and enhance the multidimensional pain management strategy. (Chapter 5 discusses cognitive and behavioral interventions in great detail.)

Relaxation techniques used by children to create a sense of relaxation and calmness can also assist with coping with painful procedures or illnesses. Imagery helps children focus on pleasant experiences, which helps them return to a state of well-being or contentment. Frequently used modalities include deep breathing, meditation, muscle relaxation, and music-assisted relaxation. Optimal response may occur when imagery and relaxation techniques are used concurrently.

Distraction is a behavioral technique children can employ to help manage pain during a procedure, injury, or chronic condition. Teaching children distraction techniques provides them with alternative therapies for pain control and management. Distractions enable children to cope during painful situations by shifting their attention and concentration from painful foci. Many different distractive techniques are available for children to use during a painful event. These include deep breathing, counting, bubble blowing, storytelling, watching television, playing music, and singing.

Biofeedback is an additional adjunctive therapy practitioners can utilize to assist children who are coping with pain needs. Biofeedback involves teaching children how to establish and maintain a sense of focus to produce a specific behavioral response. Highly trained individuals are needed to teach children specific relaxation methods enhanced by sensitive electronic equipment. A limitation of biofeedback is its lack of efficacy in children who are unable or developmentally limited in their ability to focus and target responses.

Hypnosis is another therapy children can employ to help manage their pain. Hypnosis is a therapy that can place a child in a trancelike state. This state can heighten a child's awareness and improve the ability to focus in order to manipulate pain perception. Manipulation of pain perception may help children cope better during painful procedures and limit the amount of pharmacologic intervention needed.

TEAM APPROACH

The multidisciplinary approach is the basis for the optimal pain management. This team includes highly specialized and trained practitioners. The team is generally led by a professional from the department of anesthesia, who is surrounded by pediatrics specialists. One of the key players is a clinical nurse specialist (CNS) educated in pediatric care and specializing in pediatric pain. The functions of the CNS are manifold. First the CNS acts as a liaison between the pain management service and the department of nursing. This person troubleshoots both clinical activity and interpersonal relationships with the team and the nursing department. The CNS also acts as a knowledge base for the house staff and the ancillary staff, developing educational programs and inservices for the hospital so that all may be familiar with the equipment and the signs and symptoms of pain.

The psychiatrist or psychologist is another key member of the multidisciplinary team. The psychosocial issues surrounding the acute and especially the chronic pain patient is multifactorial. This person must be well educated in pediatric psychiatry and the issues surrounding pain. Frequently the family as a whole is touched by the one child who has a pain problem, and family counseling may be necessary. The child may become withdrawn and antisocial and have emotional lability. These children may not be able to attend school; therefore their education falls behind, and they lose the friendships that have been developed in this setting.

Physical therapy is an important aspect of management of the pain patient. These patients may need the therapy for improvement of their syndrome, to keep active, and sometimes for management of the pain itself. Specialized pediatric physical therapists may be associated with major teaching institutions or can be part of a free-standing rehabilitation center. It is important to keep these patients involved in their therapy and active in the community. In addition to physical therapy, other approaches such as art therapy and TENS units may help a pediatric pain patient through a difficult period.

It is imperative that a pain management service be an organized and well-managed department with practitioners working together for the best interests of the pediatric patient. This team can also act as a resource for institutions that do not have a pain management service.

SUMMARY

Accurate assessment and measurement of pain is vital in determining the exact location and intensity of a child's or infant's discomfort. Developmentally appropriate pain assessment instruments should be utilized to measure and assess pain in these patients. Practitioners may employ pharmacologic and/or nonpharmacologic modalities to manage pain in these patients. A multidisciplinary pain management service can provide the child and family with a broad-based approach to pain management that incorporates pharmacologic and nonpharmacologic interventions into the overall pain management strategy. This comprehensive, multidimensional approach can assist children with management of their pain needs, promote healing and recovery, and return them to a state of optimal health.

References

Agarwal, R., Gutlove, D. P., & Lockart, C. H. (1992). Seizures occurring in pediatric patients receiving continuous infusions of bupivacaine. *Anesthesia and Analgesia, 75,* 284-286.

Anand, K. J. S., Sippell, W. G., & Aynsley-Green, A. (1987). Randomized trial of fentanyl anesthesia in preterm babies undergoing surgery: Effects on stress response. *Lancet, 1,* 243-248.

Apley, J. (1976). Pain in childhood. *Journal of Psychosomatic Research, 20,* 383-389.

Attia, J., Amiel-Tison, C., Mayer, M. N., Shnider, S. M., & Barrier, G. (1987). Measurement of postoperative pain and narcotic administration in infants using a new clinical scoring system. *American Society of Anesthesiology Abstracts, 67*(3A), A532.

Bailey, P., Clark, N., Pace, N., Stanley, T. H., East, K. A., van Vreeswijk, H., van de Pol, P., Clissold, M. A., & Rozendaal, W. (1987). Antagonism of postoperative opioid-induced respiratory depression: Nalbuphine versus naloxone. *Anesthesia and Analgesia, 66,* 1109-1114.

Berde, C. B. (1992). Convulsions associated with pediatric regional anesthesia. *Anesthesia and Analgesia, 75,* 164-166.

Beyer, J. E., Villarruel, A. M., & Denyes, M. (1993). *The Oucher: The new user's manual and technical report.* Evanston, IL: Judson.

Bieri, D., Reeve, R. A., Champion, G. D., Addicoat, L., & Ziegler, J. B. (1990). The Faces Pain Scale for the self-assessment of the severity of pain experienced by children: Development, initial validation, and preliminary investigation for ratio scale properties. *Pain, 41,* 139-150.

Coté, C. J. (1994). Sedation for the pediatric patient: A review. *Pediatric Anesthesia, 41,* 31-58.

Gourlay, G. K., Plummer, J. L., Cherry, D. A., Foate, L. A., & Cousins, M. L. (1989). Influence of a high-fat meal on the absorption of morphine from oral solutions. *Clinical Pharmacology and Therapeutics, 46,* 463-468.

Granu, R. V. E., & Craig, K. D. (1987). Pain expression in neonates: Facial action and cry. *Pain, 28,* 395-410.

Hester N. O., Foster R., Kristensen K., & Bergstrom, L. (1989). Measurement of children's pain by children, parents, and nurses: Psychometric and clinical issues related to the Poker Chip Tool and Pain Ladder. Final grant report. Generalizability of procedures assessing pain in children. Research funded by NIH, National Center for Nursing Research under Grant Number R23NRO1382, Sept. 1, 1986, through Aug. 31, 1988. (Available from N. O. Hester, Center for Nursing Research, School of Nursing, University of Colorado, Denver, CO 80262.)

Jacox, A., Carr, D. B., Payne, R., Berde, C. B., Breitbart, W., Cain, J. M., Chapman, C. R., Cleeland, C.S., Ferrell, B. R., Finley, R. S., Hester, N. O., Hill, C. S., Leak, W. D., Lipman, A. G., Logan, C. L., McGarvey, C. L., Miaskowski, C. A., Mulder, D. S., Paice, J. A., Shapiro, B. S., Silberstein, E. B., Smith, R. S., Stover, J., Tsou, C. V., Vecchiarelli, L., & Weissman, D. E. (1994). *Management of cancer pain. Clinical practice guideline.* AHCPR Pub. No. 94-0592. Rockville, MD: Agency for Health Care Policy and Research, PHS, USDHHS.

Johnson, M. R. (1990). Pain response in preterm infants. *Infant Behavioral Development, 67,* A440.

Korpela, R., Olkkala, K. T. (1990). Pharmacokinetics of intravenous diclofenac sodium in children. *European Journal of Clinical Pharmacology, 38,* 293-295.

Lawrence, J., Alcock, D., McGrath, P., Kay, J., MacMurray, S. B., & Dulberg, C. (1993). The development of a tool to assess neonatal pain. *Neonatal Network, 12*(6), 59-66.

Levy, G., & Garretson, L. K. (1974). Kinetics of salicylate elimination by newborn infants of mother who ingested aspirin before delivery. *Pediatrics, 53,* 201-210.

Mäkelä, A. L., Olkkala, K. T., Mattila, M. J. (1991). Steady state pharmacokinetics of piroxicam in children with rheumatoid diseases. *European Journal of Clinical Pharmacology, 41,* 79-81.

Mather, L., & Mackie, J. (1983). The incidence of postoperative pain in children. *Pain, 15,* 271-282.

Mathews, J. R., McGrath, P. J., & Pigeon, H. (1993). Assessment and measurement of pain in children. In N. L. Schechter, C. B. Berde, & M. Yaster (Eds.), *Pain in infants, children, and adolescents* (pp. 97-111). Baltimore: Williams & Wilkins.

Maunuksela, E. L., Olkkala, K. T., & Korpela, R. (1987). Measurement of pain in children with self-reporting and behavioral assessment. *Clinical Pharmacology and Therapeutics, 42,* 137-141.

McCaffery, M., & Beebe, A. (1989). *Pain: Clinical manual for nursing practice.* St. Louis: Mosby.

McGrath, P. A. (1990a). *Pain in children.* New York: Guilford.

McGrath, P. A. (1990b). *Pain in children: Nature, assessment, and treatment.* New York: Guilford.

McGrath, P. A., deVeber, L. L., & Hearn, M. T. (1985). Multidimensional pain assessment in children. In H. L. Fields, R. Dubner, & F. Cervero (Eds.), *Proceedings of the Fourth World Congress on Pain, Seattle: Vol. 9. Advances in pain research and therapy* (pp. 387-393). New York: Raven Press.

McGrath, P. J., Johnson, G. L., Goodman, J. T., Schillinger, J., Dunn, J., & Chapman, J. (1985). The CHEOPS: A behavioral scale to measure postoperative pain in children. In H. L. Fields, R. Duber, & F. Cervero (Eds.), *Advances in pain research and therapy* (pp. 395-402). New York: Raven Press.

McGrath, P. J., & Unruh, A. M. (1987). *Pain in children and adolescents.* New York: Elsevier Science.

McIlvaine, W., Chang, J. H. T., & Jones, M. (1988). The effective use of interpleural bupivacaine for analgesia after thoracic and subcostal incisions in children. *Journal of Pediatric Surgery, 23,* 1184-1187.

McIlvaine, W. B., Knox, R. F., Fennessey, P. V., & Goldstein, M. (1988). Continuous infusion of bupivicaine via intrapleural catheter for analgesia after thoracotomy in children. *Anesthesiology, 69,* 261-264.

Miser, A. W., Dothage, J. A., Welsey, R. A., & Miser, J. S. (1987). The prevalence of pain in a pediatric and young adult cancer population. *Clinical Journal of Pain, 29*(1), 73-83.

Moldenhauer, C. C., Roach, G. W., Finlayson, D. C., Hug, C. C., Kopel, M. E., Tobia, V., & Kelly, S. (1985). Nalbuphine antagonism of ventilatory depression following high-dose fentanyl anesthesia. *Anesthesiology, 62,* 647-650.

Murphy, M. R. (1989). Opioids. In P. G. Barash, B. F. Cullen, & R. K. Stoelting (Eds.), *Clinical anesthesia* (pp. 255-279). Philadelphia: Lippincott.

O'Hara, D. A., Fragen, R. J., Kinzer, M., & Pemberton, D. (1987). Ketorolac trimethamine as compared with morphine sulfate for treatment of postoperative pain. *Clinical Pharmacology and Therapeutics, 41,* 556-561.

O'Hara, M., McGrath, P. J., D'Astous, J., & Vair, C. A. (1987). Oral morphine versus injected meperidine (Demerol) for pain relief in children after orthopedic surgery. *Journal of Pediatric Orthopedics, 7,* 78-82.

Olkkala, K., & Maunuksela, E. (1991). The pharmacokinetics of postoperative IV ketorolac tromethamine in children. *British Journal of Clinical Pharmacology, 31,* 182-184.

Patel, M., Gutzwiller, F., Paccaud, F., & Marrazzi, A. (1989). A meta-analysis of acupuncture for chronic pain. *International Journal of Epidemiology, 18*(4), 900-906.

Priano, L. L., & Vatner, S. F. (1981). Generalized cardiovascular and regional hemodynamic effects of meperidine on conscious dogs. *Anesthesia and Analgesia, 60,* 649-654.

Rasch, D. K., Webster, D. E., Polard, T. G., & Gurkowski, M. A. (1990). Lumbar and thoracic epidural analgesia via the caudal approach for the postoperative pain relief in infants and children. *Canadian Journal of Anaesthesia, 37,* 359-362.

Rotenberg, F. A., & Giannini, V. S. (1992). Hyperkalemia associated with ketorolac. *Annals of Pharmacotherapy, 26,* 778-779.

Salomaki, T. E., Laitinen, J. O., & Nuutinen, L. S. (1991). A randomized, double-blind comparison of epidural versus intravenous fentanyl infusion for analgesia after thoracotomy. *Anesthesiology, 75,* 790-795.

Savedra, M. C., Tesler, M. D., Holzemer, W. L., & Ward, J. A. (1989). [Updated 1992]. *Adolescent Pediatric Pain Tool (APPT) preliminary user's manual.* San Francisco: University of California.

Savedra, M. C., Tesler, M. D., Holzemer, W. L., Wilkie, D. J., & Ward, J. A. (1989). Pain location: Validity and reliability of body outline markings by hospitalized children and adolescents. *Research in Nursing and Health, 12*(5), 307-314.

Schechter, N. L., Berde, C. B., & Yaster, M. (1993). *Pain in infants and children.* Baltimore: Williams & Wilkens.

Singleton, M. A., Rosen, J. I., & Fisher, D. M. (1987). Plasma concentration of fentanyl in infants, children and adults. *Canadian Journal of Anaesthesia, 34,* 152-155.

Sjolund, B., & Ericksson, M. (1985). *Relief of pain by TENS.* Chichester, England: John Wiley & Sons.

ter Riet, G., Kleijnen, J., & Knipschild, P. (1990). Acupuncture and chronic pain: A criteria-based meta-analysis. *Journal of Clinical Epidemiology, 43*(11), 1191-1199.

Tesler, M. D., Savedra, M. C., Holzemer, W. L., Wilkie, D. J., & Paul, S. M. (1991). The word-graphic rating scale as a measure of children's and adolescent's pain intensity. *Research in Nursing and Health, 14*(5), 361-371.

Tyler, D. C., Douthit, J., & Chapman, C. R. (1993). Toward validation of pain measurement tools for children: A pilot study. *Pain, 52,* 301-309.

Valley, R. D., & Bailey, A. G. (1991). Caudal morphine for postoperative analgesia in infants and children: A report of 138 cases. *Anesthesia and Analgesia, 72,* 120-124.

Whaley, L., & Wong, D. L. (1987). *Nursing care of infants and children.* St. Louis: Mosby.

Wood, C. E., Goresky, G. V., Klassen, K. A., Kuwahara, B., & Neil, S. G. (1994). Complications of continuous epidural infusions for postoperative analgesia in children. *Canadian Journal of Anaesthesia, 41,* 613-620.

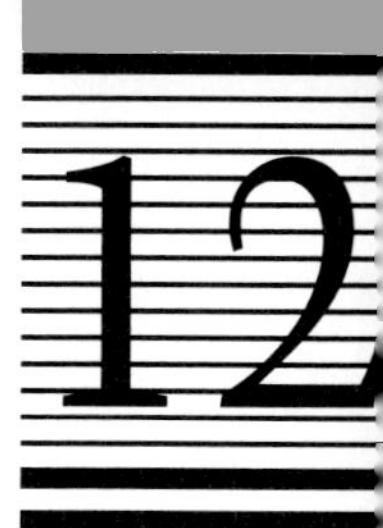

Geriatric Pain Management

Mary L. Eiman

Sharon E. Anderson

Hector Davila

Michael A. Silverman

Key Points

- The frequency of chronic pain complaints by the elderly reflects the patterns of chronic disease.
- Geriatric pain assessment is multifactorial and includes data from a history, physical examination, and functional and psychosocial assessment.
- Older adults have atypical presentation of many symptoms, including pain, which makes it more difficult to determine causation.
- Older adults may deny pain because they want to deny a decline in their health status or to avoid appearing weak.
- Older adults compose an extremely heterogeneous group; therefore assessment and management of pain must be highly individualized.
- The goal of prescribing drugs for the elderly is to achieve the maximum benefit with the lowest drug dose while causing minimal side effects.
- Nonopioid and opioid analgesics may accumulate in the body of an older adult and increase the risk of toxicity if drug doses are not titrated or reduced.
- Pharmacologic and nonpharmacologic interventions are often combined to produce higher levels of pain control.
- Members of an interdisciplinary team including the patient and family should work together in the assessment of pain and the identification of the most appropriate pain management interventions.

The management of pain in the growing geriatric population poses unique challenges to nurses and other health care providers. Caring for older patients requires recognition of the numerous complex physiologic changes associated with the process of aging and their impact on treatment for pain of acute and persistent, irreversible chronic conditions. Additionally, the demographic diversity of the older American population challenges health care providers to discover the unique needs of each individual, contradicting the misconception that this population is homogeneous.

Persons aged 65 and older currently account for 12% of the U.S. population, an estimate expected to rise to 22% by the year 2030 (Kane, Ouslander, & Abrass, 1994). As this population grows it is also aging; the "oldest old," those aged 85 and older, represent the fastest-growing segment of older adults in the United States. This heterogeneous group includes persons who are independent or well, frail community dwellers who often rely on various levels of assistance from formal and informal support networks, and individuals who are institutionalized; the last segment represents approximately 5% of the whole group.

This chapter includes a description of pain in the elderly, suggests methods of assessing pain, and identifies the physiologic changes due to aging that affect pharmacotherapy. The pharmacotherapeutic management of pain in the elderly is discussed according to the World Health Organization (WHO) analgesic ladder: nonopioid treatment of mild to moderate pain, opioid combined with nonopioid analgesics for treatment of mild to moderate pain, and opioid treatment of moderate to severe pain. A discussion of opioid tolerance and side effects is also included. Nonpharmacologic approaches to pain management are discussed. The chapter concludes by addressing the importance of the interdisciplinary team in the management of pain in geriatric patients.

DESCRIPTION OF GERIATRIC PAIN

According to McCaffery & Beebe (1989, p. 7), "pain is whatever the experiencing person says it is. . . . " The individual's perception of pain is a unique experience that includes the variables of a patient's culture, gender, past pain experience, meaning attached to pain, and physiologic alterations, including those due to aging (Ebersole & Hess, 1994).

Most elders have experienced acute pain and are familiar with its temporary nature. Acute pain is often reported following surgical operations, falls, and fractures. In contrast, chronic pain lasts longer than 6 months, often produces suffering that increases over time, and is usually not amenable to a cure (Karb, 1991). Table 12-1 lists common sites and etiologies of pain in the elderly.

The causes of chronic pain among the aged reflect the patterns of chronic disease in the population aged 65 years and older. Degenerative joint disease is identifiable in more than 80% of the geriatric population (Davis, 1988). Sixty percent of all cancers occur in this age group (Silverman & Temple, 1992). Other chronic conditions commonly producing pain in elderly patients include lumbar spinal stenosis, peripheral vascular disease, diabetic neuropathy, osteoporosis with vertebral compression, temporal arteritis, and cancer. The elderly also often suffer several conditions

Table 12-1 Common Sites and Etiologies of Pain in the Elderly

Head and neck	Occipital neuralgia
	Trigeminal neuralgia
	Cervical osteoarthritis
	Myofacial pain syndrome
	Cervical radiculopathy
	Temporal arteritis
Thorax	Postherpetic neuralgia
	Postsurgical intercostal neuralgia
	Myofacial pain syndrome
Gastrointestinal	Diabetic gastroneuropathy
	Pancreatitis
	Cancer of the pancreas
Spine	Lumbar radialopathy from:
	Spinal stenosis
	Herniated nucleus pulposus
	Peripheral neuropathies
Extremities	Sympathetically medicated pain:
	Reflex sympathetic dystrophy
	Causalgia

simultaneously, which further complicates identification of the source of the pain being reported.

Pain associated with the course of chronic conditions often produces concomitant problems that can dramatically decrease the elderly person's quality of life. Chronic pain may produce sleep disturbances, nutritional alterations, and impaired mobility. Problems with mobility may lead to social isolation and depression, which tend to enhance pain perception (Marzinski, 1991).

The sensation of pain may decrease among the aged due to changes in peripheral vasculature, skin, and pain impulse transmission through the central nervous system; however, clinical research on this question is inconclusive (Ebersole & Hess, 1994). Because aging may influence both the acuity and the severity of pain symptoms, it is essential that the nurse explore each pain complaint to its fullest extent during the assessment process.

GERIATRIC PAIN ASSESSMENT

Geriatric pain assessment is a multidimensional evaluation requiring attention to detail and the commitment of sufficient time to thoroughly explore each pain complaint. Components of the pain assessment include (a) the pain history, (b) the physical examination findings, (c) a determination of how pain interferes with functional abilities, and (d) a psychosocial evaluation to determine the impact of pain on daily life (Foley, 1994; Mosqueda, 1993).

Pain History

Assessing pain in the elderly requires thorough exploration of pain parameters and associated changes in functional status. The box on pp. 380 and 381 shows a guide to pain assessment. The cues in each of six content areas will guide the nurse toward gathering all the information necessary for a complete pain assessment. However, the patient in pain may not be able to provide all of the assessment information at the time of the complaint. Determining the intensity, location, and quality of pain may provide sufficient information for the selection of an immediate intervention. Once the pain is controlled, the nurse should plan to obtain the remaining information necessary for developing future interventions (Herr & Mobily, 1991).

The pain history of an elderly adult includes a detailed history of the patient's past and current use of prescription

GERIATRIC PAIN ASSESSMENT GUIDE

PAIN DESCRIPTION

Identify location, quality, intensity (present, worst, best), onset, duration, pattern of radiation or variation, manner of expressing pain, relationship to movement or position, time of occurrence, and related motor or sensory complaints.

AGGRAVATING AND ALLEVIATING FACTORS

Identify what intensifies or decreases the pain and what treatments, remedies, or activities relieve the pain.

PAIN TREATMENT HISTORY

List past medications taken for pain, previous treatment with local anesthetics, steroid or neurolytic (clinical or surgical) blocks, and nonpharmacologic pain interventions.

OBSERVATIONS

Note vocalizations such as groaning and facial expressions including wrinkled forehead, tightly closed or widely opened eyes or mouth, or other distorted expressions. Observe body movements noting guarding, rocking, pulling legs into abdomen, increased hand or finger movements, inability to keep still, pacing behaviors, or other restrictive motions.

IMPACT

Identify any changes in daily activities, gait, or behaviors. Note onset of new behaviors such as confusion, irritability, or increased activity; accompanying symptoms such as nausea, dizziness, sweating, or fatigue; and any changes in sleep,

GERIATRIC PAIN ASSESSMENT GUIDE—cont'd

appetite, emotions, concentration, physical activity, relationships, social interactions, and common routines.

SOCIAL HISTORY

Explore functional status prior to onset of symptoms, marital status, family or community resource network, social and leisure activities, and environmental barriers to social activity.

Modified from Herr, K., & Mobily, P. (1991). Complexities of pain assessment in the elderly: Clinical considerations. *Journal of Gerontological Nursing, 17*(4), 14.

and nonprescription medications. A format for obtaining a geriatric drug history is provided in Figure 12-1.

Additional information about the patient's pain history may be gleaned from family members and other caregivers who can verify data and provide additional insights into the patient's pain experience. When the patient is a poor historian, a family member may provide data that are of sufficient importance to change the diagnostic approach (Foley, 1994).

Interviewing elderly patients about pain complaints can pose a challenge to the nurse attempting to develop appropriate intervention strategies. Not all elderly patients are willing or able to be cooperative reporters of the extent and severity of their pain complaints. Many were socialized to the health care system in the pre-1960s era when patients viewed themselves as passive recipients of care (McCaffery & Ferrell, 1991). They may currently believe that nurses and other members of the health care team, as experts, know what is best for their pain. As a consequence, the aged may unintentionally underreport essential elements of their pain complaints.

Some aged patients fear the outcome of pain treatment and therefore decline to report increases in the severity and extent of pain. They may fear that analgesia will produce drowsiness and confusion that could lead to a fall (McCaffery

Patient's name_______________Sex____Age____Date__________

Family member contributing information______________________

Physician(s) (date last seen)________________________________

Diagnosis & past history (if relevant) :
Frequency of meals? Special diet prescribed or self –imposed?
Allergies/drug reactions: (food and/or drugs: reaction, date, action taken, outcome)
Close family members with drug allergies: (relationship, drug, reaction)
Daily consumption of alcohol: (type, amount, duration)
Smoking: (type, amount, duration)

<u>Over–the–Counter Medications</u>
List medications, dose, frequency, and when last dose taken for each of the following:
Constipation (laxatives):
Diarrhea (antidiarrheal):
Gastric upset (antacids):
Pain, headache (analgesics):
Cold medication (antihistamine, decongestants):
Cough medicine (syrups, other forms)
Drugs for sleep:
Drugs to stay awake:
Drugs for menopause (hormone replacement):
Drugs for nerves:
Drugs for fluid retention:
Do you use any salt substitutes? (Obtain name brand)
Do you use any food supplement? (name and quantity per day)
Do you buy health food store products? (Obtain listing and daily consumption)
Do you take vitamins? (Note type, strength, and amount per day)

<u>Prescription Medications</u>
Current prescribed medications: (Include name, strength, daily dose, and duration for each)

<u>Home Remedies</u>
Use of home remedies: (malady treated, compounds used, amount, frequency, duration, effects)

Prescription medications taken during the previous three months:

Nurse__________________________

Figure 12-1 Geriatric drug history.

& Ferrell, 1991), that treatment will alter their behavior or personality (Hofland, 1992), or that increased pain may herald a worsening of their condition and result in forced dependency. Others believe that pain is a natural accompaniment to old age and may stoically accept suffering (Greenlee, 1991; Herr & Mobily, 1991).

Elderly patients suffering from one of the chronic brain syndromes (CBSs), including Alzheimer's disease, exhibit memory loss and decreases in cognitive ability that may influence their ability to report pain. Parmelee, Katz, and Lawton (1993) examined pain self-reports in residential geriatric facilities and discovered that cognitively impaired persons were somewhat less likely than their cognitively intact counterparts to complain of pain. However, self-reports of cognitively impaired patients equaled those of cognitively intact persons in the presence of an identifiable physical cause for a particular complaint.

There is strong evidence to suggest that when questions are phrased simply and straightforwardly, patients with mild to moderate impairment can provide valid, reliable information about their pain. In the later stages of CBS, patients are often awake, alert, confused, and nonverbal and are able to express pain only through changes in behavior (Marzinski, 1991). As a rule, self-reports of pain by cognitively impaired geriatric patients should be believed.

Elderly patients who are unwilling or unable to verbalize information about pain need to be assessed in a manner that is supportive and considerate of their status. Interviewing patients reluctant to discuss their pain is facilitated by taking the time to establish trust and rapport in a supportive environment, communicating concern about their suffering, and educating them about pain beliefs and the consequences of intervention that may be of concern. Some patients believe that their suffering is a deserved punishment for past deeds; others may be focused on fears of addiction to analgesics (Hofland, 1992).

Patients who are confused or nonverbal are assessed by observing overt or subtle changes in behavior. With the onset of pain these patients may become either quiet and withdrawn or agitated and combative. They may also use pain cues such as grimaces (Marzinski, 1991). When knowledge of existing pain must depend on changes in behavior, observations may be validated by interviewing other staff or family members, who usually report symptoms consistent with subjective patient reports. Unlike medical professionals, caregivers tend to err by overestimating the presence of symptoms (Morris et al., 1986). Therefore, the nurse must be aware that data collected from patient caregivers may be biased. Caregivers may project their own pain experiences onto the patient when interpreting pain cues or underreport complaints that they believe are actually attention-getting behaviors.

Physical Examination

Physical examination findings provide additional information about the pain complaint. Careful observation of the patient's response to examination procedures may provide pain cues such as guarding, grimacing, head rocking, fidgeting, and attempts to cover painful areas with the hands. Objective findings of pain may also include pupillary dilation, dry mouth, pallor, diaphoresis, and changes in vital signs (Seidel, Ball, Dains, & Benedict, 1995).

Attention should be directed to the musculoskeletal, neurologic, and vascular systems as major sources of pain. Observing gait patterns, movement initiation, and the ability to transfer gives clues to both physical status and functional ability (Wolfson, Whipple, Amerman, & Tobin, 1990; Tinetti, 1986). Complaints of back pain should include assessment of the abdominal aorta for the presence of an ischemia-producing aneurysm, which may masquerade as spinal pain, especially if it is "leaking."

The use of a visual or verbal pain scale to assist the patient in rating pain intensity should be included in the examination. Using the same scale to measure repeated complaints of pain provides insights into the effectiveness of interventions. (See Chapter 1 for illustrations of pain scales.)

Functional Assessment

A clinical assessment of chronic pain in the elderly is incomplete without a functional assessment. While history and physical examination findings provide substantive insights into the patient's pain experience, the manner in which pain affects daily activities is not traditionally explored in depth in such data.

Elderly patients experiencing chronic pain often adapt to their suffering in ways that maximize independence and minimize pain. Those with impaired mobility may shop for groceries less often if they cannot rely upon someone else to perform this task. Patients whose pain is exacerbated by the movements of cooking or who are too fatigued to prepare meals may rely on whatever ready-to-eat foods are available in their homes. The impact of chronic pain on the daily life of an elderly person must be assessed in order to provide interventions that appropriately support the maintenance of that patient's independence and quality of life. The use of functional assessment instruments provides insights into the effects of the current complaint and, over time, the effectiveness of interventions.

The Katz Index of Activities of Daily Living assesses the patient's ability to perform six common daily tasks: bathing, continence, dressing, feeding, toileting, and transferring (Applegate, Blass, & Williams, 1990; Katz, Ford, Moskowitz, Jackson, & Jaffe, 1963). The Instrumental Activities of Daily Living (IADL) scale measures higher functional abilities and is an appropriate instrument for assessing elderly patients who live independently (Lawton & Brody, 1969; Mosqueda, 1993). The IADL queries patients on their abilities to shop for groceries, manage money, prepare meals, and travel, and it assists in determining the extent to which pain interferes with daily self-care and social activities.

Psychosocial Assessment

A multidimensional pain assessment also includes an examination of the psychologic and social factors affecting the patient with pain. Pain complaints can rarely be assigned to psychologic factors alone (Barsky, Frank, Cleary, Wyshak, & Klerman, 1991); however, the patient's mental status may contribute to altered perceptions of the pain experience. Conversely, chronic pain can produce feelings of loss, depression, or anxiety, particularly if the pain is interfering with daily functioning and quality of life (Kennedy, Kelman, & Thomas, 1991; Reynolds, 1994). Patients exhibiting weight loss, disturbed sleep patterns, diminished daily activities, social isolation, increased levels of anxiety, or suicidal ideation should be questioned in depth to determine the need for a full psychiatric evaluation.

A psychologic assessment beginning with a simple mini–mental-status examination provides additional data that may enhance understanding of the unique nature of the pain experience. Although the relationship between cognitive status and the pain experience is unclear, it is clear that patients with impaired cognition may be less able to report pain. Knowledge of psychologic status provides insights into patient capabilities and limitations that must be considered in developing interventions. The Folstein Mini-Mental State Examination provides a scale for screening cognitive impairment (Folstein, Folstein, & McHugh, 1979; Mosqueda, 1993).

Patients with memory deficits may be able to report present pain but may not be able to provide information concerning past pain treatments and other important historical data. Sengstaken and King (1993) found that demented or cognitively impaired elderly residents of long-term care facilities were less likely than other, more alert residents to identify pain. No assumptions, however, should be made that the self-reported symptoms of persons with cognitive deficits are of compromised reliability or validity.

The psychosocial database may be further expanded by interviewing family members and other caregivers, often overlooked as sources of pain assessment information. Caregivers are capable of making frequent observations of functional abilities and disabilities and can often provide valuable insights into changes in the patient's psychosocial status that occur as the result of pain.

PHYSIOLOGIC CHANGES IN AGING AFFECTING PHARMACOTHERAPY

The process of aging involves changes in physiology that alter drug absorption, distribution, metabolism, and excretion. Table 12-2 highlights these changes. Absorption is affected by a decrease in acid production (hypochlorhydria), slower gastric emptying, and reduced intestinal blood flow, all of which can result in decreased dissolution of some medications. Histamine (H_2) blockers such as ranitidine (Zantac) and cimetidine (Tagamet) are commonly prescribed in conjunction with pain medications, which will further decrease gastric acid secretion in elderly patients. The effects of this combination may spare the gastric lining by increasing gastric pH, but the change in pH may affect the absorption rate of a variety of medications.

Drug distribution is also influenced by the aging process. Total body water decreases in the elderly, and their percentage of body fat increases, which reduces the volume of distribution of water-soluble medications and increases the volume of distribution of fat-soluble drugs. Although

Table 12-2 Altered Pharmacokinetics in the Elderly

Absorption	Decrease in acid production with increased gastric pH
Distribution	Decrease in total body water and lean body mass
Excretion	Decrease in renal blood flow, glomerular filtration rate Increased percentage of body fat; slight decrease in serum albumin; altered protein binding; increase in α_1-glycoprotein
Metabolism	Decrease in hepatic blood flow and phase I live enzymes (oxidation hydrolysis); phase II (glucuronidation) is unchanged

Modified from McKenry, L. M., & Salerno, E. (1995). *Pharmacology in nursing.* St. Louis: Mosby.

serum albumin is minimally reduced with aging, elders with nutritional deficits may experience greater reductions in albumin that can significantly affect drug binding. For example, phenytoin (Dilantin), an anticonvulsant used to treat the chronic pain of trigeminal or postherpetic neuralgia, is highly protein-bound. In the nutritionally depleted geriatric patient, the amount of free phenytoin is increased, which could potentially lead to toxicity.

The hepatic changes that occur with aging affect drug metabolism and can lead to prolonged drug half-life and reduced total plasma clearance. Hepatic mass remains relatively stable until middle age, after which it declines slightly in relation to body weight with each decade. Regional blood flow to the liver declines with advancing years and in a 65-year-old may be 40% to 45% less than that of a person of age 25 (Vestal, 1990).

Many elderly persons experience a decline in renal function. As a consequence, pain medications (and their active metabolites) normally excreted by the kidney may have longer half-lives, which can lead to toxicity if "standard" doses are not adjusted. Salicylates, common analgesics found in many over-the-counter (OTC) pain relievers, can accumulate and lead to toxicity in older patients with reduced renal function (Stratton, 1991). Other pain medications that are excreted by the kidney may need to be administered in reduced doses.

Pharmacodynamic changes among the aged also include increased sensitivity to opioid drugs. End organ heightened sensitivity may lead to greater analgesia in the elderly than in younger patients (Foley, 1994).

THERAPEUTIC MANAGEMENT OF PAIN

Pharmacotherapy

The standard approach to pain management in the elderly includes consideration of pharmacologic and nonpharmacologic interventions. The choice of treatment depends on the findings of a comprehensive clinical assessment that focuses on the patient as the authority on his or her pain experience.

Pharmacotherapy is usually the initial choice of therapy for pain because it is low risk, produces rapid results, and is relatively inexpensive. The choice of drug for analgesia is determined by the type of pain and its intensity (Foley, 1994).

Acute pain is often relieved with pharmacologic intervention tailored to the level of pain: nonopioid analgesics for mild to moderate pain and opioid analgesics for severe pain. Chronic pain management, in its multidimensional nature, poses many significant challenges. As the duration of pain increases, depression and anxiety occur and often negatively influence the older person's social life, resulting in loneliness and hostility (Thomas, 1990). The choice of medications for chronic pain is complicated by the existence of other chronic conditions that may also require pharmacologic management.

Use of pain medication often contributes to the problem of a patient's needing several separate medications per day. Polypharmacy increases the potential for drug-drug and drug-nutrient interactions as well as the risk of adverse drug reactions. Whenever a medication is added to an already complex regimen, the potential iatrogenic complications must be considered. If not monitored properly, polypharmacy can lead to volume depletion, dehydration, and nutritional decline.

Although elderly patients may seem to be attracted to "a pill for every ill," compliance is a problematic issue. Between 25% and 50% of all geriatric outpatients fail to take medications as prescribed. Some patients fail to comprehend complex drug regimens. Others engage in "intelligent noncompliance"; they reduce or stop taking medications to lessen adverse effects but lose the beneficial effect as a result (Vestal, 1990). Patient and caregiver drug education is a critical element in enhancing compliance.

The goal of prescribing drugs for the elderly is to achieve the maximum benefit with the lowest drug dose while causing minimal side effects. Recommendations for pharmacologic therapy follow the WHO analgesic pain management ladder, which addresses treatment in three steps: mild to moderate pain treated with nonopioids, mild to moderate pain treated with nonopioid-opioid combination, and moderate to severe pain treated with opioids (Jacox et al., 1994).

Nonopioid Treatment of Mild to Moderate Pain

The first-line approach to treating mild to moderate pain includes the use of nonopioid analgesics such as acetaminophen, aspirin, and the nonsteroidal antiinflammatory drugs (NSAIDs) (Enck, 1991). Tolerance and physical dependence are not associated with these agents; however, a ceiling effect at higher doses limits their effectiveness. The ceiling effect occurs at the point that an increase in dose does not produce improved analgesia.

Acetaminophen is equivalent to aspirin as an analgesic and antipyretic, but it lacks antiinflammatory effect. Aspirin and acetaminophen do not exhibit cross-sensitivity. Low-dose acetaminophen does not risk the adverse hematologic, renal, and gastrointestinal effects of aspirin, but hepatic or renal injury can occur in higher doses. Acetaminophen can be taken regularly or on a pro re nata (prn) schedule in the treatment of mild to moderate chronic pain. The optimal single dose for acetaminophen and aspirin is commonly 650 mg (2 tablets); optimal daily doses range from 8 to 12 tablets (2600-3900 mg) (Wall, 1990). Optimal doses may be lower for patients who are frail or of diminutive size.

Aspirin use—especially prolonged—among the aged may cause gastrointestinal irritation, gradual blood loss, and ultimately anemia. Many geriatric persons have reduced stores of iron and may not be able to compensate for limited blood loss over time; the cumulative effect may be severe anemia. Diminished renal function in the elderly may lead to the accumulation of salicylates and salicylate intoxication, which can be difficult to detect. Aspirin overdose in older adults may produce vague effects of dizziness, confusion, drowsiness, or nausea and vomiting (Forman & Stratton, 1991). Tinnitus is a frequent complaint of the elderly taking higher doses of aspirin and is a sign of ototoxicity requiring dose reduction. Though aspirin is a mainstay of treatment for mild to moderate pain, studies question the advisability of its use in the treatment of frail geriatric patients (Butt, Barthel, & Moore, 1988; Maniglia, Schwartz, & Moriber-Katz, 1988).

The NSAIDs give comparable or superior pain relief to that of aspirin and are primarily useful in treating musculoskeletal, arthritic, cancer, traumatic, and soft tissue inflammation pain and pain associated with peripheral nerves (neuralgias) (Brooks & Wood, 1991). Cancer pain may also be treated with a combination of NSAIDs and opioid analgesics (Twycross, 1994).

Elderly patients receiving NSAIDs may experience side effects associated with prolonged use or overdose. All NSAIDs affect renal hemodynamics; therefore, for geriatric patients with potential or actual compromised renal function, care must be taken in the choice and dosing of these drugs. NSAIDs can worsen renal function, especially if creatinine clearance is less than 30 ml/min (Sandler, Burr, & Weinberg, 1991). Wall (1990) suggests that geriatric patients take NSAIDs with a shorter half-life, such as ibuprofen (Advil, Motrin) or fenoprofen (Nalfon), to prevent toxic accumulation of the drug. Sulindac (Clinoril) appears least likely to decrease renal blood flow and is recommended as a possible drug of choice for elderly patients with hypertension and congestive heart failure (Stratton, 1991). However, the lengthy 16.8-hour plasma half-life of sulindac may not be appropriate for frail elderly patients or patients with renal disease.

Long-term NSAID therapy in the elderly requires monitoring the patients for signs of toxicity. Forman and Stratton (1991) suggest obtaining a baseline hemoglobin and hematocrit, BUN and/or serum creatinine, and a stool guaiac sample and monitoring the patient every 3 months. Other subjective complaints and objective findings must be evaluated as they occur.

Many older adults taking NSAIDs experience gastrointestinal side effects such as nausea, abdominal pain, gastritis, and bleeding that can ultimately result in the development of severe anemia. Carson and Strom (1994) note that a number of authors commonly prescribe misoprostol (Cytotec) or an H_2 blocker to decrease the potential for NSAID-induced gastropathy. Patients should be educated about the importance of taking NSAIDs with food or milk if GI distress occurs.

Teaching patients about the potential side effects and signs of toxicity that may occur increases their compliance and facilitates individual monitoring of NSAID effectiveness (Stratton, 1991). Nonsteroidal antiinflammatory drugs can decrease the effectiveness of antihypertensive drugs and cause sodium and water retention. Both NSAIDs and H_2 blockers can cause mental status changes in the elderly including confusion, agitation, and hallucinations. Other NSAID effects may include tinnitus, blurred vision, dizziness, drowsiness, headache, prolonged bleeding time, signs of GI bleeding, weight gain due to sodium retention, or, in patients with hypertension, increased blood pressure. Other side effects and signs of toxicity may occur, depending on the particular NSAID and the individual patient's response.

In the treatment of mild to moderate pain in geriatric patients, acetaminophen or NSAID therapy should begin with the lowest possible dose. Patient response should be monitored closely before the dose is increased. In the treatment of chronic pain, NSAIDs may be taken around the clock to achieve steady-state plasma levels that permit continuous pain control (Wall, 1990). NSAIDs may also be taken as needed at the onset of pain or prophylactically in anticipation of a need for analgesia.

Although the characteristics, metabolism, and effectiveness of all NSAIDs are similar, if one NSAID fails to achieve pain control, another may work. Therapeutic levels may not be obtained for 1 to 2 weeks, so each drug must be tested for an adequate trial period before changing. Using two different analgesics of the same class is not recommended because competition for protein binding may result in reduced effectiveness. Complications from these drugs are particularly worrisome in the elderly. The use of NSAIDs in these patients, especially the very frail in whom complications could cause significant morbidity, must be weighed carefully.

Opioid Treatment of Mild to Moderate Pain

Geriatric patients who cannot tolerate or do not respond to pain treatment with nonopioid drugs often achieve pain relief with mild oral opioids. The common approach to treatment of mild to moderate pain in elderly patients includes the use of low-potency opioid analgesics including codeine (methylmorphine), oxycodone (Percodan, Tylox, Percocet), and propoxyphene (Darvon), which share the pharmacology of morphine. Mild opioids are administered regularly on a trial basis before being judged ineffective (Foley, 1994).

Codeine, a less potent morphine, is often used in combination with nonopioid analgesics to enhance pain relief in the older patient. Codeine is considered a first-line opioid in the treatment of acute pain that does not respond to nonopioid drugs. To maximize its effectiveness, codeine should be administered at the onset of pain, and oral forms should be given with milk or meals to minimize GI distress. This analgesic produces a high incidence of nausea, vomiting, and constipation and may require a change to another, less potent opioid drug (Stratton, 1991). Thirty milligrams of oral codeine has the analgesic effect of 650 mg (two tablets) of aspirin.

Oxycodone (Percodan, Tylox, Percocet), like codeine, is an opioid analgesic within the morphine series. Its action is enhanced when it is combined with a nonopioid analgesic. Percodan is an oxycodone-aspirin combination; Tylox and Percocet include oxycodone and acetaminophen. Oxycodone is a short-acting analgesic with a rapid onset and has proven to be an effective medication for moderate acute and chronic pain. Thirty milligrams of oxycodone is equivalent to 10 mg of intramuscular morphine (Wall, 1990).

Propoxyphene (Darvon), when combined with acetaminophen or aspirin, is an effective analgesic for mild to moderate pain. Propoxyphene alone has an analgesic effect equivalent to that of aspirin. Patients should be advised to take it with food or milk to minimize gastrointestinal distress.

Opioid Treatment of Moderate to Severe Pain

More potent opioid analgesics are needed when less potent opioid interventions fail to alleviate or substantially reduce pain. Addiction to these drugs (physiologic dependence) is uncommon among the elderly (Barry, 1994). Many clinicians, however, have misconceptions about the use of potent opioids and will withhold opioids needed for pain relief.

A substantial number of strong opioids are available for treating older adults in moderate to severe pain. Morphine, pentazocine (Talwin), hydromorphone (Dilaudid), meperidine (Demerol), methadone (Dolophine, Methadose), and fentanyl (Sublimaze, Duragesic) are discussed in detail in Chapter 4.

The elderly appear to be more sensitive to the analgesic effects of opioids, especially when these are given as a short-term postoperative treatment or for cancer pain. In order to achieve the maximum analgesia with minimal complications, doses need to be titrated, and the patient must be closely observed to determine drug efficacy and identify side effects. Side effects associated with opioid administration include respiratory depression, sedation, nausea and vomiting, urinary retention, and constipation (the most common side effect).

Some opioid analgesics should be avoided in the treatment of the elderly. Pentazocine (Talwin) has central nervous system effects that include confusion and agitation (Foley, 1994). Methadone has a prolonged plasma half-life, which can lead to overdose and toxicity. Meperidine (Demerol) has a low oral potency, and normeperidine, a metabolite, may accumulate and lead to central nervous system effects including seizures, agitation, and confusion (Schor et al., 1992; Williams, Urguahart, Sharrock, & Charleson, 1992).

Tolerance to opioids Patients can develop tolerance to opioids, with the same dose exhibiting a steady decline in effectiveness over time. Although tolerance develops to both analgesia and respiratory depression, tolerance to the latter develops more rapidly. Although addiction is uncommon,

Table 12-3 Side Effects of High-Risk Pharmacologic Therapy in the Elderly

Problem	Treatment
Respiratory depression (opioids)	Assess respiratory rate and depth Assess mental status Adjust medication
Constipation (opioids)	Assess bowel function Educate family/caregivers in monitoring bowel habits Adjust diet: Increase fiber Increase fruits Increase water Prescribe laxatives and stool softeners
Acute urinary retention (anticholinergics, antihistamines, opioids)	Assess urinary function Ask specific questions about loss of urine or incontinence Monitor output Assess skin for breakdown Adjust medication
Falls (confusion) (NSAIDs, phenathiazines, antidepressants, benzodiazepines, antihistamine)	Assess gait, balance (Tinetti, 1986) Employ assistive devices Adjust medication Assess safety of home environment
Delirium (opioids, corticosteroids, benzodiazepines)	Assess mental status (Folstein, Folstein, and McHugh, 1979) Monitor hydration and nutritional status Maintain skin integrity Adjust medication

physical dependence and withdrawal symptoms can occur, making it necessary to wean the patient slowly from opioid drugs (Barry, 1994).

Side effects to opioid therapy The use of opioid analgesics can produce a number of side effects in the elderly; Table 12-3 lists side effects and interventions. Respiratory depression is potentially the most serious, particularly when it occurs in geriatric patients with decreased respiratory function such as chronic obstructive pulmonary disease (COPD).

Opioid-naive patients may experience respiratory depression at the initiation of opioid therapy, but this effect can be reduced by careful titration of the drug or reversed by the titration of the opioid antagonist naloxone (Narcan). Tolerance to respiratory depression occurs only after repeated doses.

Sedation and drowsiness are also frequently reported as side effects of opioid analgesics. Older adults have diminished hunger and thirst mechanisms, which predisposes them to nutritional decline and dehydration. The swallowing mechanism and cough reflex may also be affected, thereby increasing the risk of aspiration. A reduced dose taken at shorter intervals may manage these effects. When geriatric patients are sedated by opioids, particular attention must be paid to ensure their adequate intake of food and liquids.

Constipation leading to impaction secondary to opioid analgesics can be a frequent and important side effect in the elderly patient and is believed to result from a decrease in intestinal peristalsis and secretion. Aggressive bowel regimens should be pursued to prevent this problem, which can lead to fecal impaction and its associated severe complications (Wrenn, 1989). Fecal impaction can cause obstruction, rectal prolapse, volvulus, ulceration, and perforation (stercoral ulcer). Stool softeners and laxatives are important adjuncts to opioid analgesic therapy.

Acute urinary incontinence can be caused by pharmaceuticals used in the management of pain in the elderly. This most commonly occurs with anticholinergics, antihistamines, and opioids (Dubeau & Resnick, 1991). The development of acute urinary incontinence is a significant side effect that is embarrassing to the ambulatory patient. In those patients confined to bed, incontinence can lead to skin breakdown with the formation of decubitus ulcers.

Urinary retention can be reversed by decreasing drug doses in addition to administering betanechol (Urecholine). Catheterization may also be required. This problem is manifest most often in older male patients with preexisting compromised bladder function due to prostatic hypertrophy or prior prostate surgery.

The incidence of falls and injury increases in the elderly (Rubenstein, 1993). Medications, particularly strong analgesics, phenothiazines, antidepressants, and long-acting benzodiazepines, significantly increase a patient's risk of falling. Caregivers must be aware of these complications and provide assistance in ambulation and transferring.

Nonpharmacologic Approaches to Pain Management

Nonpharmacologic interventions are commonly employed in the integrated approach to pain management in elderly adults and include both physical and psychosocial instruments. The physical approach to pain management includes exercise, cutaneous stimulation, physical therapy (PT), occupational therapy (OT), transcutaneous electrical nerve stimulation (TENS), and acupuncture. Geriatric patients with osteoarthritis are commonly treated with PT, exercise, OT, and cutaneous stimulation such as hot or cold packs and massage. Chronic back pain may respond to rest, heat, and analgesics.

Properly coordinated exercise is a mainstay in promoting the health of older adults and in treating and preventing musculoskeletal pain. Interventions requiring lengthy immobilization or the use of special devices that restrict movement should be used with caution in treating elderly patients. When immobilized, the aged can rapidly develop complications such as joint contractures, muscle atrophy, decubitus ulcers, orthostatic hypotension, depression, urinary retention, and fecal impaction. These iatrogenic complications are often avoidable if health care providers are aware of the potential problems of immobilization and cooperate with other members of the interdisciplinary team to develop appropriate interventions.

TENS is often requested by elderly patients. The value of this intervention is controversial, although those treated for mild pain with TENS claim at least temporary improvement.

TENS is used most frequently in patients with neuropathic pain, arthritis, neuralgia, and spinal pain.

Psychologic techniques are thought to be of benefit in an integrated approach to pain management in the elderly. Interventions such as relaxation, reframing, biofeedback, and imaging are receiving increasing attention as beneficial pain reduction interventions in cognitively intact older adults.

TEAM APPROACH

The interdisciplinary team approach is the contemporary model of choice in the management of geriatric pain. Interdisciplinary team interventions based upon a biopsychosocial model for diagnosis, treatment, and evaluation provide a holistic approach to pain management (Miaskowski, Jacox, Hester, & Ferrell, 1992). The core members of the team typically include a geriatric nurse practitioner or clinical specialist, a geriatrician, a physical therapist, a social worker, a pharmacist, and a chaplain. Depending on the unique needs of each patient, the team may expand to include resource persons such as dietitians or medical specialists in rehabilitation, rheumatology, orthopedics, or neurology. (See Chapter 6 for an in-depth discussion of the interdisciplinary team approach to pain management.)

The patient and family are included as members of the interdisciplinary team and participate in the decision-making process. The effectiveness of the team as a whole is often dependent on the amount and type of data collected, opportunities for sharing information and exchanging ideas, and appropriate participation of the patient and family in the selection and implementation of interventions.

Each unique combination of patient, family, and other team members yields different variables influencing pain management that must be explored in depth. The choice of an intervention can be influenced by unique patient-centered variables such as the cost of medication, religious beliefs about pain and pain relief, the effects of pharmacologic intervention on mental status, and whether or not the patient will be able to maintain or regain role function during pain treatment.

In the management of geriatric pain, the use of an interdisciplinary team approach is recommended along with case management and the development of a comprehensive plan of care. Visiting nurse agencies and other community-based resources provide additional support for patients and families and assist with compliance to the recommended intervention plan.

SUMMARY

This chapter emphasized the complex nature of pain management in geriatric patients and the importance of a multidimensional pain assessment in the selection and use of pharmacologic and nonpharmacologic interventions. The patient and family, as members of the interdisciplinary team, are important contributors to the pain management process, particularly in determining its goals.

The nurse, as the professional caregiver who spends the most time with the patient in care settings, is in a unique position to assess and intervene in the management of geriatric pain. As a key member—often the leader—of the interdisciplinary team, the nurse must use keen assessment skills to identify the subtleties of the pain experience in patients with communication deficits or reluctance to discuss their pain. Nursing interventions must be customized to the unique needs of each individual patient. Because the changing nature of pain may rapidly invalidate a once-useful intervention, nurses must constantly evaluate the effectiveness of the interventions.

References

Applegate, W. B., Blass, J. P., & Williams, T. F. (1990). Instruments for the functional assessment of older patients. *New England Journal of Medicine, 322*(17), 1207-1214.

Barry, P. P. (1994). Chemical dependency. In W. R. Hazzard, E. L. Bierman, J. P. Blass, W. H. Ettinger, J. B. Halter, & R. Andres (Eds.), *Principles of geriatric medicine* & *gerontology* (3rd ed., pp. 1125-1130). New York: McGraw-Hill.

Barsky, A. J., Frank, C., Cleary, P. D., Wyshak, G., & Klerman, G. L. (1991). The relation between hypochondriasis and age. *American Journal of Psychiatry, 148*(7), 923-928.

Brooks, P. M., & Wood, A. J. (1991). Nonsteroidal anti-inflammatory drugs: Differences and similarities. *New England Journal of Medicine, 324*(24), 1716-1725.

Butt, J. H., Barthel, J. S., & Moore, R. A. (1988). Clinical spectrum of the upper gastrointestinal effects of nonsteroidal antiinflammatory drugs: Natural history, symptomatology, and significance. *American Journal of Medicine, 84*(suppl. 2A), 5-14.

Carson, J. L., & Strom, B. L. (1994). Non-steroidal anti-inflammatory drugs. In W. R. Hazzard, E. L. Bierman, J. P. Blass, W. H. Ettinger, J. B. Halter, & R. Andres (Eds.), *Principles of geriatric medicine & gerontology* (3rd ed., pp. 947-953). New York: McGraw-Hill.

Davis, M. A. (1988). Epidemiology of osteoarthritis. *Clinical Geriatric Medicine, 4*(2), 241-255.

Dubeau, C. E., & Resnick, N. M. (1991). Evaluation of the cause and severity of geriatric incontinence: A critical appraisal. *Urologic Clinics of North America, 18*(2), 243-256.

Ebersole, P., & Hess, P. (1994). *Toward healthy aging* (4th ed.). St. Louis: Mosby–Year Book, pp. 283-300.

Enck, R. E. (1991). Pain control in ambulatory elderly. *Geriatrics, 46*(3), 49-60.

Foley, K. M. (1994). Pain management in the elderly. In W. R. Hazzard, E. L. Bierman, J. P. Blass, W. H. Ettinger, J. B. Halter, & R. Andres (Eds.), *Principles of geriatric medicine & gerontology* (3rd ed.). New York: McGraw-Hill.

Folstein, M. F., Folstein, S. E., & McHugh, P. R. (1979). Mini-mental state: A practical guide for grading the cognitive state of patients for the clinician. *Journal of the Psychiatry Record, 12,* 189-198.

Forman, W. B., & Stratton, M. (1991). Current approach to chronic pain in older patients. *Geriatrics, 46,* 47.

Greenlee, K. K. (1991). Pain and analgesia: Consideration for the elderly in critical care. *AACN Clinical Issues in Critical Care Nursing, 2,* 720-728.

Herr, K., & Mobily, P. (1991). Complexities of pain assessment in the elderly: Clinical considerations. *Journal of Gerontological Nursing, 17*(4), 12-19.

Hofland, S. L. (1992). Elder beliefs: Blocks to pain management. *Journal of Gerontological Nursing, 18*(6), 19-24.

Jacox, A., Carr, D. B., Payne, R., Berde, C. B., Breitbart, W., Cain, J. M., Chapman, C. R., Cleeland, C. S., Ferrell, B. R., Finley, R. S., Hester, N. O., Hill, C. S., Leak, W. D., Lipman, A. G., Logan, C. L., McGarvey, C. L., Miaskowski, C. A., Mulder, D. S., Paice, J. A., Shapiro, B. S., Silberstein, E. B., Smith, R. S., Stover, J., Tsou, C. V., Vecchiarelli, L., & Weissman, D. E. (1994). *Management of cancer pain. Clinical practice guideline.* AHCPR Pub. No. 94-0592. Rockville, MD: Agency for Health Care Policy and Research, PHS, USDHHS.

Kane, R. L., Ouslander, J. G., & Abrass, I. B. (1994). *Essentials of clinical geriatrics* (3rd ed.). New York: McGraw-Hill.

Karb, V. B. (1991). Pain. In Phipps, W., Long, B., Woods, N., & Cassmeyer, V. L. (Eds.), *Medical-surgical nursing: Concepts and clinical practice* (4th ed., pp. 297-326). St. Louis: Mosby.

Katz, S., Ford, A. B., Moskowitz, R. W., Jackson, B. A., & Jaffe, M. W. (1963). The index of ADL: A standardized measure of biological and psychosocial functions. *Journal of the American Medical Association, 330,* 914-919.

Kennedy, G. J., Kelman, H. R., & Thomas, C. (1991). Persistence and remission of depressive symptoms in late life. *American Journal of Psychiatry, 148,* 174-178.

Lawton, M. P., & Brody, E. M. (1969). Assessment of older people: Self-maintaining and instrumental activities of daily living. *Gerontologist, 9,* 179-186.

Maniglia, R., Schwartz, A. B., & Moriber-Katz, S. (1988). Nonsteroidal antiinflammatory nephrotoxicity. *Annals of Clinical Laboratory Science, 183,* 240-252.

Marzinski, L. R. (1991). The tragedy of dementia: Clinically assessing pain in the confused, nonverbal elderly. *Journal of Gerontological Nursing, 17*(6), 25-28.

McCaffery, M., & Beebe, A. (1989). *Pain: Clinical manual for nursing practice.* St. Louis: Mosby.

McCaffery, M., & Ferrell, B. (1991). Patient age: Does it affect your pain-control decisions? *Nursing 91, 21*(9), 44-48.

McKenry, L. M., & Salerno, E. (1995). *Pharmacology in Nursing.* St. Louis: Mosby.

Miaskowski, C., Jacox, A., Hester, N. O., & Ferrell, B. (1992). Interdisciplinary guidelines for the management of acute pain: Implications for quality improvement. *Journal of Nursing Care Quality, 7*(1), 1-6.

Morris, J. N., Mor, V., Goldberg, R. J., Sherwood, S., Greer, D. S., & Hiris, J. (1986). The effects of treatment setting and patient characteristics on pain in terminal cancer patients: A report from the National Hospice Study. *Journal of Chronic Diseases, 39,* 27-35.

Mosqueda, L. (1993). Office assessment tools. In T. T. Yoshikawa, E. L. Cobbs, & K. B. Brummel-Smith (Eds.), *Ambulatory geriatric care* (pp. 107-120). St. Louis: Mosby.

Parmelee, P. A., Katz, I. R., & Lawton, M. P. (1993). Pain complaints and cognitive status among elderly institution residents. *Journal of the American Geriatric Society, 41,* 517-522.

Reynolds, C. F. (1994). Treatment of depression in late life. *American Journal of Medicine, 97*(suppl. 6A), 395-465.

Rubenstein, L. Z. (1993). Falls. In T. T. Yoshikawa, E. L. Cobbs, & K. B. Brummel-Smith (Eds.), *Ambulatory geriatric care* (pp. 296-304). St. Louis: Mosby.

Sandler, D. P., Burr, F. R., & Weinberg, C. R. (1991). Nonsteroidal anti-inflammatory drugs and the risk for chronic renal decrease. *Annals of Internal Medicine, 115*(3), 165-172.

Schor, J. D., Levkoff, S. E., Lipsitz, L. A., Reilly, C. H., Cleary, P. D., Rowe, J. W., & Evans, D. A. (1992). Risk factors for delirium in hospitalized elderly. *Journal of the American Medical Association, 267*(6), 827-831.

Seidel, H., Ball, J., Dains, J., & Benedict, G. (1995). *Mosby's guide to physical examination* (3rd ed.). St. Louis: Mosby.

Sengstaken, E. A., & King, S. A. (1993). The problem of pain and its detection among geriatric nursing home residents. *Journal of the American Geriatric Society, 41,* 541-544.

Silverman, M. A., & Temple, J. D. (1992). Cancer in the elderly patient: Unique aspects of prevention, management, and screening. *Journal of the Florida Medical Association, 79,* 89-92.

Stratton, M. (1991). Geriatric pharmacotherapy. *Pharmguide to Hospital Medicine, 4*(3), 1-6.

Thomas, B. L. (1990). Elder care. *AORN Journal, 52*(6), 1268-1272.

Tinetti, M. E. (1986). Performance-oriented assessment of mobility problems in elderly patients. *Journal of the American Geriatric Society, 34,* 119-126.

Twycross, R. (1994). *Pain relief in advanced cancer.* New York: Churchill Livingstone.

Vestal, R. E. (1990). Clinical pharmacology. In W. R. Hazzard, R. Andres, E. L. Bierman, & J. P. Blass (Eds.), *Principles of geriatric medicine & gerontology* (2nd ed., pp. 201-217). New York: McGraw-Hill.

Wall, R. T. (1990). Use of analgesics in the elderly. *Clinics in Geriatric Medicine, 6*(2), 345-364.

Williams-Russo, P., Urguahart, B. L., Sharrock, N. E., & Charleson, M. E. (1992). Post-operative delirium: Prediction and prognosis in elderly orthopedic patients. *Journal of Gerontology, 45,* 12-19.

Wolfson, L., Whipple, R. Z., Amerman, P., & Tobin, J. N. (1990). Gait assessment in the elderly: A gait abnormality rating scale and its relation to falls. *Journal of Gerontology in Medical Science, 45,* M12-M19.

Wrenn, K. (1989). Fecal Impaction. *New England Journal of Medicine, 321,* 358.

13

Pain in Patients with HIV/AIDS

Gayle Newshan

        Treatment of Apthous Ulcers
        Painful Injections
    Nonpharmacologic Interventions
        General Comfort Measures
        Radiation and Chemotherapy
        Complementary Therapies
        Contributions of Family and Significant Others
Team Approach
Summary

Key Points

- Pain occurs at all points in the HIV to AIDS continuum.
- Pain in persons with HIV/AIDS may be caused by HIV itself, treatments for HIV, or factors unrelated to HIV.
- The etiology of pain in persons living with AIDS (PLWAs) should be identified and the underlying cause treated, since this can often eliminate the pain.
- When it is not possible to eradicate the cause of pain, pain should be treated aggressively with the appropriate pharmacologic and nonpharmacologic interventions, keeping in mind the unique considerations for their use in persons with HIV/AIDS.
- Pain management in chemically dependent persons with HIV/AIDS is complicated by staff disbelief of the patient's report of pain, the patient's fear of relapse if opioids are used, and the common myth that methadone provides analgesia.
- A major barrier to pain management in children with HIV is parental denial of the disease and thus of the child's pain.

- Because AIDS is a complex illness involving multiple diagnoses and myriad concurrent symptoms, a team approach is recommended.

The Centers for Disease Control (CDC) estimates that 1 in 250 persons in the United States is presently infected with the human immunodeficiency virus (HIV) and projects that by the end of 1994 the cumulative number of acquired immunodeficiency syndrome (AIDS) cases will be in the range of 415,000 to 535,000 (CDC, 1993a). The World Health Organization (WHO) estimates that a total of 8 to 10 million persons are currently infected with HIV worldwide (CDC, 1993b). Infection with HIV has reached epidemic proportions and is considered a chronic illness. There is no cure for HIV, and its effects can be devastating and painful.

The initial asymptomatic period of HIV infection is long, usually lasting a median of 9 or more years (Levy, 1993). Asymptomatic HIV infection usually progresses to AIDS, which is characterized by severe immunosuppression. The CDC has developed an HIV classification system (CDC, 1992) that categorizes HIV-positive persons along a continuum according to their clinical conditions, as outlined in the box on p. 408.

Pain is a common companion to persons with AIDS. Like cancer pain, pain in persons with HIV/AIDS is often underrecognized, poorly managed, and poorly documented. Pain management in this population is also complicated by a high percentage of substance abusers with AIDS. According to the CDC, 21% of persons with AIDS acquire HIV through intravenous drug use (CDC, 1994), and many persons who acquire HIV from unprotected sex may also have a substance-use history.

The purpose of this chapter is to identify common reasons that persons living with HIV/AIDS have pain, to describe the clinical features of pain in HIV/AIDS, to

CDC CLASSIFICATION OF HIV INFECTION

Category A

Asymptomatic or persistent, generalized lymphadenopathy

Category B

Symptomatic; may experience oral/vaginal candidiasis, fever, diarrhea listeriosis, idiopathic thrombocytopenia, oral leukoplakia, herpes zoster, neuropathy, pelvic inflammatory disease, or cervical displasia

Category C: AIDS Indicator Symptoms

CD4 count less than 200 or CD4% less than 14%
M. tuberculosis
Invasive cervical carcinoma
Recurrent bacterial pneumonia
Bronchial or esophageal candidiasis
Cytomegalovirus disease
Toxoplasmosis of brain
Wasting due to HIV
Kaposi's sarcoma
Lymphoma
HIV encephalopathy
Cryptosporidiosis, chronic
Pneumocystis carinii pneumonia
Salmonella sepsis
Progressive multifocal leukoencephalopathy
Mycobacterium avium or other disseminated mycobacterium
Cryptococcosis, extrapulmonary
Coccidiomycosis, disseminated
Histoplasmosis, disseminated
Isosporiasis, chronic
Herpes simplex, chronic

explore the pharmacologic and nonpharmacologic interventions available for treating their pain, and to discuss special populations for whom pain management presents unique challenges.

DESCRIPTION

Prevalence

HIV-Positive Class A and B: Pre-AIDS

Pain has been reported to occur at all points of the HIV to AIDS continuum. Among 140 ambulatory HIV-positive patients (Class A), 55% indicated they had pain other than minor day-to-day aches and pains (Zarowny, McCormack, Li, & Singer, 1992). Singer and colleagues (1993) found that 28% of HIV-positive asymptomatic and 55.6% of HIV-positive symptomatic (Class B) persons had pain. Pain in these two groups was found to be related to headaches, peripheral neuropathy, and herpes simplex.

HIV-Positive Class C: AIDS

Pain is the most common reason for persons living with AIDS (PLWAs) to be hospitalized (Lefkowitz, Lebovits, Smith, & Maignan, 1992), and pain increases with disease progression (Loveless, Bell, & Coodley, 1993; Singer et al., 1993). Reports of the prevalence of pain in PLWAs varies from 53% (Schofferman, 1988) to 97% (Singh, Fermie, & Peters, 1992). It appears that as PLWAs are surviving longer because of advances in treatment, pain is becoming more prevalent.

Etiology of Pain in PLWAs

The HIV virus infects every cell of the body. Because of this, every organ system can be affected by HIV. Because PLWAs have multiple coexisting illnesses, it is important to recognize that pain in the person with HIV/AIDS nearly always has an underlying cause. This underlying cause must be identified and appropriately treated, as treatment alone may eradicate the pain. While the cause of the pain is being determined, pain management with appropriate analgesics should be initiated (see the section on therapeutic interventions).

Pain in PLWAs may be caused by HIV infection and its complications, medical treatments for HIV, or factors unrelated to HIV. These different sources of pain will be mentioned in the discussion of pain as it occurs in each major organ system of the body.

Gastrointestinal System

Mouth pain has been found to be prevalent in up to 11% of PLWAs who have pain (Lebovits et al., 1989; Schofferman, 1988). This may be related to candidiasis, apthous ulcers, herpes simplex ulcers, Kaposi's sarcoma (KS), cytomegalovirus (CMV) ulcers, histoplasmosis, dental abscess, necrotizing gingivitis, or streptococcal infection. Mouth pain can also be related to treatments, as in the case of radiation or chemotherapy stomatitis and oral ulcers related to the antiretroviral zalcitabine. A painful tongue may be related to certain vitamin deficiencies, especially deficiency of B_{12} or B_6.

Odynophagia and dysphagia have been found to be prevalent in up to 17% of PLWAs who have pain (Moss, 1990; Newshan & Wainapel, 1993). This can be related to fungal infections, apthous ulcers, CMV ulcers, herpes simplex ulcers, gastric reflux disorders, or KS.

Abdominal pain has been found to be prevalent in up to 26% of PLWAs who have pain (Moss, 1990; Newshan & Wainapel, 1993; Schofferman, 1988). This type of pain is often related to intestinal infections such as cryptosporidia, shigella, salmonella, *Mycobacterium avium* complex, *Giardia lamblia,* cryptoccocus, *Entamoeba histolytica, Isospora belli,* and *Clostridium difficile.* Other causes of abdominal pain include CMV colitis/ileitis, lymphoma, KS, HIV enteropathy, and pelvic inflammatory disease. Non–HIV-related causes of abdominal pain, such as peritonitis, ectopic pregnancy, small bowel obstruction, perforated ulcer, ruptured ovarian cyst, and acute appendicitis, must also be considered.

Biliary tract pain is usually related to obstruction, which can be caused by cryptosporidia, KS, lymphoma, CMV, campylobacter, *Mycobacterium avium* complex, or gallstones. Pancreatitis is related to intravenous pentamadine, CMV infection, toxoplasmosis, alcohol, or some antiretrovirals, such as didanosine and zalcitabine.

Anorectal pain has been found to be prevalent in 6% of PLWAs who have pain (Moss, 1990). This is often related to perirectal abscess formation, perirectal fistulas, herpes simplex ulcers, anorectal carcinoma, hemorrhoids, and foreign objects. Some patients insert foreign objects rectally for sexual pleasure, and traumatic injury can often result, especially when breakable objects are used. Proctitis occurs commonly in men and can be related to herpes simplex, *Chlamydia trachomatus, Neisseria gonorrhoeae,* or CMV.

Genitourinary System

Genitourinary pain can be related to cystitis, herpes simplex, epididymitis, renal calculi, or bartholinitis.

Neurologic System

Headaches have been found to be prevalent in up to 17% of PLWAs with pain (Newshan & Wainapel, 1993; Schofferman, 1988). There are multiple causes of headaches, such as central nervous system toxoplasmosis, central nervous system nocardia, and meningitis due to cryptococcus, histoplasmosis, *Mycobacterium tuberculosis,* or syphilis. Headaches can also be related to sinus infections, herpes encephalopathy, progressive multifocal leukoencephalopathy, and lumbar punctures. Other causes of headaches are stress (tension), migraines, and medications. Many medications commonly used to treat HIV and HIV-related infections can cause headaches, including zidovudine, interferon, acyclovir, nizoral, amphotericin, atovaquone, and sulfonamides.

Peripheral neuropathy has been found to be prevalent in up to 59% of PLWAs in pain (Singer et al., 1993). Causes of neuropathy include HIV, CMV, and medications such as vincristine, isoniazide, didanosine, zalcitabine, and stavudine.

Less commonly, vitamin deficiency or diabetes can be a factor in causing peripheral neuropathy.

Spinal or back pain occurs in about 5% of PLWAs who have pain (Newshan & Wainapel, 1993). Causes include spinal abscess formation, lymphoma, and *Mycobacterium avium* complex. Lumbar punctures can also cause pain.

Dermatologic System

Skin pain is prevalent in up to 15% of PLWAs in pain (Newshan & Wainapel, 1993; Schofferman, 1988). This can be related to herpes zoster, cutaneous KS, burns, postherpetic neuralgia, bacterial abscesses, decubitus ulcers, allergic dermatitis, cellulitis, and folliculitis.

Musculoskeletal System

Bone, joint, and muscle pain is prevalent in up to 33% of PLWAs in pain (Singh et al., 1992). Joint pain may be related to HIV arthropathy, avascular necrosis, *Mycobacterium avium* complex, a reactive process such as Reiter's syndrome, or psoriatic arthritis. Fibromyalgia and polymyositis may be related to chronic HIV infection, depression, or abuse of cocaine, crack cocaine, or alcohol. They can also be caused by medications such as zidovudine and isoniazide (Simms et al., 1992).

Cardiopulmonary System

Chest pain is reported in up to 22% of PLWAs in pain (Lebovits et al., 1989). This type of pain can be related to pericarditis, endocarditis, *Pneumocystis carinii* pneumonia, bacterial pneumonia, pneumothorax, pleural effusion, KS, lymphoma, costochondritis, rib fracture, and trauma. Procedure-related pain includes pain due to chest tubes and postoperative pain.

Other

Singh and colleagues (1992) report that 56% of PLWAs who have pain describe "diffuse pain," and Moss (1990) reports that 10% of PLWAs with pain describe "total body pain." Moss suggests that this kind of nonspecific report indicates the patient's response to overwhelming emotional distress.

Clinical Features

Little is known about the experience of pain in PLWAs. Some of the reported clinical features described here only hint at the full impact of pain on the quality of life for PLWAs.

Peripheral neuropathy is described as "pins and needles," burning, numbness, throbbing, cramping, tingling, and aching (Newshan & Wainapel, 1993; Schofferman, 1988). Patients with neuropathy usually experience progressive difficulty with walking and performing other activities of daily living. For some PLWAs even the weight of a blanket can be extremely uncomfortable.

Esophagitis is described as a sharp, retrosternal burning (Newshan & Wainapel, 1993). Patients with esophagitis often report painful and difficult swallowing. This problem can also interfere with their ability to eat and take medications and can have a major impact on overall well-being.

Arthralgia in HIV/AIDS is described as polyarticular by 62% of patients, with the knee, ankle, and elbow typically affected (Saraux et al., 1994). It is also often associated with morning stiffness and sleep disturbances (Saraux et al.). It has been described as being dull and aching in character (Newshan & Wainapel, 1993).

Pain intensity is reported to range from moderate to severe in most studies. Anand, Carmosino, and Glatt (1994) found that pain was graded as more than 7 on a 0 to 10 scale in all PLWAs who were evaluated ($N = 24$), and Hoyt, Nokes, Newshan, Staats, and Thorn (1994) found that mean pain intensity was 5 on a 0 to 10 scale in a sample of 71 PLWAs.

Pain has been found to contribute to disability in PLWAs; patients with more pain typically have lower Karnofsky scores (Loveless et al., 1993). As the disease progresses and pain increases, patients often become weaker, are forced to give up their jobs, and require more assistance with personal tasks and household functions.

Special Populations

Children with HIV

Adults are not the only group affected by HIV. The World Health Organization projects that by the year 2000, 10 million children and adolescents worldwide will be infected with the virus (WHO, 1993). Czarniecki, Boland, and Oleske (1993) provide one of the few reports of pain in children with HIV. They found that pain was related to headaches, cellulitis, herpes infections, bacterial abscesses, otitis media, esophagitis, and procedures such as venipuncture and lumbar puncture. In addition, children with HIV encephalopathy experience painful muscle spasms and spasticity.

A major barrier to pain management in children with HIV is parental denial of the disease and thus of the child's pain (Czarniecki et al., 1993; Well-Halpern, Debre, & Griscelli, 1993). Czarniecki and co-workers also report that many families are reluctant to have their children treated with opioids because of their own negative experiences with drug abuse. Development of a trusting relationship between staff and family and education about commonly held myths are key components to providing comfort to children infected with HIV.

Chemically Dependent Patients

As mentioned earlier, nearly one in four persons living with HIV/AIDS became infected with HIV because of intravenous drug use. Many are either actively using drugs such as cocaine, crack cocaine, alcohol, and heroin or are former users of these substances.

There are three major factors complicating pain management in persons with a chemical dependence history. First, health care providers often hold negative and prejudicial attitudes toward persons with chemical dependence (Forrester & Murphy, 1992). Because of this, health care providers often disbelieve reports of pain in the chemically dependent, labeling them "drug-seeking." In fact, several studies (Lebovits et al., 1989; Newshan & Wainapel, 1993; Schofferman, 1988) have found no significant difference in etiology of pain in PLWAs who are chemically dependent compared with PLWAs who are not chemically dependent. In addition, Hoyt and colleagues (1994) report no significant difference in patient perception of pain when comparing chemically dependent PLWAs and non–chemically dependent PLWAs.

Second, some drug users may be using methadone to stem heroin craving. Many health care providers mistakenly believe that methadone maintenance provides analgesia, though the opposite is true: persons on methadone require additional opioids to control pain (Hicks, 1989; Payne, 1989). Anand and colleagues (1994) found that PLWAs on methadone maintenance were able to achieve pain relief when given supplemental opioids for pain and that substance-using PLWAs exhibited no difference in response to pain medications when compared with non–substance-using PLWAs.

The same principles of pain management that apply to non–chemically dependent PLWAs should be applied to the chemically dependent. Both pharmacologic and nonpharmacologic methods are as useful in the chemically dependent patient as they are in the non–chemically dependent patient. Health care providers should believe the complaint of pain, in spite of the possibility of being duped (McCaffery & Vourakis, 1992). Abuse behaviors do occur (see the box on p. 416), presenting a great challenge to health care providers and often resulting in frustration. Suggested responses to abuse behaviors are outlined in the box on p. 417.

Finally, many former substance users are reluctant to use opioid analgesics because of fear of relapse. They may have spent many months or years battling addiction and may share the commonly held myth that using opioids for pain will cause addiction. Family members of these patients

DRUG ABUSE BEHAVIORS

1. Attempting excessive negotiations for pain medications
2. Selling drugs to or buying drugs from other patients
3. Testing positive in urine toxicology for nonprescribed substances
4. Frequently alleging loss or theft of prescriptions
5. Failing to keep clinic appointments while arriving only to pick up prescriptions
6. Refusing to undergo diagnostic tests to determine cause of pain
7. Making excessive emergency room visits for opioids
8. Borrowing pain medicine from friends or family members
9. Engaging in nonprescribed use of opioids such as chewing fentanyl patches or dissolving opioid pills in water for mainlining
10. Nodding out or coming to clinic or office high or disoriented

may share and contribute to this fear. The health care provider should be sensitive to the concerns of the patient and family, explaining that now the patient is taking the opioid for a medically prescribed reason, not to get "high" (Vallerand, 1994). It is also often helpful to enlist the support of substance abuse counselors who can assure the patient that they will be available should abuse behavior occur.

Patients with Dementia

Approximately 75% of PLWAs have mild to severe clinically detectable dementia at the time of death (Sotrel & Multani, 1992). *AIDS dementia complex* (ADC) is a term describing a constellation of signs and symptoms manifested by progressive cognitive impairment with accompanying motor and behavioral disturbances. Price and Sidtis (1992) describe ADC as having four stages (see the box on p. 418). Pain management in patients with ADC is complicated by

INTERVENTIONS FOR DRUG ABUSE BEHAVIORS

1. Address the issue directly with patient.
2. Consult with clinical experts such as drug counselors or pain specialists for support.
3. Develop a contract with the patient that limits opioid prescriptions to 1 week's worth at a time with no refills. Be consistent and inform the patient that he or she will be sent to the ER if the prescription is "lost" or "stolen." Consider escorting the patient to the pharmacy to get the prescription filled.
4. Explore the option of restricting the patient to one pharmacy if he or she is on Medicaid or another state-regulated prescription program.
5. Avoid a power struggle; stay calm; be consistent.

difficulties in assessment and communication. Very little is known about the relationship between pain and neurocognitive decline. It is likely that patients with ADC suffer pain, especially if they have coexisting conditions known to be painful. Considerations for assessment of persons with ADC are discussed in the next section.

THERAPEUTIC MANAGEMENT

Assessment

The guidelines for assessment of pain given in Chapter 1 should be followed for pain in PLWAs. All PLWAs should be asked if they are experiencing pain or discomfort. Any new pain should be evaluated to determine its etiology. Key points to remember include: assessment of pain and response to treatment are continuous processes; pain is a subjective phenomenon, its most reliable indicator being patient self-report; and pain assessment should be clearly documented.

Assessment of pain in the person with ADC is particularly challenging and requires knowledge of the patient, understanding of pain etiology in PLWAs, and clinical sensitivity. It is important to know the patient so that behavioral

STAGES AND ASSOCIATED SYMPTOMS OF AIDS DEMENTIA COMPLEX

Stage 0	No symptoms
Stage 1	Mild symptoms: loss of train of thought, difficulty with memory, need to keep lists, fatigue
Stage 2	Moderate symptoms: difficulty with reading and concentration, inability to work, need for increasing help with household and personal tasks, cognitive decline, apathy, and withdrawal
Stage 3	Severe symptoms: greatly diminished intellect; psychomotor slowing; progressive difficulty with balance, coordination, and fine motor skills
Stage 4	Terminal stage: near vegetative state, vacant stare, paraparesis, incontinence

Modified from Price, R., & Sidtis, J. (1992): The AIDS dementia complex. In G. Wormser (Ed.), *AIDS and other manifestations of HIV infection.* (2nd ed., pp.373-382). New York: Raven Press.

changes can be identified. For example, a patient who becomes restless or who stops eating may be experiencing pain. Continue any pain medications the patient has been taking, even if ADC causes the patient to give a confusing picture of the pain. For example, it is not uncommon for a patient with ADC who reports pain to say only a few minutes later that there is no pain. Although such inconsistencies can be difficult to interpret, the health care provider should err on the side of compassion by promoting comfort through pharmacologic and/or nonpharmacologic means.

Assessment of patients with ADC should be unhurried. It is important to be assured of having the patient's attention before initiating the conversation. The health care provider should use clear, concise statements and ask only one question at a time. When possible, it is often best to ask questions requiring simple "yes" or "no" responses.

Pharmacologic Interventions

The pharmacologic approaches to pain management were thoroughly discussed in Chapter 4. This section is designed to provide an overview of specific analgesic considerations for PLWAs and to provide recommendations for the treatment of certain painful AIDS-related conditions.

Nonsteroidal Antiinflammatory Drugs

Nonsteroidal antiinflammatory drugs (NSAIDs) play an important role in the pharmacologic management of pain in persons with HIV/AIDS. They can be used to relieve throbbing or aching pain, joint pain, and sinus headaches. They are also used to boost the effectiveness of opioid therapy. Several precautions, however, must be taken before prescribing them to PLWAs. First, many PLWAs have thrombocytopenia or renal insufficiency, and for these patients NSAIDs should be avoided. Salsalate and tolmentin produce less inhibition of platelet aggregation than do other NSAIDs and can therefore be considered for patients with only mild thrombocytopenia (DiGregorio et al., 1994).

Second, toxicity from NSAIDs is greater in persons with low serum albumin levels, a common consquence of HIV infection. Therefore, caution is indicated when these agents are used in persons with wasting syndrome and cachexia, which are often associated with low albumin levels. Third, because NSAIDs should be taken with food, the health care provider must evaluate the patient's dietary intake to determine whether an antacid is required to prevent gastric irritation. Persons with gastric Kaposi's sarcoma are at increased risk for gastrointestinal bleeding and should therefore either always take the NSAID with an antacid or avoid NSAIDs completely.

Finally, indomethacin should be avoided when a patient is taking zidovudine, an antiviral medication. Theoretically, concurrent use of these two medications can result in indomethacin or zidovudine toxicity (USP DI, 1994), although clinical data to support this are lacking.

Opioids

Opioids are the mainstay of pain management in PLWAs. The box on p. 421 lists tips that the nurse should give patients taking opioids. As with all patients, optimal doses are determined by individual titration. Although many PLWAs experience diarrhea, a bowel regimen to avoid constipation and obstruction must still be considered.

When using long-acting oral opioid preparations, it is important that the pill not be crushed, chewed, or broken. In addition, the medicine, which is activated by fluids, may be ineffective if the patient is dehydrated and unable to drink sufficient liquid. Because PLWAs have high metabolic rates, a dosage interval of 8 hours is often more effective than the 12-hour interval commonly used with cancer patients.

When using fentanyl transdermal patches, it is important to remember that PLWAs often experience fevers and sweats. Fevers will cause the fentanyl to be more quickly absorbed, which will result in shorter duration of effectiveness as well as possible sedation during the febrile episode. Diaphoresis can make it difficult for the patch to adhere to the skin; some patients find using an Ace bandage or terrycloth sports band helpful to keep the patch in place. The patch should be applied only to intact skin. It should not be applied to thick, cutaneous Kaposi's sarcoma lesions, where the skin lacks penetrability. Nor should it be applied to irradiated or inflamed skin.

It is generally recommended that medications metabolized by hepatic glucuronidation not be given together (USP DI, 1994). Two such medications are zidovudine and morphine. It is theoretically possible that concurrent administration of these drugs could result in zidovudine toxicity. However, this has never been clinically reported to occur in PLWAs. To date, no studies have discussed the effect of the concurrent use of zidovudine and morphine. Several studies (Dixon & Higginson, 1991; Newshan & Wainapel, 1993) have documented successful morphine use by PLWAs, but concurrent administration of zidovudine was not reported in these cases.

PATIENT EDUCATION: TIPS FOR PATIENTS TAKING OPIOID ANALGESICS

Storage: Keep out of reach of children; store away from heat and moisture; keep suppositories refrigerated but not frozen; discard outdated medicine.

Travel: When traveling, always carry the opioid in its original, labeled package. If traveling internationally, ask your health care provider to write a letter on official stationery stating your medical condition and listing medications prescribed to avoid confiscation at customs.

Renewals: Anticipate your opioid needs and give your health care provider several days' notice to write a prescription before you run low; do not wait until you have taken your last dose to call for a prescription.

Administration: Opioids can be taken with or without food. Long-acting preparations should be taken with a full glass of liquid and should not be crushed, chewed, or broken. Suppositories should be moistened with water and the flat end inserted first into the rectum. Transdermal patches should be applied to intact skin; avoid broken or inflamed areas.

Communication: Talk to your health care provider if you feel the medicine is not working properly or if you are having unacceptable side effects, such as nausea or excessive sedation. Do not increase the dose without checking with your health care provider.

Routes of Administration

Persons living with AIDS often suffer from dehydration, malnourishment, and electrolyte imbalances due to vomiting, diarrhea, and anorexia. In such cases, alternative routes to oral administration of medication need to be considered. In the patient who is vomiting, rectal and topical routes should be considered. In the patient who is having diarrhea and vomiting, the topical route is preferred. In the patient who has difficulty swallowing, liquid or rectal preparations may be tried. Health care providers often forget that some NSAIDs are available in liquid or suppository form, as are morphine and hydromorphone. Few PLWAs, however, require parenteral opioids if the appropriate analgesics are administered in adequate doses via the most suitable route (Anand et al., 1994; Newshan & Wainapel, 1993).

Treatment of Peripheral Neuropathy

Peripheral neuropathy in persons with HIV/AIDS usually requires a combination approach. If the pain is described as "pins and needles," burning, or tingling, a tricyclic antidepressant is suggested. Any of the following can be tried: amitriptyline, doxepin, imipramine, or desipramine, in doses beginning at 10 mg and titrated to desired effect. Patients need to be reminded that it can take up to 2 weeks for the effect to be noticed. If the pain is described as aching or throbbing, an NSAID is recommended. If the patient reports a cramping quality, then quinine sulfate at bedtime can be tried. Patients with neuropathy will often require a mild opioid in addition to any one or more of the preceding medications to control pain. An investigational drug, peptide T, used by some PLWAs to decrease the symptoms of neuropathy, is available only through clinical trials or underground buyer's clubs. Its clinical efficacy has not been proven.

Certain anticonvulsants have traditionally been used to treat neuropathy, including phenytoin, clonazepam, and carbamazepine. Phenytoin and carbamazepine must be used with caution in PLWAs because of their neutropenic effect.

Topical use of capsaicin ointment is practical only if a small area, such as fingertips or toes, is affected, because it must be used several times a day for analgesia to be achieved.

There are several nonpharmacologic interventions that are helpful in the treatment of neuropathy, including acupuncture, support stockings, massage, and exercise.

Treatment of Apthous Ulcers

Apthous ulcers are painful idiopathic ulcers with deeply eroded bases found in the mouth or esophagus and are usually responsive to treatment with glucocorticosteroids (Glick, 1993). If they are in the oral cavity, the steroid can be applied topically with Kenalog in Orabase several times a day. If the ulcers are in the esophagus, dexamethasone elixir or prednisone pills can be prescribed in a tapering dose. The ulcers usually resolve in 5 to 10 days of treatment, although they commonly recur. While the ulcers are being treated with steroids, taking a stomatitis elixir before meals or medications is suggested. This is commonly a mixture of Benadryl elixir, viscous lidocaine, and an antacid. Many patients will also require an opioid until the ulcers have completely resolved.

Painful Injections

Many PLWAs who develop anemia and neutropenia require Epogen injections three times a week or Neupogen injections daily. For PLWAs who have muscle wasting and cachexia, these repeated injections can be uncomfortable. One solution to the discomfort is to use a topical preparation of lidocaine or prilocaine for providing localized anesthesia prior to the injections. This preparation was developed to decrease painful venipunctures in children and is therefore safe to use in treating the pediatric population as well as adults.

Nonpharmacologic Interventions

Nonpharmacologic approaches are reviewed in Chapter 5. This section will provide specific recommendations for PLWAs.

General Comfort Measures

It is surprising how comforting an egg crate–type foam mattress can be for a PLWA, especially if that patient is wasted and cachectic. These mattresses are typically available in hospitals and can usually be ordered for the home.

Similarly, a foam or gel cushion for a chair or wheelchair can allow a PLWA to sit for longer periods with greater comfort.

Radiation and Chemotherapy

Radiation and chemotherapy can be remarkably palliative, especially for patients with pain from KS. With treatment, the Kaposi's tumor will shrink, and the debulking can help tremendously to decrease pain. It is often helpful to tell patients who are reluctant or afraid to undergo radiation or chemotherapy that doing so can greatly ease their pain.

Complementary Therapy

Several complementary therapies have been used to decrease pain in PLWAs. Aroma therapy has been used to reduce muscle aches and generalized pain in PLWAs (Teopista, 1993). Therapeutic touch (Newshan, 1989) and relaxation and imagery techniques (Newshan & Wainapel, 1993) have been used to decrease abdominal pain, joint pain, headache, and pain due to KS in PLWAs.

Contributions of Family and Significant Others

Involvement of family and significant others in the treatment of pain in the PLWAs can have a beneficial effect on the treatment outcome. These persons can provide concrete help, such as prepouring a patient's medications or massaging sore muscles. They may also provide psychologic support by reinforcing that it is beneficial, not harmful, to take pain medication.

TEAM APPROACH

Human immunodeficiency disease is a complex illness with an unpredictable course. Patients living with HIV/AIDS often have overwhelming social and financial needs as well as emotional, physical, and spiritual difficulties. Because of this, it is unlikely that one health care provider alone can respond to all these needs, and so a team approach can be helpful.

For example, when painful swallowing and mouth sores are a problem, the dietitian can be consulted for recommendations in meal preparation. For musculoskeletal pain and neuropathy, a physical therapist can initiate an exercise program, treat the pain with ultrasound or transcutaneous electrical nerve stimulation, or create a splint or brace for support. For housing difficulties, such as when patients can no longer negotiate stairs or when they begin to require help at home, a social worker can be of assistance. For patients who experience anxiety, depression, relationship problems, or other emotional problems, the expertise of a psychologist or psychiatrist can be invaluable. For chemically dependent patients, substance abuse counselors can provide counseling and referrals to treatment programs. In the amelioration of the myriad of other symptoms experienced by PLWAs, such as nausea, diarrhea, dyspnea, itching, vomiting, fatigue, and cachexia, the physician plays a crucial role. The pharmacist can be consulted for help in identifying drug interactions and formulations. For coordination of the team as a whole, the nurse is a pivotal team member who is often the first to identify problems and evaluate responses to treatment.

It must be remembered that the most important member of the team is the patient. PLWAs are usually highly knowledgeable about their disease and typically demand active involvement with all aspects of treatment. This should be respected and encouraged.

SUMMARY

In summary, it is clear that pain is a common companion of persons living with HIV/AIDS. It is also clear that, with drug therapy as the mainstay of the treatment program, there are many interventions that can ameliorate this pain. Pain in PLWAs is often complicated by polypharmacy, multiple concurrent diagnoses, chemical dependence history, or dementia. It is crucial for the health care provider to know and understand the etiology of pain as well as the pharmacologic considerations of analgesic use in PLWAs. Although we cannot cure AIDS, we can provide comfort and care to patients living with HIV/AIDS.

References

Anand, A., Carmosino, L., & Glatt, A. (1994). Evaluation of recalcitrant pain in HIV-infected hospitalized patients. *Journal of Acquired Immune Deficiency Syndromes, 7,* 52-56.

Centers for Disease Control (CDC). (1992). 1993 revised classification system for HIV infection and expanded surveillance case definition for AIDS among adolescents and adults. *MMWR: Morbidity and Mortality Weekly Report, 41* (RR-17), 1-19.

Centers for Disease Control (CDC). (1993a). Statistical projections/trends. *AIDS Information* (Document 320210).

Centers for Disease Control (CDC). (1993b). International projections/statistics. *AIDS Information* (Document 320220).

Centers for Disease Control (CDC). (1994). HIV/AIDS surveillance report. *6* (1), 1-27.

Czarniecki, L., Boland, M., & Oleske, J. (1993). Pain in children with HIV disease. *PAACNOTES: Newsjournal of the Physicians Association for AIDS Care, 5*(12), 492-495.

DiGregorio, G., Barbieri, E., Ferko, A., Sterling, G., Camp, J., & Prout, M. (1994). *Handbook of pain management* (4th ed.). West Chester, PA: Medical Surveillance.

Dixon, P., & Higginson, I. (1991). AIDS and cancer pain treated with slow release morphine. *Postgraduate Medical Journal, 67*(suppl. 2), S92-S94.

Forrester, D., & Murphy, P. (1992). Nurses' attitudes towards patients with AIDS and AIDS-related risk factors. *Journal of Advanced Nursing, 17,* 1260-1266.

Glick, M. (1993). Oral pain. *PAACNOTES: Newsjournal of the Physicians Association for AIDS Care, 5*(6), 226-230.

Hicks, R. (1989). Pain management in the chemically dependent patient. *Hawaiian Medical Journal, 48*(11), 491-494.

Hoyt, M., Nokes, K., Newshan, G., Staats, J., & Thorn, M. (1994). The effect of chemical dependency on pain perception in persons with AIDS. *Journal of the Association of Nurses in AIDS Care, 4*(3), 33-38.

Lebovits, A., Lefkowitz, M., McCarthy, D., Simon, R., Wilpon, H., Jung, R., & Fried, E. (1989). The prevalence and management of pain in patients with AIDS: A review of 134 cases. *Clinical Journal of Pain, 5,* 245-248.

Lefkowitz, M., Lebovits, A., Smith, G., & Maignan, M. (1992). The prevalence and management of pain in patients with AIDS: A second look three years later. In *Proceedings of the VIII International Conference on AIDS* (Abstract PuB 7304), Amsterdam.

Levy, J. (1993). The transmission of HIV and factors influencing progression to AIDS. *American Journal of Medicine, 95,* 86-98.

Loveless, M., Bell, L., & Coodley, G. (1993). Pain associated with HIV disease and its complications. In *Proceedings of the IX International Conference on AIDS* (Abstract WS-B31-6), Berlin.

McCaffery, M., & Vourakis, C. (1992). Assessment and relief of pain in chemically dependent patients. *Orthopedic Nursing, 11*(2),13.

Moss, V. (1990). Palliative care in advanced HIV disease: Presentation, problems and palliation. *AIDS, 4*(suppl. 1), S235-S242.

Newshan, G. (1989). Therapeutic touch for symptom management in persons with AIDS. *Holistic Nursing Practice, 3*(4), 45-51.

Newshan, G., & Wainapel, S. (1993). Pain characteristics and their management in persons with AIDS. *Journal of the Association for Nurses in AIDS Care, 4*(2), 53-59.

Payne, R. (1989). Pain in the drug abuser. In R. Payne & K. Foley (Eds.), *Current therapy of pain* (pp. 47-53). Philadelphia: Decker.

Price, R., & Sidtis, J. (1992). The AIDS dementia complex. In G. Wormser (Ed.), *AIDS and other manifestations of HIV infection* (2nd ed., pp. 373-382). New York: Raven Press.

Saraux, A., Taelman, H., Clerinx, J., Batungwanayo, J., Kagame, A., Kabagabo, L., Bogaerts, J., Van der Perre, P., & Le Goff, P. (1994). Persistent arthralgia and its association with HIV infection in Rwanda. *Journal of Acquired Immune Deficiency Syndromes, 7,* 158-162.

Schofferman, J. (1988). Pain: Diagnosis and management in the palliative care of AIDS. *Journal of Palliative Care, 4,* 46-49.

Simms, R., Zerbini, C., Ferrante, N., Anthony, J., Felson, D., & Craven, D. (1992). Fibromyalgia syndrome in patients infected with human immunodeficiency virus. *American Journal of Medicine, 92,* 368-374.

Singer, E., Zorilla, C., Fahy-Chandon, B., Chi, S., Syndulko, K., & Tourtellotte, W. (1993). Painful symptoms reported by HIV-infected men in a longitudinal study. *Pain, 54,* 15-19.

Singh, S., Fermie, O., & Peters, W. (1992). Symptom control for individuals with advanced HIV in a subacute residential unit: Which symptoms need palliation? In *Proceedings of the VIII International Conference on AIDS* (Abstract PuB 5248), Amsterdam.

Sotrel, A., & Multani, P. (1992). Pathology of the nervous system in HIV-infected patients. In G. Wormser (Ed.), *AIDS and other manifestations of HIV infection* (2nd ed., pp. 543-584). New York: Raven Press.

Teopista, N. (1993). The use of aroma therapy in the management of people with AIDS. *Proceedings of the IX International Conference on Aids* (Abstract PuB 29-2171), Berlin.

USP DI (1994). *Drug information for the health care professional* (14th ed.). Rockville, MD: U.S. Pharmacopeial Convention.

Vallerand, A. (1994). Street addicts and patients with pain: Similarities and differences. *Clinical Nurse Specialist, 8*(1), 11-15.

Well-Halpern, F., Debre, M., & Griscelli, C. (1993). Efficacy of pluridisciplinary approach to the best care of pain in AIDS children. In *Proceedings of the IX International Conference on AIDS* (Abstract PuB 38-2396), Berlin.

World Health Organization (WHO). (1993). *Global progress on AIDS.* Geneva: WHO.

Zarowny, D., McCormack, J., Li, R., & Singer, J. (1992). Incidence of pain in ambulatory HIV patients. In *Proceedings of the VIII International Conference on AIDS* (Abstract PuB 3551), Amsterdam.

14

INVASIVE INTERVENTIONS

Donna M. Jasinski

Cassandra J. Snyder

Key Points

- Comprehensive patient assessment, selection, education, and management are crucial to successful treatment.
- Nerve blocks are used to make diagnoses, predict effects of other therapies, prevent chronic pain syndromes, and provide anesthesia and postoperative analgesia.
- Intraspinal opioids are useful for the management of acute and chronic pain.
- For chronic pain, noninvasive treatments should be tried before invasive interventions are considered.
- Intrathecal opioids can be used for chronic, malignant pain for short or long durations.
- Members of the team caring for the patient must possess the knowledge base and expertise relative to the therapy.

Invasive interventions may be used for the management of both acute and chronic pain. Acute pain, especially postoperative or that associated with trauma, may be controlled optimally with intravenous or intraspinal drug infusions. Patient-controlled analgesia (PCA), continuous epidural infusions, and patient-controlled epidural analgesia (PCEA) have revolutionized acute pain management. Proper therapies applied to pain of limited duration usually resolve acute pain within a few days or weeks.

Chronic pain, which has been defined as pain lasting for greater than 6 months, may require invasive interventions when noninvasive treatment modalities have proven unsuccessful. Jacox and colleagues (1994) recommend that, with rare exceptions, noninvasive analgesic treatments should precede invasive approaches to chronic cancer pain. However, should invasive treatments be necessary, various therapies (nerve blocks, spinal cord stimulation, long-term opioid infusions via external or internal pump) can provide patients with otherwise elusive pain relief and increase their quality of life.

Crucial to the success of therapy involving invasive interventions are the care provider's extensive skill, experience, and in-depth knowledge. Adherence to general and specific rules of patient selection criteria, coupled with patient education on the risks and benefits of the proposed therapies, will greatly enhance patient satisfaction and therapeutic outcome.

DESCRIPTION

This chapter provides an overview of three specific invasive approaches to pain management: nerve blocks, intravenous and spinal infusions, and spinal cord stimulation. Continuous or patient-controlled analgesia (PCA) infusions of opioids via intravenous or intraspinal (epidural or intrathecal) routes are often utilized for the relief of acute and chronic pain. These modalities provide continuous analgesia, thereby avoiding the peaks and troughs of traditional pro re nata (prn) dosing of either oral or intramuscular opioids.

Nerve blocks often successfully control acute pain associated with operative procedures and acute pain that is neuropathic in origin, as with acute reflex sympathetic dystrophy and acute herpes zoster. In chronic pain syndromes, nerve blocks are utilized for diagnosis, prognosis, and therapy.

Spinal cord stimulation involves the painless electrical stimulation of large afferent nerve fibers in the dorsal column of the spinal cord to inhibit the transmission of pain. Though invasive, it is nondestructive in nature, causing no permanent interruption of nerve pathways.

THERAPEUTIC MANAGEMENT

Assessment

Comprehensive assessment is critical to the aggressive management of pain. In assessing a patient's suitability for invasive treatment modalities, it is critical that all information about the patient's condition be integrated. The overall assessment of the patient is essential to appropriate patient selection and to the relative success of the invasive therapy. The reader is referred to Chapter 1 for an overview of general assessment techniques. Key components of the assessment of patients with chronic pain include a detailed history, a neurologic examination, a psychologic evaluation, pain measurement data, and results of previous trial procedures. Chapter 9 discusses in greater detail the assessment of a patient suffering from chronic nonmalignant pain. Assessment information specific to each invasive therapy will be addressed in more detail in the description of each modality.

Nerve Blocks

Therapeutic use of local anesthetics to produce an interruption of sensory and nociceptive pathways is a longstanding practice in treating both acute pain secondary to operative procedures and chronic pain of many different origins. Regional nerve blocks serve to anesthetize a select area—usually an extremity—for certain operative procedures. The use of these blocks is usually restricted to the operative setting; therefore the discussion of regional blockade for acute pain will be limited to this use.

Nerve blocks are very useful in the diagnosis and treatment of chronic pain, although the degree to which they relieve chronic pain varies (Abram, Anderson, & Maitra-D'Cruze, 1981; Arnhoff, Triplett, & Pokorney, 1977). Bonica (1990) has outlined the indications for and usefulness of nerve blocks. Jacox and colleagues (1994) have developed recommendations for clinicians considering nerve blocks for the treatment of chronic pain:

1. The mechanism of the patient's pain must be thoroughly assessed in order to select the most appropriate nerve block.
2. Patients should be screened for coexisting medical conditions, ability to understand the risks associated

with the nerve block, and ability to cooperate during the block.

3. The person performing the block should be experienced, skillful, and able to provide follow-up assessment and treatment.
4. The person performing the block should be prepared to deal with side effects and provide emergency treatment as necessary.
5. Radiographic control should be used when safety and ease depend on precise anatomic guidance.

Nerve blocks may be utilized for diagnostic, prognostic, prophylactic, or therapeutic purposes. Table 14-1 summarizes the indications for each use. Neuronal blockade, used as a diagnostic tool, can determine the anatomic source of the pain and ascertain specific nociceptive pathways. Nerve blocks are particularly valuable in determining whether the pain originates from a peripheral site, from the central nervous system, or from emotional, psychologic, or behavioral problems.

Prognostic blocks achieved by neurolytic blocks and neuroablative procedures can predict and allow patients to experience the expected results of prolonged interruption of neuronal pain transmission. Neurolytic blocks produce prolonged destruction of axons or cell bodies of peripheral somatic and sympathetic nerves by the injection of a

Table 14-1 Indications for Nerve Blocks

Type	Indication
Diagnostic	Determine the anatomic source of pain
	Ascertain specific nociceptive pathways
	Differentiate central from peripheral pain
Prognostic	Predict effects of neuroablative procedures
	Allow patients to experience effects of permanent therapies
Prophylactic	Prevent development of chronic pain syndromes
Therapeutic	Provide optimal relief of pain in self-limiting disorders
	Permit more effective application of definitive therapy

chemical agent. Neuroablative procedures are surgical operations in which the nerve, nerve root, or portions of the spinal cord may be resected. They are destructive surgical operations usually reserved for patients with chronic pain who have a life-shortening malignancy.

Prevention of the development of certain chronic pain syndromes (reflex sympathetic dystrophy, phantom limb pain) can be accomplished with prophylactic nerve blocks. Therapeutic nerve blocks provide relief in self-limiting disorders and permit more effective application of definitive therapy (Bonica, 1990).

Drugs Used for Nerve Blocks

Local Anesthetics

Local anesthetics are utilized for all types of nerve blocks. Neurolytic agents are utilized for therapeutic nerve blocks following successful results with a diagnostic local anesthetic agent. The type, volume, and concentration of drug varies with the site of neural blockade, the technique, and the duration of anesthesia needed.

Local anesthetics prevent the development of an action potential in a nerve by preventing movement of sodium ions into the cell through the sodium channels. The resting membrane potential is normally −90 mV. When an impulse passes along a nerve the membrane becomes permeable to sodium and the inside of the membrane becomes +40 mV with respect to the outside, generating an action potential. When local anesthetic is present the membrane is stabilized. Because the anesthetic binds to sodium channels and prevents their opening, an action potential cannot be generated.

Local anesthetics are composed of hydrophilic and lipophilic components linked by either an ester or amide intermediate chain. This linkage is the basis for classification of the local anesthetics (Wood & Wood, 1990). The hydrophilic component is usually a secondary or tertiary amine, and the lipophilic component is usually an unsaturated aromatic ring. Lipid solubility is essential to the anesthetic activity of the local anesthetics. Examples of local anesthetics in the ester group include procaine, chloroprocaine, and tetracaine. Local anesthetics in the amide group are lidocaine, mepivacaine, bupivacaine, and etidocaine. The type of linkage determines the site of biodegradation; esters are hydrolyzed in the plasma, and amides are more slowly metabolized in the liver.

The action of local anesthetics depends on their lipid solubility, protein binding, and dissociation constant. Generally, high-lipid-solubility, high-protein-binding agents have longer durations of action and potency. Those with pKa values close to physiologic pH have a more rapid onset. Table 14-2 illustrates the duration, potency, and onset time of the local anesthetics. The resulting blood levels after administration depend on dose, absorption from the site, biotransformation, and elimination of the drug.

Nerve fiber size and conduction velocity vary. There is a positive relationship between the diameter of the nerve fiber and the concentration of the drug that is required to produce blockade of the nerve. Peripheral nerves are composed of myelinated A and B fibers and unmyelinated C fibers. Pain impulses are carried on myelinated A-delta and unmyelinated C fibers and are blocked by similar concentrations of local anesthetic (Stoelting, 1991). Low concentrations of

Table 14-2 Local Anesthetic Duration and Potency

Drug	Duration	Potency	Onset
Procaine	Short	Low	Slow
Chloroprocaine	Short	Low	Fast
Lidocaine	Intermediate	Intermediate	Fast
Mepivacaine	Intermediate	Intermediate	Slow
Prilocaine	Intermediate	Intermediate	Slow
Cocaine	Intermediate	Intermediate	Fast
Bupivacaine	Long	High	Slow
Tetracaine	Long	High	Slow
Etidocaine	Long	High	Slow

local anesthetics block preganglionic sympathetic nervous system B fibers. Slightly higher concentrations block conduction in C fibers and small A fibers. Blocking these fibers causes loss of pain and temperature sensation. Touch, proprioception, and motor function are preserved.

Nursing care of patients receiving local anesthetics via nerve block involves postblock assessment of vital signs, motor and sensory function, pain status, and side effects. Potential side effects of local anesthetic administration are detailed in Table 14-3.

Allergic reactions are rare with either type of local anesthetic, occurring more frequently with the ester-type local anesthetics. Systemic toxicity associated with local anesthetic administration results from inadvertent arterial injection of the drug, which elevates the level of the drug in the blood. The blood level of the drug is affected by total dose, site of injection, tissue binding, tissue perfusion, drug-induced vasodilation, and use of vasoconstrictors. Patients may initially experience tinnitus or a metallic taste on the tongue when systemic toxicity occurs. Higher blood levels of local anesthetics produce seizures and may even cause circulatory collapse. Monitoring and resuscitative equipment should always be available.

Epinephrine added to local anesthetics can produce beneficial results. By producing local vasoconstriction, it can decrease absorption, thus lowering peak blood levels. A second effect of a decreased rate of absorption is an increase in the duration of action.

Table 14-3 Side Effects of Local Anesthetic Administration

System	Side Effects
Nervous	Fainting, convulsions, headache
Cardiovascular	Hypotension, rapid pulse, respiratory depression
Gastrointestinal	Nausea, vomiting
Other	Urticaria, pruritus

Neurolytic Drugs

The use of neurolytic drugs to destroy peripheral nerve pathways has declined with the development of other invasive treatment modalities for chronic pain. This technique is still used for pain relief in advanced incurable cancer (Cousins & Bridenbaugh, 1988), certain ischemic vascular conditions, and sympathetic dystrophies. Patients are given two or three prognostic blocks with local anesthetic before the nerve is actually destroyed with a neurolytic drug such as alcohol, phenol, or glycerol. Phenol produces a sensation of warmth followed by numbness. Alcohol is more difficult for the patient to tolerate because it produces an intense burning sensation. This may be alleviated by prior injection of a local anesthetic. Neurolytic blocks have also been associated with the risk of paresis, bowel and bladder dysfunction, and painful neuritis.

Corticosteroids

Corticosteroids can be effective in reducing inflammation and have been widely utilized in epidural injections. They can provide relief of neuralgic pain associated with low back pain. Other inflammatory conditions such as facet or sacroiliac joint syndromes may also respond well to steroid injections. Steroids have a tendency to worsen the pain for anywhere from a few days to several weeks before providing relief (Gregg, 1991). Patients must be informed of this along with the other side effects that a particular block may produce.

Types of Nerve Blocks

The types of nerve blocks useful for the treatment of acute and chronic pain are somatic peripheral nerve blocks, central neural blocks, and sympathetic blocks.

Peripheral Nerve Blocks

The box on p. 438 shows the different types of somatic peripheral nerve blocks. Somatic peripheral nerve blocks are

TYPES OF SOMATIC PERIPHERAL NERVE BLOCKS

Cranial nerve blocks
- Trigeminal nerve block (gasserian ganglion block)
- Block of the ophthalmic division or block of the maxillary nerve (and its branches)
- Mandibular nerve block
- Facial nerve block
- Block of the glossopharyngeal and vagus nerves

Cervical plexus block

Brachial plexus (and its branches) block

Lumbosacral plexus (and its branches) block

very useful in conditions such as causalgia, acute reflex sympathetic dystrophy, certain neuropathies or plexopathies, or chronic cancer pain in which nociceptive stimulation contributes to the pain (Bonica, Liebeskind, & Albe-Fessard, 1979).

Blocks of the cranial nerves are utilized to diagnose and treat pain syndromes associated with cancer and cancer treatment radiation therapies. The trigeminal nerve and its branches may be blocked by performing a gasserian ganglion block. The crescent-shaped gasserian ganglion lies lateral to the internal carotid artery and cavernous sinus and occupies Meckel's cave, located just posteromedial to the foramen ovale. Radiography is used to confirm needle position in performing the technically difficult gasserian ganglion block. The procedure is usually painful, and patients usually require a great deal of sedation. After two or three prognostic blocks with a long-lasting local anesthetic have determined that the block can provide complete relief, a neurolytic block with alcohol can be performed to provide continuous pain relief. Block of individual nerve branches is technically less difficult than block of the gasserian ganglion. It is essential to have a thorough knowledge of the anatomy of the target nerve and adjacent structures with which the solution might come in contact.

A brachial plexus block may be indicated for surgery, postoperative pain relief, or relief of chronic pain of the upper extremities in certain conditions. Raj (1994) has found indications for brachial plexus block if pain relief is not adequate after stellate ganglion blocks for causalgia, reflex sympathetic dystrophy, peripheral neuropathies, or Raynaud's syndrome.

The brachial plexus, which is formed by the ventral rami of C5, C6, C7, C8, and T1, can be blocked by four approaches: interscalene, supraclavicular, infraclavicular, and axillary. Because the nerves lie within a vascular area, intravascular injection, and a toxic response to it, are always possibilities. Resuscitation equipment and drugs must be available for treatment of central nervous system (CNS) toxicity. Complications associated with supraclavicular and interscalene approaches include pneumothorax (which may produce chest pain), respiratory difficulty, and a cough. Paralysis of the diaphragm has also occurred with the interscalene approach. Patients should be observed for respiratory difficulty and given support of respiration if it develops.

Peripheral nerve blocks of the lower extremities may be accomplished by blocking the lumbosacral plexus or its branches, which are the sciatic nerve, the femoral nerve, the obturator nerve, and the lateral femoral cutaneous nerves. These localized blocks may produce loss of sensation around the painful area; motor function is not usually impaired.

Central Nerve Blocks

Injection of local anesthetics into the subarachnoid or epidural space is a long-standing practice for the relief of acute pain associated with surgery or childbirth. Chronic low back pain has been relieved by injection of local anesthetic and steroids into the epidural space and subarachnoid space

(Benzon, 1986). Neurolytic blocks have been used to treat chronic cancer pain when there is a short life expectancy (Swerdlow, 1983). Knowledge of the spinal anatomy is important to the practitioner's understanding of how intraspinal drugs work and to providing the care necessary to patients who receive this type of therapy.

Spinal Anatomy

The spinal canal extends from the foramen magnum to the sacral hiatus. The bony structures include 7 cervical, 12 thoracic, and 5 lumbar vertebrae. Three interlaminar ligaments bind together the vertebral processes of these vertebrae: the supraspinous ligament, the interspinous ligament, and the ligamentum flavum, which joins the laminae of the vertebrae. Figure 14-1 shows the spinal anatomy.

The spinal cord is enclosed in three meninges. The pia mater lies closest to the spinal cord and is attached to it. The dura mater is a fibrous sheath that runs the length of the spinal cord and is fixed caudally at S2. The arachnoid mater lies between the pia mater and the dura mater. At birth the spinal chord ends at L3, moving progressively cephalad until age 2. In adults and children 2 two years of age the spinal cord ends at L1. Nerve roots branch out distally from the end of the spinal cord to form the cauda equina. Below the level of L2 the nerves are mobile.

The subarachnoid (also called intrathecal) space is the space between the pia mater and the arachnoid mater. It contains the spinal cord, the nerves, the cerebrospinal fluid, and the blood vessels that supply the spinal cord. It extends from S2 to the cerebral ventricles. The cerebrospinal fluid, which is clear and colorless, has a volume in the subarachnoid space that is approximately 30 ml.

The epidural space extends from the base of the skull to the sacrococcygeal membrane. It is a potential space located between the ligamentum flavum and the dura mater. The epidural space is filled with connective tissue, fatty tissue, and blood vessels.

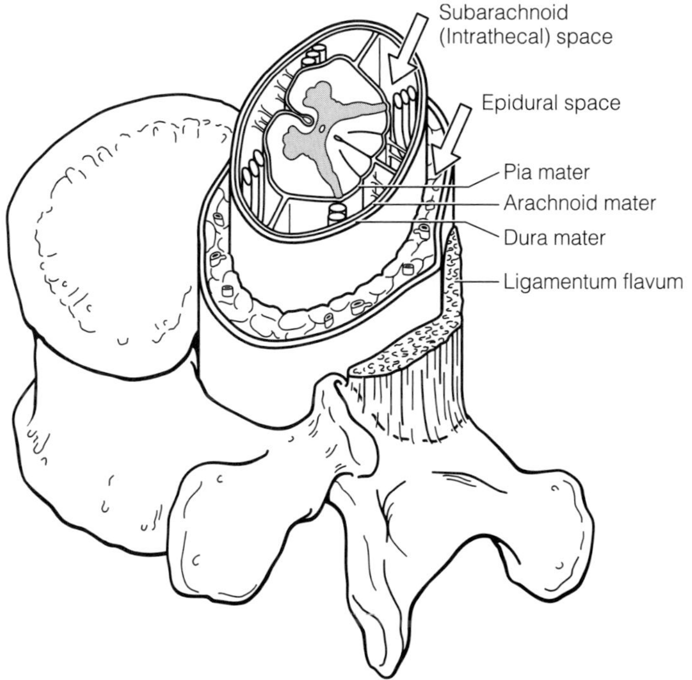

Figure 14-1 Spinal anatomy.

Spinal and Epidural Blocks

Because the spinal cord ends at L1, the needle is usually placed below L2 to avoid injury to the spinal cord. The interspaces between L3 and L4 and between L4 and L5 are the most commonly used. The patient is placed in the lateral or sitting position. In the lateral position the patient's knees are drawn up toward the chest and the chin is flexed down to maximally flex the spine, which is horizontal to the table. When the sitting position is used the patient's head and shoulders are flexed downward, the feet rest on a stool, and the patient's back is close to the edge of the table.

The skin is prepared and draped, and local anesthetic is injected into it at the intended site of needle insertion. For a spinal block, a 22- or 25-gauge needle is used. After passing through the skin and subcutaneous tissue, the needle penetrates the supraspinous ligament, interspinous ligament, ligamentum flavum, and dura mater. Figure 14-2 shows a needle entering the epidural space.

Local anesthetic introduced into the epidural space produces analgesia by two mechanisms. First, the local anesthetic acts directly on the nerve roots after it diffuses across the dura. Then, once it has diffused into the paravertebral area through the intervertebral foramina, it produces paravertebral blockade. Because the local anesthetic must diffuse before it can reach its site of action, the onset of an epidural

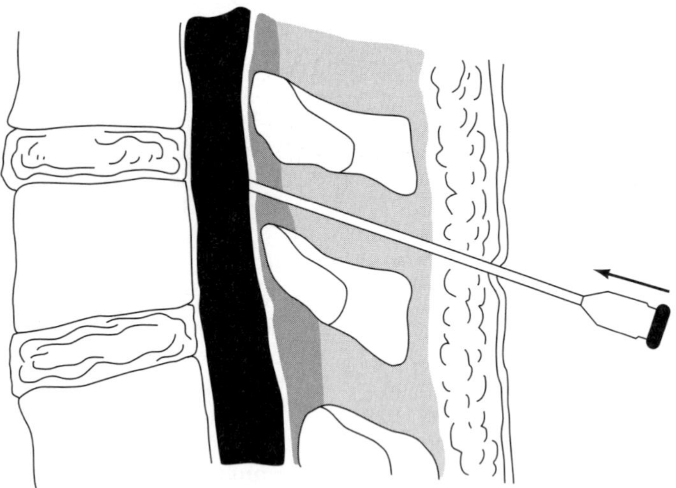

Figure 14-2 Needle entering epidural space.

block is slower than that of a spinal block. Typically, sensory anesthesia is not apparent for at least 15 minutes.

Most commonly, a 17-gauge Touhy needle is used for performing an epidural block. Once the needle passes the ligamentum flavum, the epidural space is identified by a loss of resistance to syringe-plunger displacement. Epidural anesthesia requires larger drug volumes than does spinal anesthesia to diffuse through the surrounding nerves and block neural transmission.

When the needle pierces the dura to enter the subarachnoid space, it comes in contact with cerebrospinal fluid. A small volume of drug (e.g., 100 to 150 mg procaine, 50 to 100 mg lidocaine, 5 to 15 mg bupivicaine) is used in the subarachnoid space to produce pain relief. Local anesthetic injected into the cerebrospinal fluid acts on the superficial layers of the spinal cord, but most of the action occurs at the preganglionic fibers where they leave the anterior rami of the spinal cord (Stoelting, 1991). Preganglionic sympathetic nervous fibers are blocked at lower concentrations than are necessary to produce sensory or motor block. Therefore using the spinal technique for pain relief results in an accompanying sympathetic blockade. Physiologic alterations include reduced venous return and increased vascular capacitance.

Possible complications associated with spinal and epidural nerve block techniques include neurologic changes, headache, backache, hematoma, infection, and cardiac arrest. Hypotension is a common side effect of excessive subarachnoid or epidural block. Treatment consists of infusion of fluids and a small dose of vasopressor (ephedrine). When these procedures are carried out, the patient should be monitored and resuscitative equipment should be available. An excessive level of spinal anesthesia can block preganglionic cardiac accelerator fibers (T1 to T4). Respiratory depression can also result from excessively high central nerve blockage.

Sympathetic Nerve Blocks

Bonica (1990) has noted that sympathetic hyperactivity can contribute to or cause pain by any of the following mechanisms: (a) sensitization of peripheral nociceptor, (b) production of vasoconstriction, (c) reflex changes involving afferent and efferent fibers, (d) liberation of norepinephrine, (e) sensitization of neurons in the dorsal horn, (f) maintenance of trigger points, and (g) inhibition of gastrointestinal and genitourinary tracts, causing ileus and decreased urine output.

The sympathetic nervous system can be blocked by three methods: block of the somatic nerve and consequently of the corresponding sympathetic nerves, intravenous (IV) regional infiltration, and intraspinal block. Blockade can be achieved at several levels: the subarachnoid space, the epidural space, the paravertebral or prevertebral regions, peripheral nerves, and the endings of postganglionic axons. The best location for diagnostic block is at the sympathetic chain, where it will affect only sympathetic nerves (Raj, 1994).

Sympathetic blockade of the lower cervical and upper thoracic chain is usually referred to as a *stellate ganglion block.* It is commonly used in the management of pain in the upper limbs, neck, and thoracic viscera. The stellate ganglion chain is located in the neck at C6 level. Performance of this block involves extension of the head, lateral retraction of the carotid sheath, insertion of a needle at C6 level in the peritracheal space, and injection of between 5 and 10 ml of local anesthetic. Figure 14-3 shows the anatomic placement of this block. Signs of a successful block include ptosis of the eyelid on the blocked side followed by miosis; the sensation of a lump in the throat with slight difficulty swallowing, lasting 3 to 4 hours; flushing of the face on the blocked side; hoarseness; nasal congestion of the blocked side; and warmth, anhidrosis (absence of sweating), and vasodilation of the arm on the blocked side. Complications include pneumothorax, hematoma, hemoptysis, seizure, and potential cerebrospinal fluid (CSF) injection with an associated respiratory arrest.

Sympathetic blockade of the lumbar chain is indicated for causalgias, reflex sympathetic dystrophies, postamputation syndromes, and peripheral vascular disease. The lum-

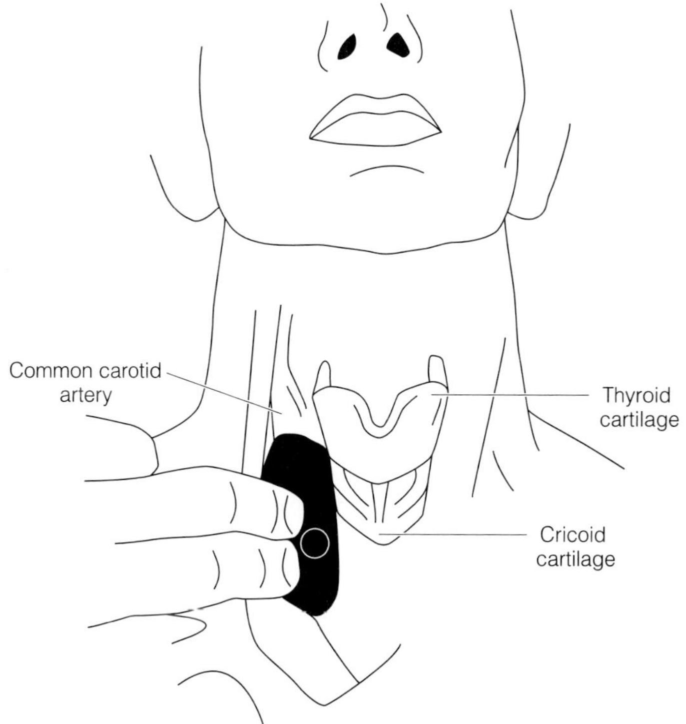

Figure 14-3 Stellate ganglion block.

bar sympathetic ganglia lie along the anterolateral surface of the lumbar vertebral body. To perform this block, a spinal needle is inserted laterally, using fluoroscopic guidance, between the subcostal margin and the top of the iliac crest at L3, as shown in Figure 14-4. Signs of a successful block are an increase in skin temperature and flushing of the blocked side. Complications include puncture of the kidney with resulting hematuria, hypotension, abdominal pain, and persistent weakness in the legs.

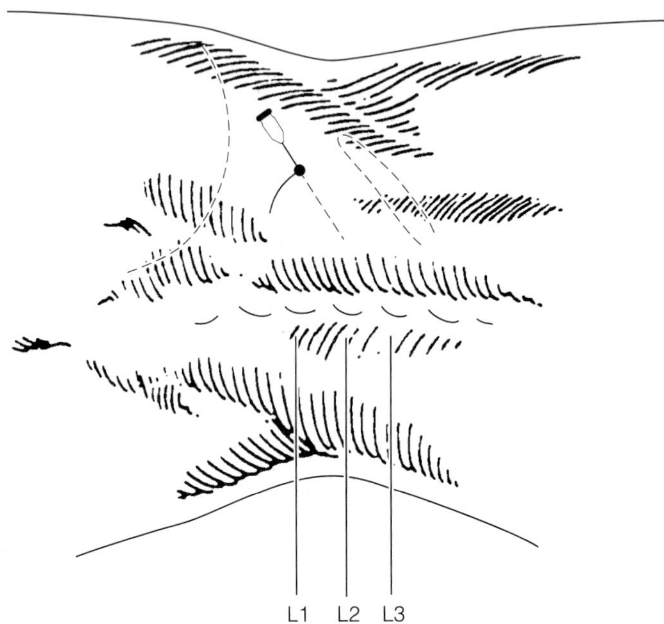

Figure 14-4 Lumbar sympathetic block.

Spinal Cord Stimulation

Utilizing electricity to test the gate control theory, Melzack and Wall (1965) proposed that the nervous system can inhibit pain by "closing the gate" that is located in the dorsal horn of the spinal cord. This gate can be closed by stimulation of large afferent fibers or their collaterals in the dorsal columns, which suppresses small-fiber input (pain) at the presynaptic or postsynaptic level in the spinal cord. The reader is referred to Chapter 1 for further detail on the gate control theory.

The work of Melzack and Wall provided the scientific rationale for the use of spinal cord stimulation. Spinal cord stimulation involves the selective use of painless electrical stimulation of large afferent fibers in the dorsal columns of the spinal cord to inhibit transmission of painful stimuli to the brain.

The first spinal cord stimulator was placed by Shealy, Mortimer, and Reswick (1967). Their initial results were excellent, but long-term results were poor. Minimal control of parameters and poor patient selection contributed to these results. Significant advances have been made since the introduction of spinal cord stimulation. Electrodes with multiple contact points that allow optimal stimulation have been developed. Success rates of 60% to 70% have been reported in the relief of chronic pain (Long, North, & James, 1981; North et al., 1991; Spiegelman & Friedman, 1991).

Spinal cord stimulation has an advantage over neurosurgical and neurolytic procedures in that it is nondestructive, causing no permanent interruption of nerve pathways. Furthermore, its effects are reversible. Any side effects cease after the stimulation is discontinued. Trials allow for patient screening before implantation of a permanent system.

Patient selection is of utmost importance to the success of spinal cord stimulation as a treatment for chronic pain. Medtronic, Incorporated (Minneapolis), a manufacturer of spinal cord stimulators, recommends that the following general criteria be met before a patient is treated with spinal cord stimulation: (a) there is a demonstrated pathology—i.e., an objective cause of the pain; (b) more conservative therapies have failed; (c) the patient is not a candidate for further surgical intervention; (d) no serious drug habituation problems exist untreated; (e) psychiatric clearance has been obtained; and (f) the patient's predominant pain complaint is radiating extremity pain. Patients with adhesive arachnoiditis, failed back surgery syndrome, peripheral causalgia, ischemic limb pain, and phantom limb pain are the most likely to benefit from this treatment modality because they generally meet the aforementioned criteria. Finally, the patient needs to be willing and motivated to work with the treatment team. Spinal cord stimulation will reduce pain, but it will not eliminate it or cure its underlying cause. Patients need to understand this, and if trial stimulation meets the pain relief goals, they should participate in the determination of whether to proceed with the treatment.

To stimulate the spinal cord, electrodes may be placed into the epidural space either through a thoracic laminectomy or percutaneously through a special needle that allows multiple passes of the electrode. In either technique the patient is awake but sedated. Patient cooperation is needed to determine optimal localization of the electrode. A trial stimulation should produce a fine, tingling sensation in the area where the pain is usually felt. Temporary placement with the option of converting to a permanent implant has value for patients with complex pain syndromes when the effectiveness of spinal cord stimulation is questionable (Raj, 1994). If stimulation produces appropriate relief, the battery pack and cable that attach to the electrode to deliver stimulation may be surgically implanted.

Because the patient's cooperation is essential to the success of spinal cord stimulation, patient education is a critical component. Table 14-4 summarizes the components of patient education.

Intravenous Drug Delivery

Intravenous (IV) analgesia has become widely accepted as a convenient and effective mode of pain relief. The IV route provides the most rapid onset of analgesia (usually within 6 to 10 minutes) with the shortest duration of action. Intravenous opioids most commonly used for pain control are morphine, hydromorphone, and meperidine. (For further information on these drugs, refer to Chapter 4.) Administration of intravenous analgesia may be via bolus, continuous drip, or patient-controlled analgesia (PCA) mode.

Intravenous Bolus

Intravenous bolus administration allows for small amounts of opioid to be given frequently, providing for faster onset and greater ease in titration. An IV bolus can provide immediate pain relief, but this relief diminishes quickly

Table 14-4 Patient Education for Spinal Cord Stimulation

Time Frame	Education Topics
Review the goals	Focus on decreasing, not eliminating, the pain.
Product review	Allow patient to handle the equipment. Provide product literature for patient and family to read.
Preoperative education	Hold patient and family teaching session with time for questions and answers. Discuss surgery workup routine.
Intraoperative education	Review plans for the day of surgery. Describe what to expect in the operating room.
Immediate postoperative period	Explain any restrictions. Describe how stimulation will feel. Discuss stimulation needs and how they will vary with activity.
Discharge planning	Review instruction sheets. Involve the family in postoperative care. Discuss follow-up care and activities.

due to the short duration of analgesia (45 to 60 minutes). The major limitation of bolus administration is that blood levels of the drug rise after administration and then fall, providing periods of relief and possibly sedation followed by periods of breakthrough pain. Therefore, IV boluses are appropriate for rapid control of severe pain on a short-term basis (see Chapter 8 for more information about IV boluses for acute pain) and for establishing the hourly dose for continuous IV infusion.

Continuous IV Infusion

For pain that is of longer duration, continuous IV infusion is almost always preferred over intermittent boluses of opioid. Continuous IV opioid administration provides the patient with a constant level of pain relief by delivering a continuous dose of medication into the patient's bloodstream. This route may be appropriate for relief of acute pain from various causes (surgery, trauma, burn); it should not be reserved only for end-stage conditions. With this route, titration is of great importance in establishing a balance between sedation and analgesia.

Intravenous Patient-Controlled Analgesia

Patient-controlled analgesia (PCA), a relatively new method for the delivery of intravenous analgesia, allows patients to find their own levels of pain relief by self-administering the opioid via a preprogrammed intravenous infusion device. As with bolus and continuous modes of administration, PCA therapy needs to be titrated to achieve a balance between analgesia and sedation. The use of small, patient-controlled doses of opioid, coupled with the option of providing the patient with a continuous background, or "basal," rate, individualizes parenteral pain management. (For a detailed discussion on PCA, refer to Chapter 8.)

Intraspinal Drug Delivery

The benefit of intraspinal opioid administration as a pain treatment modality was made apparent by the discovery of opiate receptors in the central nervous system (Pert & Snyder, 1973). It was subsequently reported that opioids administered by the epidural or intrathecal route can act on these receptors to produce analgesia. Wang, Nauss, and Thomas (1979) first reported the use of intrathecal morphine for pain relief in chronic cancer patients, and Behar, Olshwang, Mazola, and Davidson (1979) reported pain relief with morphine injected into the epidural space.

Early clinical applications were not without side effects (sedation, respiratory depression, pruritus, nausea, and urinary retention). More refined patient selection and dosing practices have produced the same benefits with a higher degree of safety. Consequently, opioid administration via the intrathecal or epidural route is becoming a widely accepted therapy for the management of obstetrical pain, acute postoperative pain, and chronic pain of malignant origin.

Intraspinal opioid therapy has numerous benefits. First, good to excellent overall analgesia is typically maintained with lower doses of opioid (Cousins & Mather, 1984; Rawal et al., 1984). Patients are subsequently more alert and can participate to a greater degree in their care. Second, side effects are typically minimized. Effective pain relief with minimized sedation and other adverse side effects is typically associated with better patient satisfaction, improved maternal-newborn bonding after cesarean section (Belzarena, 1992; Cohen & Woods, 1983), and earlier postoperative mobilization. Intraspinal analgesia has also been shown to reduce physiologic stress after major surgery as well as reducing the incidence of some very serious complications, thereby improving surgical outcome (Shulman, 1984; Rawal et al.; Torda & Pybus, 1984). A clear advantage of intraspinal opioids over local anesthetics is that they block pain pathways but do not block sympathetic, sensory, and motor pathways. Physiologic alterations that occur with local anesthetics are avoided.

Despite the many advantages, there are contraindications to the use of intraspinal therapies. These are detailed in the box on p. 452. These must be identified when epidural or intrathecal administration is being contemplated so that alternative pain relief measures can be employed if necessary.

The following discussion of patient and catheter assessment and management outlines general nursing considerations in the care of patients receiving intraspinal analgesic therapy. As with other therapies, the reader should consult specific institutional or state nurse practice regulations and professional organizational guidelines for standards of care.

Catheter Placement and Management

Treatment of acute and chronic pain may be achieved with infusion of opioids via an epidural or intrathecal catheter. For patients undergoing a surgical procedure, the anesthesiologist or nurse anesthetist will usually place the

CONTRAINDICATIONS TO THE USE OF INTRASPINAL ANALGESIA

- Musculoskeletal or spinal deformities that prohibit the placement of a needle or catheter
- Clotting disorder or deficiency
- Coagulopathy that has not been reversed
- History of severe respiratory problems
- Infection
- Increased intracranial pressure
- Drug allergy

catheter preoperatively in anticipation of intraoperative as well as postoperative use. As described earlier in this chapter, the patient is placed in the lateral or sitting position; the skin is prepared, draped, and anesthetized; and an appropriate needle is then carefully inserted into either the epidural or intrathecal space. Once the presence of the needle in its intended location is verified, a catheter is inserted through the needle and advanced to the appropriate level. The needle is then carefully removed over the outside of the catheter so as not to damage the catheter or cause puncture of the dura. Many catheters are marked with black "hash marks" to identify centimeters. The number of marks showing as the catheter exits the patient's back should be noted after insertion and with each site check to ensure that the catheter has not moved. The distal end of the catheter is then inserted into a tubing adaptor, and a 0.22-μm filter is then attached. At this time, a test dose of local anesthetic is usually given to further confirm catheter placement. The catheter is then secured in place at the insertion site with a clear, occlusive dressing; the edges of the dressing are further secured with a dressing retention sheet or with tape. The catheter is then "taped" along the patient's back and up over the shoulder, where it can be easily accessed for bolus administration or attachment of administration tubing. It is imperative to ensure that the catheter and connections are secure to prevent accidental catheter displacement. A color-coded label identifying the catheter as either epidural or intrathecal should be placed at the catheter adaptor-tubing connection to prevent inadvertent injection of medication intended for systemic therapy. Medications for epidural or intrathecal use must not contain preservatives because these may damage neural tissue. Tubing with injection ports should not be used with epidural analgesia administration.

When the catheter is in place, it is essential to inspect the insertion site at least every 8 hours to ascertain that the catheter and dressing remain patent and that there are no signs of infection. Catheter displacement should be suspected if the number of "hash marks" showing has changed or if bloody or clear fluid is present under the dressing at the insertion site. An epidural catheter can migrate into the subarachnoid or intravascular space or out of the epidural space completely. The presence of 0.5 ml or more of clear or bloody fluid upon catheter aspiration indicates catheter migration and warrants discontinuation of the therapy. Nerve root irritation and hematoma are other adverse effects that could occur while the catheter is in place; therefore motor and sensory assessments should be performed during routine monitoring.

Clinical Pharmacology of Epidural Opioids

The choice of epidural opioid is often influenced by the site of epidural catheter placement, the technique of administration, and physician preference. Table 14-5 lists the clinical pharmacology of commonly used intraspinal opioids, and Table 14-6 lists dosage information for PCEA.

Morphine and hydromorphone are hydrophilic (water soluble) in nature. Thus they spread extensively in the cerebrospinal fluid before slowly diffusing into the spinal cord tissue, where they reach the opioid receptor sites in the substantia gelatinosa. This diffusion process explains why hydrophilic opioids have a slow onset of action. However, once these opioids bind to opiate receptors in the substantia

Table 14-5 Clinical Pharmacology of Intraspinal Opioids

Opioid	Lipid Solubility	Recommended Dose Range	Onset (minutes)	Duration (hours)
Morphine	Low	2-4 mg	30-60	12-24
Hydromorphone	Low	1.0-1.5 mg	20-30	6-18
Fentanyl	High	50-200 μg	4-6	2-3
Sufentanil	High	20-50 μg	5-10	2-4

Modified from Cousins, M. J., & Mather, L. E. (1984). Intrathecal and epidural administration of opioids. *Anesthesiology, 61,* 276.

Table 14-6 Opioid Doses for Patient-Controlled Epidural Analgesia

Drug Mixture	Bolus (ml)	Dose (ml)	Delay (min)	Basal Rate (ml/hr)
Morphine, 0.2 mg/ml	10	0.2-0.5	10	1-2
Fentanyl, 10 μg/ml	2.5-10	2-5	10	1-4
Fentanyl, 5 μg/ml, and bupivicaine, 0.0625%	6-12	2-4	10	2-4
Sufentanil, 2 μg/ml	5-10	2-4	10	2-4

Modified from Grass, J. A. (1993). *Epidural analgesia for acute pain management.* Deerfield, Ill.: Bard MedSystems Division.

gelatinosa, subsequent diffusion out of the spinal cord tissue is also slow, which equates to a long duration of action (Cousins & Mather, 1984; Willens & Myslinski, 1993). This offers the patient a relatively long period of analgesia, even with single-dose administration. Disadvantages of hydrophilic opioids include the long onset prior to analgesia, unpredictable duration of action, and an increased chance of side effects because of the extensive rostral spread (Cousins & Mather; DeCastro, Meynadier, & Zenz, 1991).

Highly lipophilic opioids, such as fentanyl and sufentanil, have a very high solubility and spread minimally through the CSF prior to uptake in the spinal cord tissue, resulting in rapid-onset analgesia. However, this rapid uptake is associated with rapid diffusion out of the spinal cord tissue and into the systemic vasculature. Therefore fentanyl and sufentanil have a shorter duration of action than morphine, thus requiring continuous infusions to maintain a significant analgesic level in the patient. The use of these opioids is also associated with a decreased side-effect profile (Cousins & Mather, 1984; DeCastro et al., 1991) due to the limited rostral spread of the drug in the CSF. Disadvantages of lipophilic opioids include systemic absorption with prolonged administration and limited effectiveness as a single-dose analgesic.

Patient Assessment and Management

Frequent and thorough assessment of the patient receiving intraspinal analgesia is critical to ensure a positive patient outcome. Nurses caring for these patients must be educated in the pharmacokinetics of intraspinal opioids, spinal anatomy, epidural catheter placement and verification, appropriate monitoring parameters, and recognition of potential side effects and complications (Lubenow & Ivankovich, 1991; Olsson, Leddo, & Wild, 1989). The box on pp. 456 and 457 summarizes patient assessment, monitoring parameters, and general guidelines that must be followed in the care of the patient receiving intraspinal analgesia. Frequent assessment of the patient's respiratory status is crucial to ensure prompt recognition of the most serious side effect, respiratory depression. Respiratory depression can occur early (within 2 hours) or late (up to 24 hours into the therapy). Early respiratory depression, seen with both hydrophilic (morphine) and lipophilic (fentanyl) opioids, occurs as a result of the rapid vascular uptake of drug from the epidural space and subsequent redistribution to the central respiratory center (Kafer, Brown, & Scott, 1983). Late respiratory depression, usually seen with morphine, is due to cephalic diffusion of the opioid in the CSF and distribution into the respiratory center. Several risk factors have

PATIENT ASSESSMENT AND MANAGEMENT GUIDELINES

A. Pain
   1. Perform consistent patient assessment.
   2. Perform assessments at least every 4 hours.
   3. Use supplemental techniques and medications.

B. Respiratory
   1. Assess rate and depth every hour, at least for the first 24 hours.
   2. Recognize early or late respiratory depression.
   3. Keep naloxone available on the unit.
   4. Keep resuscitation equipment (oxygen, ambu-bag, suction and intubation equipment) available.

C. Sedation
   1. Check patient's ability to be aroused and level of consciousness every hour while patient is awake.
   2. Avoid any sedative medications (antihistamines, antiemetics).
   3. Elevate head of bed to prevent rostral spread.

D. Cardiovascular
   1. Check blood pressure and pulse every 4 hours when a local anesthetic is used (because of possible sympathetic blockade) and every 8 hours otherwise.
   2. Keep fluids and vasopressors available to treat hypotension if necessary.

E. Nausea and vomiting (caused when rostral spread of drug triggers vomiting center in the medulla)
   1. Provide antiemetics.
   2. Prevent aspiration.

F. Urinary retention
   1. Monitor intake and output.
   2. Assess for discomfort, distension, urgency.

G. Pruritus (may be related to stimulation of CNS opiate-sensitive receptors or result when opioid moves

PATIENT ASSESSMENT AND MANAGEMENT GUIDELINES—cont'd

rostrally in the CSF to the trigeminal nerve (Scott & Fisher, 1982))

1. Watch for it on face and upper abdomen, where it usually occurs; it is not a segmental response.
2. Use a nonsedative antihistamine.

H. Catheter

1. Keep catheter and connections intact and securely taped.
2. Keep insertion site clean and dry; watch for redness, drainage, or hematoma.
3. Use an occlusive dressing.
4. Change bag, tubing, and dressing according to institutional protocol.

I. Discontinuation of catheter

1. Inspect tip of catheter to ensure that the entire catheter was removed and that no shearing occurred.
2. Cover site with an adhesive bandage.
3. Assess for drainage from site.

J. Patient-family education

1. Discuss purpose and benefits of epidural analgesia.
2. Discuss catheter placement and management.
3. Mention duration of infusion and management.
4. Discuss relief of pain.
5. List potential side effects and management.
6. Review postinfusion care and pain management.

been identified that predispose patients to the occurrence of clinically relevant respiratory depression. These include (a) the elderly, (b) residual effects of other CNS depressants, (c) relative lack of tolerance, (d) large epidural doses given postoperatively, and (e) intrathecal technique and thoracic epidural catheters (Cousins & Mather, 1984; Gustafsson, Schmidt, & Jacobsen, 1982; Kafer et al., 1983).

Implanted Intraspinal Delivery Systems for Chronic Pain

Patients with chronic pain due either to malignancy or to other causes who are referred for intraspinal drug therapy usually have an implanted delivery device that can be maintained on a long-term basis. Several types of continuous-delivery systems exist. Epidural catheters can be tunneled beneath the skin and connected to external access ports. This system is usually used only in patients with a short life expectancy because it carries an increased risk of infection and the risk of cerebrospinal fluid leakage associated with external ports. A safer alternative is the use of subcutaneous ports into which the drug can be injected as a bolus or given continuously via pump. Patients can routinely be maintained safely at home with these systems for long periods of time, which adds to their comfort level and quality of life.

Totally implanted infusion systems, programmed to deliver small doses of opioid intrathecally, are more expensive but represent a safe and reliable alternative for patients who will require long-term (greater than 3 months) opioid therapy.

The most commonly used implanted infusion system consists of a spinal catheter, an extension catheter, and an 18-ml reservoir infusion pump. Insertion of the pump and components requires a surgical procedure and close follow-up care by the pain management team caring for the patient.

Adherence to patient selection criteria contributes to the success of this therapy. Patient selection for continuous implanted intraspinal opioid delivery includes a comprehensive pain assessment, an opioid and nonopioid use history, and a functional assessment. In addition, the patient needs to be examined for physiologic abnormalities (coagulopathies, electrolyte imbalance) and must have a comprehensive psychologic examination. Other considerations include cost to the patient (insurance coverage) and the availability of support systems for constant care. Table 14-7 lists patient selection criteria for intraspinal drug delivery.

A positive patient outcome depends on patient education. A comprehensive plan, similar to the educational plan

Table 14-7 Patient Selection Criteria for Implanted Intraspinal Drug Delivery

○ Objective evidence of pathology	○ Lack of coagulopathy and sepsis
○ Failure of more conservative therapy	○ Absence of drug-seeking behavior
○ Favorable response to trial procedures	○ Absence of hypersensitivity to opioids
○ Psychologic clearance	○ Absence of spinal cord tumor
○ Life expectancy greater than 3 months	○ Absence of hepatic or renal failure

outlined for patients being treated with spinal cord stimulation, should be put into effect (see Table 14-4). In addition to being comprehensive, the plan must be ongoing. Follow-up care and instruction for the patient are as important as the initial familiarization with the device, the surgery, and the postoperative care. This education involves not only the patient but also the family and other caregivers. Jacox and colleagues (1994) emphasize the importance of patient education and recommend that patients be active participants in their care. They specifically recommend that patients be educated about the use of opioids as part of the treatment plan. Recommendations include (a) telling patients that opioid analgesics will not lead to addiction, (b) dealing with tolerance to opioids by using higher drug doses, and (c) correcting myths about the use of opioids as part of the treatment plan.

TEAM APPROACH

To optimize the application of invasive interventions for the management of acute pain, the various members of the health care team must cooperate throughout the patient's course of hospitalization and treatment. (Chapter 6 discusses the team approach to management of pain in greater detail.) The institutional process of managing acute pain should begin with a commitment to providing the best level of pain relief that may safely be administered. Each institution must develop an effective pain control plan that includes all resources needed (Jacox et al., 1994) and assigns responsibility to interested individuals and groups. This will ensure a high quality of pain care for patients. To this end, multidisciplinary acute pain services have been established in many institutions to manage patients with intravenous and intraspinal analgesic therapies. Because institutions vary widely in size, complexity, volume of surgical procedures, and patient populations, various types of pain management teams exist. Jacox and colleagues state that responsibility for pain management care should be assigned to those most knowledgeable, experienced, interested, and available to deal with patients' needs in a timely fashion. In many facilities, though, this service is performed primarily by physicians (anesthesiologists, surgeons), nurse anesthetists, nurses, and pharmacists, with other members (physical therapists, social workers, biomedical engineers, and administrators) taking supporting roles when needed. The main goals of the team should be to provide improved patient care and analgesia through education of staff, employment of progressive pain management techniques, and careful, consistent management with thorough follow-up care. Pain management involving invasive interventions requires skilled decision making. Decision making is enhanced by effective communication among representatives of all disciplines involved in the patient's care. Patients who are referred for invasive interventions have usually been "in the system" for quite some time and are typically being seen by many practitioners. The success of any intervention depends on a consistent treatment plan agreed on by all involved, especially the patient and his or her family.

The makeup of the chronic pain team will vary according to the treatment plan and setting (outpatient clinic, inpatient, or operative). It is imperative that every member of the team be familiar with any equipment or device that is to be used and be able to explain to the patient its purpose and use. This is especially true for the nurse, who is often the individual playing the primary role in the education and follow-up processes.

Establishing a trusting relationship with patients and their families is of utmost importance. Chronic pain patients are often dealing with a myriad of other issues in their lives; understanding and reassurance can alleviate many of the fears and misconceptions they might be experiencing. Patients also need to be active participants in their own care. This fosters a greater level of understanding and increases patient satisfaction. Treatment does not end once a nerve block has been performed or a device implanted. Follow-up care is as crucial as the intervention itself. Patients and families should have a telephone contact and should be given clear, concise instructions; written information is helpful. Long-term care includes continual pain assessment, pharmacologic adjustment, lifestyle adjustment, and consideration of social, emotional, and financial matters. The entire interdisciplinary team is involved throughout the course of therapy.

SUMMARY

Patient assessment, selection, and education are crucial to the succcss of invasive interventions utilized for the management of acute and chronic pain. Members of the team caring for the patient must possess a thorough knowledge base and demonstrate the skills necessary to provide optimal pain care. The relief of pain can, at times, seem like the ultimate challenge to the caregiver. Invasive interventions, when utilized properly, serve as a progressive, timely, and comprehensive approach to this challenge.

References

Abram, S. E., Anderson, P. A., & Maitra-D'Cruze, A. M. (1981). Factors predicting short-term outcome of nerve blocks in the management of chronic pain. *Pain, 10,* 323.

Arnhoff, F. N., Triplett, H. B., & Pokorney, B. (1977). Follow-up status of patients treated with nerve blocks for low back pain. *Anesthesiology, 46,* 170.

Behar, M., Olshwang, D., Mazola, G., & Davidson, J. T. (1979). Epidural morphine in treatment of pain. *Lancet, 1,* 527.

Belzarena, S. D. (1992). Clinical effects of intrathecally administered fentanyl in patients undergoing Cesarean section. *Obstetric Anesthesia, 74,* 653–657.

Benzon, H. T. (1986). Epidural steroid injections for low back pain and lumbosacral radiculopathy. *Pain, 24,* 277.

Bonica, J. J. (1990). *The management of pain* (2nd ed.). Philadelphia: Lea & Febiger.

Bonica, J. J., Liebeskind, J. C., & Albe-Fessard, D. G. (1979). *Second world congress on pain, proceedings, advances in pain research and therapy* (Vol. 3). New York: Raven Press.

Cohen, S. E., & Woods, W. A. (1983). The role of epidural morphine in the postcesarean patient: Efficacy and effects on bonding. *Anesthesiology, 58*(6), 500–504.

Cousins, M. J., & Bridenbaugh, P. O. (Eds.). (1988). *Neural blockade in clinical anesthesia and management of pain* (2nd ed.). Philadelphia: Lippincott.

Cousins, M. J., & Mather, L. E. (1984). Intrathecal and epidural administration of opioids. *Anesthesiology, 61,* 276–310.

DeCastro, J., Meynadier, J., & Zenz, M. (1991). *Regional opioid analgesia.* Dordrecht, Netherlands: Kluwer Academic.

Gregg, R. V. (1991). Should nerve blocks be used for chronic noncancer pain? *American Pain Society Bulletin, 1*(3), 1.

Gustafsson, L. L., Schmidt, B., & Jacobsen, K. J. (1982). Adverse effects of extradural and intrathecal opiates: Report of a nationwide survey in Sweden. *British Journal of Anaesthesia, 53,* 479–486.

Jacox, A., Carr, D. B., Payne, R., Berde, C. B., Breitbart, W., Cain, J. M., Chapman, C. R., Cleeland, C. S., Ferrell, B. R., Finley, R. S., Hester, N. O., Hill, C. S., Leak, W. D., Lipman, A. G., Logan, C. L., McGarvey, C. L., Miaskowski, C. A., Mulder, D. S., Paice, J. A., Shapiro, B. S., Silberstein, E. B., Smith, R. S., Stover, J., Tsou, C. V., Vecchiarelli, L., & Weissman, D. E. (1994). *Management of cancer pain. Clinical practice guideline.* AHCPR Pub. No. 94-0592. Rockville, MD: Agency for Health Care Policy and Research, PHS, USDHHS.

Kafer, E. R., Brown, J. T., & Scott, D. (1983). Biphasic depression to ventilatory responses to CO_2 following epidural morphine. *Anesthesiology, 58,* 418–427.

Long, D. M., North, R., & James, C. S. (1981). Electrical stimulation of the spinal cord and peripheral nerves for pain control. *Applied Neurophysiology, 44,* 207–217.

Lubenow, T. R., & Ivankovich, A. D. (1991). Postoperative epidural analgesia. *Critical Care Nursing Clinics of North America, 3*(1), 25–32.

Melzack, R., & Wall, P. D. (1965). Pain mechanisms: A new theory. *Science, 150,* 108.

North, R., Campbell, J. N., James, C. S., Conover-Walker, M. K., Wang, H., Piantadosi, S., Ryback, J. D., & Long, D. M. (1991). Failed back surgery syndrome: 5-year follow-up after spinal cord stimulator implantation. *Neurosurgery, 28*(5), 692–699.

Olsson, G., Leddo, C., & Wild, L. (1989). Nursing management of patient receiving epidural narcotics. *Heart and Lung, 18*(2), 130–137.

Pert, C. B., & Snyder, S. H. (1973). Opiate receptor: Demonstration in nervous tissue. *Science, 179,* 1011.

Raj, P. P. (1994). *Practical management of pain* (2nd ed.). St. Louis: Mosby.

Rawal, N., Sjostrand, U., Christoffersson, E., Dahlstrom, B., Arvill, A., & Rydman, H. (1984). Comparison of intramuscular and epidural morphine for postoperative analgesia in the grossly obese: Influence on postoperative ambulation and pulmonary function. *Anesthesia and Analgesia, 63,* 583–592.

Scott, P. V., & Fisher, H. B. J. (1982). Intraspinal opiates and itching: A new reflex? *British Medical Journal, 284,* 1016–1017.

Shealy, C. N., Mortimer, J. T., & Reswick, J. (1967). Electrical inhibition of pain by stimulation of the dorsal column: Preliminary clinical reports. *Anesthesia and Analgesia, 46,* 489–491.

Shulman, M. (1984). Post thoracotomy pain and pulmonary function following epidural and systemic morphine. *Anesthesiology, 61,* 569–575.

Spiegelmann, R., & Friedman, W. (1991). Spinal cord stimulation: A contemporary series. *Neurosurgery, 28,* 1.

Stoelting, R. K. (1991). *Pharmacology & physiology in anesthesia practice.* Philadelphia: Lippincott.

Swerdlow, M. (1983). *Relief of intractable pain.* New York: Elsevier.

Torda, T., & Pybus, D. (1984). Extradural administration of morphine and bupivacaine. *British Journal of Anaesthesia, 56,* 141–146.

Wang, J. K., Nauss, L. A., & Thomas, J. E. (1979). Pain relief by intrathecally applied morphine in man. *Anesthesiology, 50,* 149.

Willens, J. S., & Myslinski, N. R. (1993). Pharmacodynamics, pharmacokinetics, and clinical uses of fentanyl, sufentanil, and alfentanil. *Heart & Lung, 22*(3), 239–251.

Wood, M., & Wood, A. (1990). *Drugs and anesthesia* (2nd ed.). Baltimore: Williams & Wilkins.

15

Pain Management in Special Situations

Neal Weinreb

Key Points

- The assessment and treatment of pain in special populations, such as substance abusers, patients with concurrent organ dysfunction, and patients with phantom pain, presents a clinical challenge to the nurse and other health care professionals.
- Proper management of pain in these populations requires patient involvement and additional clinical knowledge and expertise from the pain management team.
- Patients in special situations are usually very heterogenous; therefore, their pain management must be highly individualized.
- Pseudoaddiction is an iatrogenic syndrome of uncontrolled pain, inadequate therapy, and increased patient suffering that may result in severe distress and mistrust between the patient and health care providers. This is preventable.
- Effective pain management requires interdisciplinary collaboration and the use of both pharmacologic and nonpharmacologic interventions as appropriate.

This chapter is devoted to a discussion of a variety of clinical problems in pain assessment and management that are related to one another solely in the difficulty their solutions pose to the palliative care team. In a certain sense, the chapter title's reference to "special situations" might well be regarded as outdated and regressive; every patient represents a unique clinical circumstance and requires an *individualized* pain control plan developed and agreed on by themselves, their families, and the health care team (Jacox et al., 1994). Therapeutic interventions are not prescribed by rigid, cookbooklike formulas and protocols; they are adjusted and titrated to individual needs based on the goals of maximal pain relief and prevention at the cost of minimal toxicity. In this sense, every person is a "special situation."

Nevertheless it is useful for didactic reasons to identify certain discrete problems in pain management that demand additional knowledge and expertise from the health care team. This chapter will discuss several of these areas, including treatment of pain in current and former abusers of opioids or other substances; pain control in patients with concurrent hepatic, renal, or pulmonary dysfunction; procedural pain; pain management in pregnancy; and approaches to the treatment of intractable pain, including pain associated with reflex sympathetic dystrophy and phantom pain.

INTRACTABLE PAIN

"Intractable" can be defined as "stubborn," "persistent," or "difficult to alleviate, remedy, or cure." In applying this concept to pain, there are two elements that must be satisfied to establish intractability: chronicity and relative refractoriness to "standard" therapeutic interventions.

Acute pain is characterized by a well-defined temporal pattern of onset usually associated with a clearly identifiable etiology. Because acute pain is a consequence of and a response to a specific tissue insult or injury, it may be regarded as being physiologically meaningful. Acute pain is generally reversible: as the injured tissue undergoes repair, the pain tends to regress in a linear fashion (Payne & Gonzales, 1993). Acute pain is generally associated with subjective and objective physical signs and hyperactivity of the autonomic nervous system, including such manifestations as tachycardia, elevated blood pressure, vasoconstriction, and sweating (refer to Chapter 1). Assuming appropriate assessment, diagnosis, natural history, and intervention, acute pain cannot be intractable, although patients with intractable, chronic pain certainly may suffer from periodic acute exacerbations. On the other hand, prolonged acute pain associated with delayed diagnosis or inadequate therapy, or acute pain repeatedly provoked by incidents of abuse or injury (Drossman, 1994), may induce plastic changes within the peripheral and central nervous system that create and perpetuate a state of intractable, chronic pain (Portenoy, 1993).

Chronic pain differs from acute pain in that it usually results from irreversible pathophysiologic processes, persists longer than several months, and tends to progress in concert with the natural evolution of the disease. It is characterized by cyclic fluctuations in pain intensity, but unless it is modulated by therapeutic maneuvers, it is a constant unwanted visitor. Because of the way the autonomic nervous system adapts to chronic pain, patients with chronic pain lack the objective symptoms common with acute pain and are often apathetic, withdrawn, noncommunicative, sleepy, and depressed. Confounding even the sensitive observer, they often deny the presence of pain. Because of the lack of expression of the classical symptomatology of acute pain, patients with intractable chronic pain are frequently misdiagnosed and misunderstood. As shown in Figure 15-1, these patients can become trapped in a self-perpetuating cycle of pain, insomnia, depression, and fatigue, to the extent that some look to early death or suicide as the only way out (Quill, 1993). However, when properly recognized and acknowledged, chronic pain is generally, although rarely easily, amenable to treatment. Therefore, for a substantial majority of patients, even chronic pain should not be intractable.

The standard principles and specifics of chronic pain assessment and management were reviewed in Chapter 9. Some key points in assessment are as follows (Enck, 1994):

1. Believe the patient's complaint of pain.
2. Elicit a comprehensive history of the pain.
3. Use a standard pain intensity scale.
4. Assess for emotional, spiritual, and social factors.
5. Perform a thorough physical examination.
6. Evaluate the extent of disease.
7. Anticipate and treat "procedural pain."
8. Diagnose the cause of the pain.
9. Define, explain, and, with consent, initiate treatment.

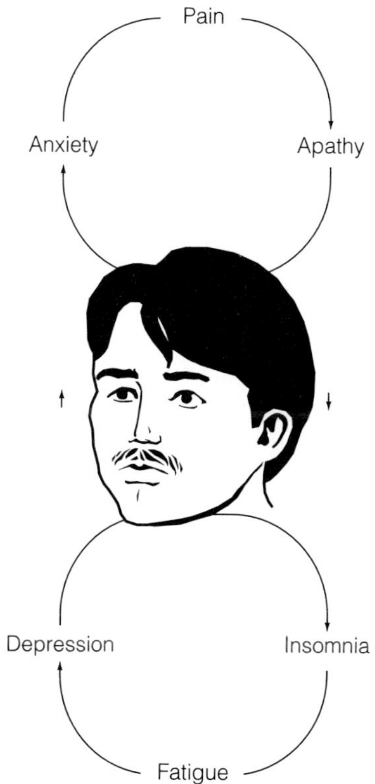

Figure 15-1 "Behind the eight ball": the cycle of chronic, intractable pain.

10. Continuously reassess patient response and adjust the plan accordingly.

Upon achieving initial relief of pain, the key objectives in the treatment of chronic pain become pain prevention and the optimization of the patient's sense of well-being. The latter goal is usually enhanced by minimizing sedation and choosing the least invasive, most effective analgesic techniques. Pharmacologic intervention should incorporate the concepts of the analgesic ladder and appropriate use of adjuvant medications. Non–ceiling-effect opioid analgesics should be used in functionally effective doses, titrated according to individual need and response, and prescribed on a regular schedule with provision for additional pro re nata (prn) doses for "breakthrough" pain. Nonpharmacologic modalities should be integrated into the plan of care as indicated in Chapter 5, and parenteral, epidural, and intrathecal analgesics (refer to Chapter 14) should be offered to refractory patients with appropriate clinical and prognostic indications. Figure 15-2 shows a hierarchy of these various pain management strategies.

With the successful application of these concepts and principles, it may be theoretically possible to reduce the percentage of patients with truly intractable pain to between 1% and 5% of the total population at risk. However, the estimates depicted here apply only to the management of chronic cancer pain, may not reflect all other settings and populations, and represent only a range of current opinion as to what represents optimal therapy (Jacox et al., 1994). Furthermore, it is not clear how close each pain management strategy represented in the pyramid actually came to the goal of total pain relief. In fact, one study suggests that in 5% to 25% of cancer patients, vigorous pharmacotherapy relieves symptoms only at the cost of profound sedation (Ventafridda, Ripamonti, DeConno, Tamburini, & Cassileth, 1990). Until data are available from further research and investigation and, more significantly, until the basic, well-founded principles of chronic pain management are widely disseminated and effectively applied, intractable pain will continue to be a major source of suffering for patients and their loved ones.

GUIDELINES FOR PAIN MANAGEMENT IN ABUSERS OF OPIOIDS OR OTHER SUBSTANCES

One of the major impediments to achieving adequate pain control continues to be fear of addiction. Concern among the lay public about the addictive potential of opioid analgesics is

Antineoplastic therapy
Palliative radiation therapy
Adjuvant drugs
Physical modalities
Psychosocial modalities

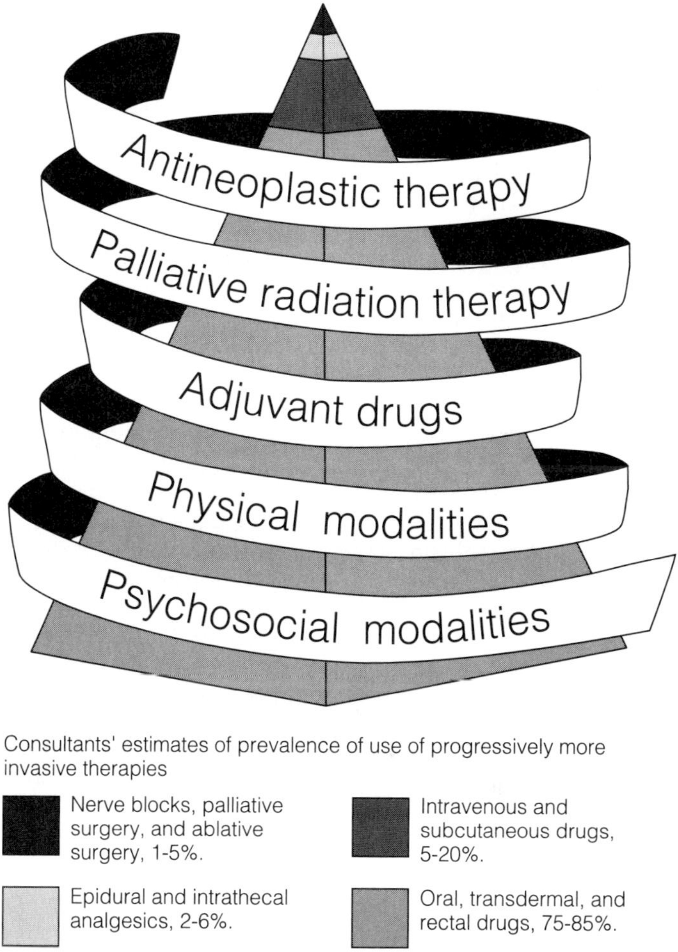

Consultants' estimates of prevalence of use of progressively more invasive therapies

Nerve blocks, palliative surgery, and ablative surgery, 1-5%.

Intravenous and subcutaneous drugs, 5-20%.

Epidural and intrathecal analgesics, 2-6%.

Oral, transdermal, and rectal drugs, 75-85%.

Figure 15-2 Pain management strategies: a hierarchy. (From Jacox, A., Carr, D. B., Payne, R., Berde, C. B., Breitbart, W., Cain, J. M., Chapman, C. R., Cleeland, C. S., Ferrell, B. R., Finley, R. S., Hester, N. O., Hill, C. S., Leak, W. D., Lipman, A. G., Logan, C. L., McGarvey, C. L., Miaskowski, C. A., Mulder, D. S., Paice, J. A., Shapiro, B. S., Silberstein, E. B., Smith, R. S., Stover, J., Tsou, C. V., Vecchiarelli, L., & Weissman, D. E. (1994). *Management of cancer pain. Clinical practice guideline.* AHCPR Pub. No. 94-0592. Rockville, MD: Agency for Health Care Policy and Research, PHS, USDHHS.)

so pervasive that patients and their families often resist their use, believing that chronic pain, especially that associated with cancer, is inevitable and untreatable. This irrational fear that the medically indicated use of opioid analgesics will inevitably have a negative effect has been termed "opiophobia" (Morgan, 1986). The national preoccupation with the battle against illicit drug use has greatly contributed to the development of this phenomenon, with the unfortunate result that thousands of patients with uncontrolled pain become casualties of "friendly fire" in the war on drugs (Blum, Kleinman Simpson, & Blum, 1990; Enck, 1991).

Health care providers are equally misinformed and uneducated about proper techniques for the management of pain and are no less opiophobic than the general population (Cleeland et al., 1994; Von Roenn, Cleeland, Gonin, Hatfield, & Pandya, 1993). Unwillingness to use opioids is irrational in light of well-established medical indications and the risk-to-benefit ratio (Blum et al., 1990). Uninformed physicians often withhold opioids as a weapon of last resort because they do not want to see their patients "hooked" on these drugs (Enck, 1991). When prescribed, analgesic doses are often too small to provide patients with sufficient pain relief (Blum et al.). Nurses compound the problem by underadministering analgesic drugs prescribed on a prn basis and by pressuring physicians to rescind standing narcotic orders (Lander, 1990). Caregivers also tend to doubt the honesty of patient reports of the frequency or severity of pain, with the result that unpopular or difficult patients are suspected of not having real pain and may even be subjected to "placebo tests" to prove that their complaints of pain are fictitious or exaggerated (Lander).

One of the more striking examples of this phenomenon is the widespread stereotyping of patients with sickle cell disease as manipulative and addiction prone. Chronic pain exacerbated by severe painful crises continues to be one of the major morbidities and causes for hospitalization in sickle cell disease. Traditionally, patients are treated only when crises ensue, most commonly with short-acting analgesics such as meperidine administered on a prn basis, based on the erroneous belief that crises are manifestations of reversible vasoocclusion. In fact, much of the pain is chronic and sustained because of an irreversible process of infarction (Brookoff & Polomano, 1992) and is thus more comparable to intractable cancer pain than to transitory, acute pain. The discontinuous provision of analgesia to sickle cell disease patients generates the pain avoidance behaviors that are characterized as signs of drug addiction and that have earned individuals with sickle cell disease the label of "problem patients." In contrast, when a study population of adult patients with sickle cell disease was treated with a pain control program modeled on regimens used to treat chronic cancer pain, including sustained courses of orally administered, controlled-release morphine and patient education sessions, this provision of adequate pain control resulted in decreased hospital visits and admissions for sickle cell pain (Brookoff & Polomano).

The vicious circle created by the combination of uncontrolled pain, ever-increasing suffering, and inadequate therapy often leads to a breakdown of the relationship between the patient and the health care team, as illustrated in Figure 15-3. Paradoxically, this scenario, whose roots emanate from the desire to avoid addiction, sometimes brings about an iatrogenic syndrome that has been termed "pseudoaddiction" (Weissman & Haddox, 1989). The natural history of this syndrome includes three characteristic phases:

1. Inadequate prescription of analgesics to meet the primary pain stimulus, resulting in persistent uncontrolled pain.
2. Escalation of analgesic demands by the patient associated with behavioral changes to convince others of the pain's severity. Patients in this phase are often characterized as craving or seeking drugs and stigmatized as drug addicts.

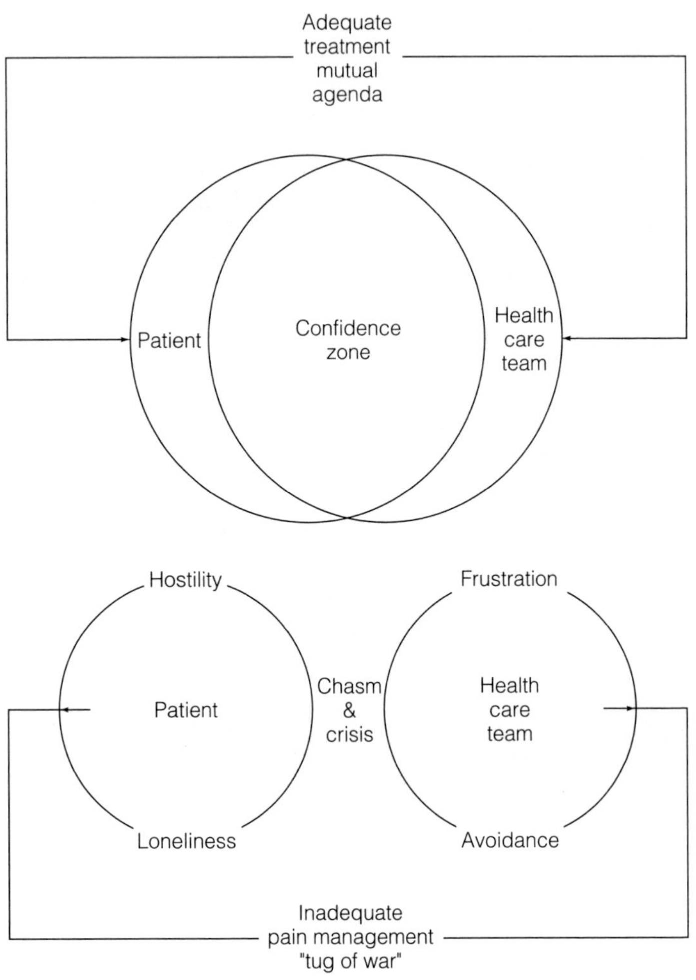

Figure 15-3 Inadequate pain management "tug of war."

3. A crisis of mistrust between the patient and members of the health care team, leading inevitably to alienation and therapeutic failure.

The consequences to the patient of inadequate pain treatment include loss of trust; feelings of anger, isolation, and loss of self-worth; depression; and, possibly, suicidal ideation. Additionally, pain and stress have been shown to inhibit immune function and enhance tumor growth in animals, suggesting that it may be physically deleterious to withhold analgesic drugs from patients with cancer pain (Sees & Clark, 1993). Opiophobia is a major cause of unrelieved pain worldwide. Even in developed countries, nearly 25% of all cancer patients still die with severe, unrelieved pain (Blum et al., 1990).

The fear of opioid addiction has perpetuated a situation in which patients in pain are made to suffer because of the barriers that have been created to prevent addiction. This suffering might conceivably be rationalized if the medical use of opioids did indeed bring about a significant risk of addiction. In reality, published reports (Kanner & Foley, 1981; Porter & Jick, 1980) indicate that the risk of addiction in patients not previously identified as substance abusers who are treated appropriately for pain with opioid analgesics is extremely low—perhaps as low as 0.01% (Blum et al., 1990). Nevertheless, despite the scientific evidence to the contrary, fallacious beliefs about the addiction liability of narcotics persist among health care professionals (Lander, 1990). The needless suffering caused by the underuse of medically indicated opioid analgesics will be overcome only via intensive educational efforts directed at patients, their families, physicians, nurses, and all other members of the health care team.

This is not to say that the problem of substance abuse and addiction is an inconsequential medical and societal issue. Alcoholism is the most common form of addiction to a psychoactive substance in our culture. There is a 3% to 16% incidence of alcoholism and a 5% to 6% lifetime prevalence of other forms of drug addiction in the United States (Savage, 1993). It is currently estimated that there are approximately 500,000 opioid addicts in the United States alone (Friedman, 1990). Cross-addiction is common. Thirty-six percent of individuals diagnosed as actively drug dependent are concurrently diagnosed as alcohol dependent. Thirty-seven percent to 84% of cocaine, opioid, marijuana, and amphetamine addicts have a history of alcoholism, and 80% to 90% of alcoholics are addicted to nicotine. The rate of alcoholism among smokers is 10 to 14 times higher than among nonsmokers. These data suggest that the propensity for addiction, regardless of the substance, reflects the influence of biological or environmental determinants (Savage).

The relevance of these observations to problems in pain management is clear. Although the incidence of iatrogenic addiction in patients with no prior personal or family history of substance abuse is negligible, significant numbers of patients in need of pain management may already be active or recovered substance abusers. For example, it is estimated that 19% to 25% of hospitalized patients requiring treatment for acute pain can be expected to have problems with alcohol abuse and that the prevalence of addiction among patients with chronic pain of nonmalignant origin is 3% to 19%. In patients with cancer pain, the incidence of alcoholism and other substance abuse probably parallels that of the general population. However, in patients whose cancers are associated with chronic use of alcohol or tobacco (e.g., lung, esophageal, head and neck, and pancreatic cancer), the incidence of prior addiction may be even higher (Savage, 1993).

Alcoholism and other addictions are usually underdiagnosed, even in pain clinics. Reasons for underdiagnosis include lack of training and skill in recognition, belief that the condition is untreatable, and moral judgmentalism (Savage, 1993). Additionally, because of problems such as opiophobia, pain specialists often underemphasize or downplay the possibility of addiction among their patients (Wesson, Ling, & Smith, 1993). It is particularly important to be aware of a history of previous or current substance abuse in patients with chronic pain because it may be necessary to modify their pharmacologic interventions to achieve effective pain control and avoid toxicity. For example, the use of acetaminophen may have to be restricted in known alcoholic patients in whom chronic liver disease is suspected, and larger-than-usual opioid dosages may be necessary to control chronic pain in opioid abusers, as will be discussed later.

The similarities between the behavioral patterns that characterize substance abusers and patients suffering chronic pain suggests the presence of an interrelationship between the neurophysiologic pathways that mediate pain and those that mediate addiction. These behaviors, including sleep disturbance, anxiety, and affective disorders and depression, are common in both addictive disease and in patients with chronic pain. A number of observations support the hypothesis that addictive disease and chronic pain are different clinical manifestations of related neurophysiologic disorders (Savage, 1993).

Chronic use of opioids, alcohol, cocaine, and other drugs has been observed to induce changes in central opioid receptors and in norepinephrine, serotonin, dopamine, and γ-aminobutyric acid (GABA) availability. As described by Savage (1993), these receptor and neurotransmitter changes might potentially affect modulation of nociception as well. Central α-receptors play a role in both pain and addiction, as evidenced by the efficacy of clonidine in treatment of neuropathic pain and as an inhibitor of withdrawal symptoms from opioids. Cocaine is believed to provide its intense reward stimulation through enhancement of dopamine action on opioid-mediated receptors in the limbic system. GABA agonists such as baclofen have analgesic properties, whereas other GABA agonists reinforce the addictive properties of alcohol and benzodiazepine drugs. Sympathetic arousal plays a role in the mediation of many types of pain and is also characteristic of chemically dependent individuals. Sympathetic stimulation in substance abusers may alter nociceptive pathways and pain-inhibitory mechanisms in ways that may potentiate the pain experience. A syndrome of pain facilitation or disinhibition, whose mechanism is unknown, has been described in patients with chronic pain and concurrent active addiction (Savage, 1993). In patients with this syndrome, pain is frequently decreased or even resolved following detoxification from drugs of dependency. The complex neurophysiologic interplay between pain and addiction pathways illustrates how important it is that the pain management team be sensitive to the presence of substance abuse in chronic pain patients, familiar with the diagnostic features of addiction, and prepared to make necessary modifications in the treatment plan when treating chronic pain in the addicted patient.

Assessment for Addiction

Figure 15-4 shows a clinically useful classification of chronic pain patients with regard to usage of drugs and potential for substance abuse. The first step involves distinguishing those patients with no history of medication or substance abuse

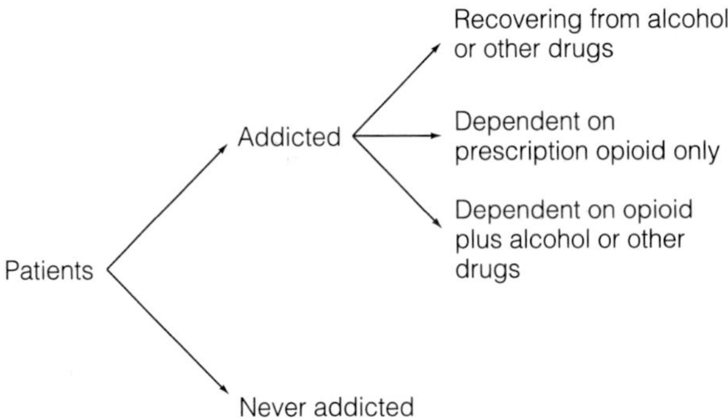

Figure 15-4 Classification of patients by their addiction status. (Reprinted by permission of Elsevier Science Inc. from "Prescriptions of Opioids for Treatment of Pain in Patients with Addictive Disease" by D. R. Wesson, W. Ling, and D. E. Smith, *Journal of Pain and Symptom Management,* Vol. 8, No. 5, p. 292. Copyright 1993 by the U.S. Cancer Pain Relief Committee.)

from those who currently are or ever have been addicted to recreational drugs, medications, or other substances. The classification further attempts to identify those patients with no past or current history of drug abuse who may have a higher risk of developing addictive-type behaviors while undergoing therapy for chronic pain. It should be remembered that addictive disease develops as a result of complex interactions among biologic predisposition, psychosocial and environmental factors, and chemical exposure. The course of the disease varies from individual to individual, and people who have led long, addiction-free lives can develop an addictive pattern of abuse at any time. The object of addiction may change or remain constant (Savage, 1993). Some predisposing factors to be considered in the assessment of pain patients for potential opioid abuse include:

1. Family history, particularly parental, of alcoholism or other substance abuse
2. Physical or sexual abuse or abandonment in childhood
3. Concomitant habituation or abuse of other substances such as tobacco, alcohol, benzodiazepines, or cocaine
4. Close environmental proximity to family members or other associates who are themselves substance abusers or who are involved with the use of street drugs or with the "drug culture"

In these patients, the standard protocols and guidelines for administration of analgesic medications may need to be modified to provide a greater degree of structure and control, as will be discussed in the section regarding the previously addicted patient at risk for relapse.

In assessing patients for opioid substance abuse, it is essential to distinguish clearly among the concepts of tolerance, physical dependence, and addiction (Enck, 1991). Opioid pain tolerance is defined as the need for escalating opioid doses to maintain adequate analgesia in a patient whose increased pain cannot be attributed primarily to progression of the underlying disease process. Data from tests performed on animals suggest that patients may be expected to develop tolerance to opioids after as little as one week of exposure, although the rate of development of tolerance may vary from patient to patient. Cross-tolerance between different opioid drugs is common but often incomplete, a point of importance when switching from one analgesic to another. Tolerance to opioid side effects such as sedation, euphoria, dysphoria, respiratory depression, and constipation develops at a different rate from tolerance to analgesia (Enck). Despite the phenomenon of tolerance, once chronic pain is controlled, most patients can be maintained on stable opioid doses for weeks to months provided there is no progression of the underlying disease process. Although distinguishing between analgesic tolerance and increased pain as a reason for dose escalation can sometimes be difficult, it is essential to remember that tolerance alone does not equal addiction, and its existence does not justify withholding adequate analgesic doses from patients with chronic pain (Sees & Clark, 1993).

Physical dependence is defined as an altered physiologic state produced by repeated administration of a drug to the extent that sudden cessation results in withdrawal symptoms (Enck, 1991). Withdrawal symptoms include anxiety, nervousness, irritability, chills, hot flashes, excessive salivation, tearing, rhinorrhea, sweating, nausea, vomiting, abdominal cramps, insomnia, and multifocal myoclonus. The severity of withdrawal is a function of the duration and the dose of the opioid administered, and the onset of symptoms is a function of the elimination half-life of the opioid on which the patient has become physically dependent. Like tolerance, physical dependence is a pharmacologic effect seen in response to the repeated administration of opioids in humans and laboratory animals and is distinctly different from the psychologic phenomenon of drug addiction (Enck). When starting patients on opioid analgesics, it is important to explain that both tolerance and physical dependence will occur and to reassure the patient and their families that these effects are expected and are not expressions or manifestations of drug addiction.

In contrast to tolerance and physiologic dependence, opioid addiction is a maladaptive state of psychologic dependence characterized by a continued, single-minded craving for opioids, manifesting in compulsive drug-seeking behavior and an overwhelming involvement in drug procurement and use (Enck, 1991). Additionally, addiction is characterized by loss of control over the use of the drug in terms of both dose and frequency and by continued use of the drug despite adverse consequences (Sees & Clark, 1993). The addict's focus is on the next episode of use or on memories of past experiences (Wesson et al., 1993). Further characterization of addictive behavior includes:

1. Overwhelming concerns about continued drug availability
2. Unsanctioned dose escalation
3. Continued use despite significant side effects
4. Manipulation of physicians and others in the health-care team to obtain additional drug supplies (e.g., "losing" drugs)
5. Alteration of prescriptions
6. Acquisition of drugs from multiple medical or non-medical sources
7. Drug hoarding or selling
8. Unapproved use of coaddictive substances during opioid therapy (Portenoy, 1990)

For patients with chronic pain, the preceding criteria are considerably more useful than the DSM-III-R (American Psychiatric Association, 1994) diagnostic criteria definition of addiction for patients without underlying medical problems requiring opioids. According to the DSM-III-R criteria, shown in Table 15-1, three of nine diagnostic criteria are sufficient to support a diagnosis of psychoactive substance use disorder, but only four of the criteria (numbers 3 through 6) relate to level of function and dysfunctional use of medications (Sees

Table 15-1 Comparison of DSM-III-R Criteria for Drug Dependence Applied to Opioid Abusers and Chronic Pain Patients Who Are Not Addicted but Being Maintained on Opioids for Treatment of Pain

Diagnostic Criteria	Pain Patient	Opioid Abuser
Requires at least three of the following:		
(1) Opioids often taken in larger amounts or over a longer period than the person intended	Patient is able to ration medication between planned visits to prescribing physician	Unable to store some away and ration use over days or weeks
(2) Persistent desire or one or more unsuccessful efforts to cut down or control opioid use	May want to decrease use, but when pain becomes worse, reluctantly agrees to continue medication	Relapses to drug use after detoxification
(3) A great deal of time spent in activities necessary to get the opioids, taking opioids, or recovering from their effects	May spend large amounts of time going to physicians; is generally cooperative with physician about nonopioid pain control strategies; is more disabled without medication	Life is consumed with acquiring money to purchase drugs, drug use, and drug-related activities; most recreational time is spent with other drug users
(4) Frequent intoxication or withdrawal symptoms when expected to fulfill major role obligations at work, school, or home	Rarely, if ever, occurs	Common occurrence

(5) Important social, occupational, or recreational activities given up or reduced because of opioid use	Activities given up primarily because of pain. May be more active on opioid medication	Activities not relating to drug use cease to be interesting or important
(6) Continued opioid use despite knowledge of having a recurrent social, psychological, or physical problem	May continue medication despite concerns about addiction expressed by family or friends	Drug use continues despite arrests, family fights, divorce, loss of children, loss of job, and adverse health consequences
(7) Marked tolerance: need for markedly increased amounts of the opioid (i.e., at least 50%) in order to achieve intoxication or desired effect, or markedly diminished effect with continued use of the same amount	May be present	Usually present
(8) Opioid withdrawal symptoms	Present when opioids stopped abruptly	Present when opioids stopped abruptly
(9) Opioids often taken to relieve or avoid withdrawal symptoms	Opioid use primarily in response to pain	Opioid withdrawal symptoms precipitate frantic drug-seeking behavior

USEFUL QUESTIONS FOR PROBING ADDICTION IN CHRONIC PAIN PATIENTS

Drug-taking reliability
- Does the patient take opioids or other psychoactive medications as prescribed?
- Frequency? Dose?

Loss of control of drug use
- Does the patient have partially used bottles of medications at home?
- Will the patient bring them in for verification?

Indications of drug-seeking behaviors
- Frequently reports losing medications?
- Demands drugs of high street value?
- Has prescriptions from multiple doctors?
- Has prescriptions filled at multiple pharmacies?

Abuse of drugs other than those prescribed
- Alcohol? Cocaine? Marijuana? Heroin? Amphetamines?
- Opioids? Benzodiazepines?

Contact with the street-drug culture
- Friends or family members who are street-drug users?
- Does the patient buy street drugs for any purpose?

& Clark, 1993). Five of the nine diagnostic criteria (1, 2, and 7 through 9) are essentially related to physical dependence or tolerance and will generally be easily met by any patient who has been receiving long-term opioid therapy for treatment of chronic pain (Sees & Clark). Therefore, according to these criteria, virtually every chronic pain patient taking opioid analgesics according to accepted management protocols would be considered to be addicted. Wesson and colleagues' (1993) adaptation of the DSM-III-R criteria (Table 15-1) illustrates how these criteria can be interpreted and applied in assessing addiction in patients with chronic pain. The box on pp. 484 and 485 (Sees & Clark) provides

USEFUL QUESTIONS FOR PROBING ADDICTION IN CHRONIC PAIN PATIENTS—cont'd

Adverse life consequences not due to chronic pain, but due to the effects of opioids or other drugs

- Inability to work?
- Loss of friends or alienation of family?
- Decreased interest in recreational activities?
- Adverse health consequences?

Cooperation with full treatment plan and alternative pain management techniques

- Avoiding situations that induce pain?
- Using nonnarcotic medications?
- Using physical therapy?
- Using TENS* units if indicated?
- Meditation or biofeedback?

Reprinted by permission of Elsevier Science Inc. from "Opioid Use in the Treatment of Chronic Pain: Assessment of Addiction," by K. L. Sees and H. W. Clark, *Journal of Pain and Symptom Management,* Vol. 8, No. 5, p. 261. Copyright 1993 by the U.S. Cancer Pain Relief Committee.
**TENS,* Transcutaneous electrical nerve stimulation.
These questions should also be asked of family members to validate the history given by the patient.

a list of questions based on the patient's behavior and level of function that are useful for detecting addiction in chronic pain patients.

Pain Management in Substance Abusers

As indicated by the different classifications in Figure 15-4, the approach to pain management in patients with addiction problems varies according to the state of activity of the abusive disorder. Thus, for patients who are actively addicted, treatment guidelines differ somewhat depending on whether the addiction is to prescription drugs alone or to multiple agents, including alcohol and street drugs. Treating former addicts requires distinguishing among those who are recovered (although never cured), those who are participants in a recovery program, and those who are newly drug free but still wrestling with the problems of abstinence. A distinction also needs to be made among addicts suffering from the pain of cancer, AIDS, or other terminal diseases; those with pain of chronic, nonmalignant illnesses; and those with acute or subacute, reversible pain. The management of intravenous drug abusers suffering from AIDS and associated neuropathic pain is a particular challenge, though one that can be met given sufficient expertise and attention to detail (Anand, Carmosino, & Glatt, 1994). In all circumstances, consultation and collaboration between teams of experts in pain management and addiction should be encouraged; pain specialists need to increase their sensitivity to the possibility of addiction among their patients, and addiction specialists, especially those whose primary treatment philosophy is "drug free," must accept that controlled opioid maintenance is mandatory for many patients with chronic, intractable pain (Wesson et al., 1993). All members of the health care team need to remember that pain can function as an obstacle to the individual's recovery from addiction and that addiction will complicate the treatment of chronic pain (Savage, 1993).

Treatment of Currently Addicted Patients

Currently addicted patients who are the most problematic for the health care team are those who are addicted to multiple agents including alcohol, cocaine, and other street drugs. For guidelines on treating this population, see the box on pp. 488 and 489. These patients are often increasingly manipulative, irrational, demanding, and angry, and they tend to generate feelings of frustration and hostility in physicians, nurses, and other caregivers. It is a challenge to care for some of these patients in a private medical office or in a pain clinic. Hospice teams, which in the United States tend to focus on home care delivery, may find their mission in caring for these patients literally impossible and even dangerous. In some patients, successful pain treatment is possible only in the context of an addiction treatment program.

Pain Management in Recovered and Recovering Addicts

Pain management in patients who are recovered or recovering addicts is complicated by concerns about relapse and recidivism that are shared, to one extent or another, by the patient, the family, and the health care team. Patients fear that the history of prior substance abuse will irrevocably alter their reputation and standing with the health care team to the extent that their complaints of persistent or escalating pain will be ignored, doubted, and attributed to drug craving. Furthermore, recovered patients, who have been taught that addiction is incurable, worry that they may again become drug dependent. As a result, patients themselves may reject adequate analgesic doses and appropriate escalations necessary to achieve pain control. Concerns of the health care team include the risk of reinducing dependent or abusive behavior and uncertainty as to how to accurately distinguish appropriate requests for increased opioids in response to increased pain from inappropriate requests reflecting reversion to drug-seeking behavior (Gonzalez & Coyle, 1992). Some guidelines for treatment of this population appear in the box on pp. 490 and 491.

Unfortunately, there are few objective data in the literature regarding the outcome of chronic pain treatment, including cancer pain, in the patient with a history of opioid abuse (Gonzalez & Coyle, 1992). There may be reason to suspect that the rarity of iatrogenic addiction in patients without a history of substance abuse may not apply to recovered opioid addicts. Opioid receptors appear to retain their avidity for opioids even after prolonged periods of abstinence (Savage, 1993). Individuals who are recovering or abstinent are at life-long risk of relapse (Savage). Many addiction experts believe that craving or relapse can be triggered by pain or by exposure to opioids (Wesson et al., 1993), although no clear documentation that opioid exposure predisposes the individual to relapse exists (Savage). On the other hand, clinical experience suggests that patients

GUIDELINES FOR TREATMENT OF CURRENTLY ADDICTED PATIENTS

- Encourage open communication with the patient.
- Avoid charting comments about drug use behaviors unless you have discussed your concerns with the patient.
- Remember that denial is a cardinal feature of addiction (Savage, 1993).
- Obtain information about the patient's drug use from sources other than the patient (Wesson et al., 1993).
- Do not withhold opioids from patients with moderate or severe pain; doing so will only encourage craving and drug-seeking behavior.
- Accept and respect the report of pain in spite of the possibility of being duped.
- Assure patients that they will receive as much medication as needed to relieve pain.
- For certain patients with chronic pain unrelated to cancer, consider a trial period free of opioids to determine whether the medications themselves may be acting to facilitate or disinhibit pain. Explain the ways in which chemical dependency may reinforce the cycle of chronic pain. During the withdrawal period, administration of clonidine may be helpful in minimizing physiologic stress (Savage, 1993).
- Establish a written treatment plan or contract, negotiated with and agreed to by the patient. Elements in the plan include: allowable medications and doses; amounts of medication to be dispensed; policies regarding refills and "lost medications"; frequency of office, clinic, or home care visits; commitment to addiction therapy if appropriate in the clinical context; and the consequences of failure to follow the plan (Wesson et al., 1993).
- Arrange for all opioids and other adjunctive and psychotropic medications to be prescribed by the same physician.

GUIDELINES FOR TREATMENT OF CURRENTLY ADDICTED PATIENTS—cont'd

- Encourage participation of nurse addiction and pain specialists and designate a nurse as coordinator for the management team.
- Remember that these patients have often developed drug tolerance and thus may require much larger doses of opioids than the average patient. Titrate to effect. Estimate the patient's usual daily intake and provide therapeutic dosing above this baseline dose to obtain effective analgesia.
- Attempt to use regularly scheduled, long-acting opioids for baseline pain management. Avoid prn schedules except as indicated for intermittent or breakthrough pain.
- Use adjunctive medications (e.g., NSAIDs) liberally, but do not use them as replacements for opioids.
- Encourage the use of alternative tools for pain control such as relaxation, exercise, and physical therapy consistent with the underlying medical condition, and productive activity including work, occupational therapy, creativity, and social interactions. Pace activities to avoid exacerbation of pain (Savage, 1993).
- Utilize nonpharmacologic pain control techniques including meditation, mental imagery, breathing techniques, stretch exercises, application of ice or heat, massage, and immobilization.
- Should the patient demand rapid or unexpected escalation in dosage requirements disproportional to the apparent extent or progression of the underlying disease, do not be too hasty to attribute this to the coexistent addictive disorder. Take the time to identify other potential areas of distress and suffering, including emotional, social, and spiritual pain, and intervene appropriately.
- Remember that, as in all patients with chronic pain, realistic restoration of function and maximization of quality of life are the common goals that should motivate the patient, family, caregivers, and health care team alike.

GUIDELINES FOR MANAGING PAIN IN RECOVERED AND RECOVERING PATIENTS

- Distinguish between abstinence and recovery. The abstinent person who is struggling with his or her abstinence is often still in denial, isolated, socially dysfunctional, unable to derive pleasure from other sources, and actively fighting drug craving. It is usually best to manage pain in these patients in a manner similar to that used for actively addicted patients (Savage, 1993).
- Believe the patient's complaint of pain.
- Determine whether pain control techniques (pharmacologic and nonpharmacologic) other than opioids are preferable.
- Address patient and family concerns about dependence and relapse. Explain that physical dependency, which will occur, is not the same as addiction.
- Reassure the patient and family that opioid use will be structured. Formulate and obtain patient agreement to a treatment plan contract.

with a history of substance abuse who develop cancer-related pain, either while on methadone maintenance or while entirely drug free, can successfully have their pain managed in a manner similar to that used in patients without a history of abuse (Gonzalez & Coyle, 1992). Indeed, undertreatment of pain and the risk of iatrogenic "pseudoaddiction" is common in this population, leading to the general consensus that no medication is contraindicated when it is the only reasonable option for treatment.

INFLUENCE OF CONCURRENT MEDICAL CONDITIONS ON PAIN MANAGEMENT

Many patients with chronic pain, including nearly all with advanced metastatic cancer (see Chapter 10) or terminal nonmalignant conditions (see Chapter 9), suffer from con-

GUIDELINES FOR MANAGING PAIN IN RECOVERED AND RECOVERING PATIENTS—cont'd

- One caretaker should be designated as responsible for pain management.
- Use drugs in effective doses and titrate the doses to achieve adequate analgesia. Do not underdose, as this may lead to anxiety and drug craving.
- Prescribe on a scheduled (around-the-clock) basis.
- Limit quantities per prescription and do not allow refills.
- Have spouse, friend, other caregiver, or pharmacist dispense each dose.
- Maintain frequent contact with the patient and the caregiver.
- Urge increased involvement in a recovery program or other support group.
- Remember that stress may increase the patient's request for analgesics.
- Be alert for and address aberrant drug use behavior suggestive of true addiction, such as acquisition of drugs from multiple sources, repeated claims of lost medications, unsanctioned dose increases, and prescription fraud.

current medical and metabolic disorders that alter the pharmacokinetics of commonly prescribed analgesics, thus leading to toxic drug side effects at doses that would normally be easily tolerated. Additionally, the clinical manifestations of these disorders frequently mimic the signs and symptoms of drug toxicity, leaving the patient, family, and health care team unsure about how best to proceed. For example, hypercalcemia, commonly noted in patients suffering pain from metastatic bone disease, is associated with lethargy, disorientation, constipation, anorexia, nausea, and vomiting—symptoms that are common side effects of opioid administration. Complaints associated with renal failure and uremia, including weakness, nausea, lethargy, pruritus, neuromuscular irritability, and twitching, can also be caused by opioids, and uremic gastrointestinal bleeding can be attributed to the concurrent use of nonsteroidal antiinflammatory drugs (NSAIDs). Asterixis, personality changes, intellectual deterioration, delirium, stupor, and unresponsiveness caused by the onset of hepatic encephalopathy may be attributed to or provoked by the concurrent use of opioids, anxiolytics, or other psychotropic medications in patients with advanced liver dysfunction. Clinically significant drug interactions may also provoke toxic side effects, as is the case, for example, between opioids and alcohol (Jacox et al., 1994), opioids and cimetidine (Glare & Walsh, 1991), alcohol and benzodiazepines, and monoamine oxidase inhibitors and either tricyclic antidepressants or meperidine (Mehta, 1995). None of these coexisting conditions obviates the obligation to adequately control pain, which for the actively dying patient may be the only significant consideration, regardless of concurrent side effects. In earlier phases of disease, however, recognition of the significance of these comorbid states may prompt choices and doses of analgesics that will minimize toxicity and enhance overall palliation.

Renal Impairment

Most opioids, including morphine, meperidine, methadone, and levorphanol, are metabolized by the liver into active and inactive metabolites, which are then excreted by the kidney (Hammack & Loprinzi, 1994). The elimination of free morphine is unchanged in patients with impaired renal function, but there is marked prolongation of the elimination of the major metabolites morphine-3-glucuronide (M3G) and morphine-6-glucuronide (M6G). Although M3G is pharmacologically inactive, M6G is pharmacologically more potent than free morphine and accumulates in patients with renal insufficiency, sometimes causing adverse opioid effects. Another metabolite, normorphine (NM)—which, like normeperidine, is potentially neurotoxic and proconvulsant—is also excreted renally, but it is not known whether this metabolite accumulates in patients with renal impairment (Glare & Walsh, 1991). In view of the critical contribution of renal function to opioid excretion, it is recommended that initial opioid doses be lowered or given less frequently in patients with renal insufficiency (Jacox et al., 1994). Similar caution is advised with elderly patients, some of whom may have decreases in glomerular function (Jacox et al.) (see Chapter 12). For patients with severe renal impairment, the lack of accumulation of toxic metabolites may make hydromorphone preferable to morphine as the opioid of choice. Once steady-state pain control is achieved, most patients with slowly progressive deterioration of renal function can be accommodated by the usual practice of titration of dose against effect. However, should well-controlled patients develop sudden exacerbation of renal failure—as in acute obstructive uropathy, for example—opioid toxicity may occur, necessitating temporary drug withdrawal and downward dose adjustment (Inturrisi & Hanks, 1993).

For patients on hemodialysis, supplemental dosing of opioids is not required during or following dialysis, except for patients on pentazocine, which, being a mixed agonist-antagonist, is usually not a recommended agent for patients with chronic pain. Postdialysis supplemental dosing is necessary for acetaminophen, aspirin, and salsalate, but not for other NSAIDs or for tricyclic antidepressants (Simmons & Johnson, 1991). In patients with renal insufficiency who are not on dialysis, NSAIDs are usually contraindicated because of additional nephrotoxic potential. Renal syndromes with NSAIDs include fluid retention, interstitial nephritis, and papillary necrosis (Rawlins, 1993).

Liver Impairment

Although the liver is the principal site of morphine metabolism in humans, glucuronidation is rarely impaired in hepatic failure, as supplemental glucuronidation occurs in the bowel (Twycross, 1993). For the majority of patients with impaired liver function, no special precautions are required in the use of morphine, and the dose should be titrated against effect as usual (Inturrisi & Hanks, 1993). Morphine is well tolerated in patients up to the point of hepatic precoma (Twycross).

However, with severe hepatic dysfunction, morphine may provoke or exacerbate hepatic encephalopathy, which suggests that patients should be carefully monitored and doses reduced in the face of severe hepatic dysfunction (Glare & Walsh, 1991). Other opioids, including methadone, levorphanol, pentazocine, propoxyphene, and meperidine, have increased bioavailability in patients with impaired hepatic function and can cause CNS depression mimicking hepatic encephalopathy (Jacox et al., 1994). For this reason, morphine is the opioid of choice in patients with hepatic dysfunction. Meperidine has also been reported to cause neuroexcitatory toxicity in a patient with alcoholic hepatitis and cirrhosis (Danziger, Martin, & Blum, 1994).

In patients with even mild liver disease, acetaminophen doses need to be reduced below the accepted total daily allowance of 4 g, and patients need to monitored carefully for evidence of hepatotoxicity (Whitcomb & Block, 1994). Because of the prevalence and easy availability of multiple over-the-counter acetaminophen-containing medications, acetaminophen overdosing is quite common and is a significant cause of morbidity. NSAIDs rarely have significant hepatotoxicity. However, due partly to coagulation abnormalities and partly to other factors associated with chronic liver disease, the risk of gastrointestinal bleeding is increased in patients with cirrhosis and chronic hepatic dysfunction. Tricyclic antidepressants are primarily metabolized by the liver and should be used cautiously in patients with significant hepatic dysfunction.

Pulmonary Insufficiency

Pulmonary insufficiency, even when associated with chronic obstructive lung disease and hypercarbia, should not be an insurmountable obstacle to effective pain management. Frequently, physicians are reluctant to use opioid analgesics for pain relief in patients with chronic lung disease, just as many physicians are resistant to using opioids for the relief of terminal dyspnea because of their reflexive avoidance of any drug with the potential for respiratory depression (Johansen,

1990). Many physicians, influenced by work in the 1950s demonstrating the potential hazards of opioid administration in patients with respiratory failure, are also convinced that the use of morphine in patients with pulmonary impairment hastens death and is tantamount to murder—or, at the very least, euthanasia. However, more recent clinical experience shows that when low doses of morphine are gradually titrated upward, the risk of respiratory depression is small because of the rapid development of tolerance. With the possible exception of patients with severe chronic hypoxia whose ventilatory drive depends heavily on the response to CO_2, or of opioid-naive patients treated precipitously rather than gradually, opioid analgesics can be used in the management of chronic pain without significant risk of respiratory depression (Inturrisi & Hanks, 1993; Jacox et al., 1994; Johansen). Furthermore, cautious use of opioids in patients with chronic obstructive lung disease may also alleviate breathlessness and even increase exercise tolerance (Woodcock et al., 1981). In dying patients, the use of morphine for palliation of terminal dyspnea is well established (Bruera, MacEachern, Ripamonti, & Hanson, 1993).

Procedural Pain

It is well recognized that, in children with cancer, more than half of all painful experiences are related to diagnostic procedures and invasive treatments. Even in adults, up to 15% of "cancer" pain is actually procedural or iatrogenic in nature, usually resulting from the side effects of surgery, radiotherapy, or chemotherapy. However, for patients suffering from chronic pain and other disabling symptoms associated with intractable disease, even relatively innocuous procedures may exacerbate pain and anxiety, adding significantly to their discomfort. Imagine the discomfort and pain experienced by patients with bony metastatic disease each time they are transported for diagnostic radiography or transferred from stretcher to table to stretcher to bed while receiving palliative radiotherapy. Bone marrow biopsies, lumbar punctures, paracenteses, thoracenteses, chest tube insertions, frequent venipunctures, and even fecal disimpactions are all bedside procedures capable of causing both fear and severe discomfort. Magnetic resonance and computed tomography imaging procedures often provoke extreme claustrophobic anxiety. By anticipating and preventing procedural pain and discomfort, the health care team can significantly improve patient well-being and ability to cope with the other symptoms and manifestations of disease.

Before performing a procedure, clinicians should develop a plan to prevent or reduce pain that takes into account the nature of the procedure, the degree of pain expected, and the needs of the patient. Strategies for dealing with procedural pain start with informed consent. The patient should know the following: why the procedure is being performed; how much pain or discomfort will be associated with the procedure and how long the pain or discomfort will last; what other risks are associated with the procedure; when the results will be available; and whether the procedure will have to be repeated, and if so, how often. Anticipated procedure-related pain or anxiety should be treated prophylactically while preexisting pain is managed as optimally as possible. Even if the procedure itself is inherently painless, remember that moving the patient may provoke pain. Stabilize or immobilize painful extremities before transportation and administer appropriate analgesics with sufficient lead time to allow for full therapeutic effect. Delays can escalate pain and anxiety and should be avoided. Anxiolytic agents such as lorazepam or other benzodiazepines are often necessary to increase relaxation and decrease unwanted movements during the procedure. Imagery and hypnosis may sometimes be helpful.

Pharmacologic agents for the management of procedural pain include local anesthetics, opioids, and benzodiazepines. Local anesthetics, such as xylocaine, can be administered by local infiltration or by topical application. Eutectic mixture of local anesthetics (EMLA), which is often used in children before venipuncture or accessing infusaports, must be applied 60 to 90 minutes before the procedure (see Chapter 11). Opioids can be given either intravenously or orally, but the intravenous route has the advantage of rapid onset and ease of titration. Prior to performing bone marrow biopsies in adults, it is common to intravenously administer 5 mg of morphine or 50 to 75 mg of meperidine (in opioid-naive patients) and 0.5 to 2 mg of lorazepam. For procedures of longer duration in adults, 2 to 4 mg of morphine can be administered every 5 minutes and titrated to analgesic effect. Of course, if patients are already receiving larger maintenance doses of opioids for chronic pain, larger procedure-associated doses will be necessary, calculated according to accepted formulas for "rescue" doses (see Chapter 10). Benzodiazepines provide sedation, muscle relaxation, and, in higher doses, amnesia; however, they do not provide analgesia, which is why they should be used along with opioids for painful procedures. An alternative to lorazepam is midazolam IV, titrated in increments of about 0.5 mg. The combination of opioid and benzodiazepine, especially in opioid-naive patients, significantly increases the risk of respiratory depression, and geriatric patients should be monitored particularly closely. Should respiratory depression occur, stimulation of the patient and administration of small, frequent doses of intravenous naloxone (0.04-mg doses for adults) may be adequate to reverse mild degrees of hypoventilation. Assisted ventilation and repeated doses of naloxone may be needed for more profound degrees of respiratory depression.

Other pharmacologic agents that are sometimes useful include nitrous oxide, ketamine, thiopental, propofol, and methohexital, contingent on the availability of trained personnel. Skilled supervision is necessary whenever systemic pharmacologic agents are used for conscious sedation, and appropriate resuscitative equipment and at least one health care professional proficient in airway management and advanced life support should be available. During the procedure, a health care professional not involved in performing the procedure or restraining the patient should monitor the patient's heart rate, respiratory rate and effort, blood pressure, level of consciousness, and arterial oxygen saturation by pulse oximetry. Monitoring should continue after the procedure until the patient is fully awake and restored to the former level of function. Take the time to speak to the patient and/or family after the procedure to determine whether the pain prevention strategies were successful and to identify and treat any painful or uncomfortable sequelae (Jacox et al., 1994).

MANAGEMENT OF PAIN IN PREGNANCY

This section will address pain in pregnancy from the same perspective that should be applied to the definition of all other pain, which insists on the credibility of patient reports of pain. The fact that the usual pains of pregnancy emanate from a natural process whose outcome is generally regarded as among the most uplifting of human experiences does not lessen the intensity of those pains. Childbirth pain is commonly used as the extreme against which other painful events are measured, and parous women, when providing pain judgments, often say that nothing compares to labor pain (Hapidou & DeCatanzaro, 1992).

Low back and posterior pelvic pain account for the majority of sick leave among pregnant women (Ostgaard, Zetherstrom, Roos-Hansson, & Svanberg, 1994), and some degree of abdominal pain is virtually physiologic in pregnancy (Epstein, 1994). Differentiation between low back and posterior pelvic pain is important, as posterior pelvic pain can frequently be reduced by a nonelastic pelvic support (Ostgaard et al., 1994). Good physical fitness prior to pregnancy reduces the risk of development of back pain, whereas low socioeconomic class, prior history of low back pain, and certain ultrasonographic and obstetric data are predictive of a higher risk of developing back pain (Orvieto, Achiron, Ben-Rafael, Gelernter, & Achiron, 1994). No correlation has been observed between back pain during and after pregnancy, nor between the need for pain relief in labor and birthweight or Apgar score (Ostgaard, Andersson, & Wennergren, 1991). Sacroiliac subluxation, a common cause of low back pain in pregnancy, is amenable to treatment with rotational manipulation of the sacroiliac joints (Daly, Frame, & Rapoza, 1991).

Back pain usually disappears in the first 6 months postpartum, except in women with recurrent back pain from previous pregnancies, in whom back pain may persist considerably longer (Östgaard et al., 1991).

Most recommended interventions for back pain due to pregnancy are nonpharmacologic and emphasize physical techniques such as the aforementioned rotational manipulation and exercise programs designed to enhance overall physical fitness. Early intervention may limit or prevent low back pain later in pregnancy (Orvieto et al., 1994). Pharmacologic interventions are often discouraged and/or avoided by women who wish to minimize drug exposure during pregnancy. Acetaminophen, one of the WHO step 1 analgesics, has not been reported to cause birth defects or other problems in pregnant women or nursing babies, even though it does pass into breast milk in small amounts (USP DI, 1993).

The use of NSAIDs during pregnancy is more problematic. Studies on birth defects with these medications have not been done in humans. Data from animal trials have shown that birth defects did not occur with commonly used NSAIDs such as ibuprofen, ketoprofen, naproxen, piroxicam, or tolmetin but did occur with various other NSAIDs such as diflunisal and indomethacin. However, many NSAIDs did cause other harmful or toxic effects in animal fetuses and, when administered late in pregnancy, sometimes prolonged pregnancy or labor or caused other problems during delivery. Even in humans there is a chance that NSAIDs may cause unwanted effects on the heart or blood flow of the fetus or newborn baby if they are taken regularly during the last few months of pregnancy (USP DI, 1993). In one study (Dildy, Moise, Smith, Kirshon, & Carpenter, 1992), 100 mg of indomethacin administered daily for a mean duration of 12 days for opioid-"resistant" pain associated with carneous degeneration of uterine leiomyomata was associated with abnormalities in three of seven patients. There were two aborted pregnancies, and one fetus had transient constriction of the ductus arteriosus and transient oligohydramnios.

However, five term deliveries were of healthy, normal infants. In women with ankylosing spondylitis, ibuprofen may be the preferred treatment during pregnancy and lactation (Gran & Husby, 1992), but in general, a prudent course in pregnancy would seem to be avoidance of NSAIDs whenever possible. It would also seem advisable for nursing mothers to avoid NSAID use because many NSAIDs pass into the breast milk, and some, such as indomethacin, phenylbutazone, and meclofenamate, cause unwanted effects in nursing babies (USP DI).

Opioid therapy for severe, acute pain may be indicated during pregnancy and, at times, during the labor process. However, the perinatal use of opioids (even meperidine 75 to 100 mg IM) just before and during delivery can cause central nervous system and respiratory depression in the newborn baby (Viegas, Khaw, & Ratnam, 1993). Furthermore, in experimental animals, the neonatal use of morphine and related compounds has altered developmental processes, inducing changes that endure into adulthood (Harrison, Zadina, Banks, & Kastin, 1993). In terms of efficacy, single doses of both IM meperidine (50 to 100 mg) and IM ketorolac were relatively ineffective in relieving labor pain, although ketorolac had a superior safety profile (Walker, Johnston, Fairlie, Lloyd, & Bullingham, 1992). Furthermore, particularly with regard to the effectiveness of meperidine (and, indeed, as regards all obstetric pain relief), medical professionals commonly believe that they are providing adequate pain relief whereas women report the relief as unsatisfactory (Rajan, 1993). Sublingual buprenorphine (a mixed agonist-antagonist opioid) administered during the first stage of labor produced analgesia up to 9 hours after administration, did not delay the progress of labor, and had no adverse effect on the fetal heart rate or Apgar scores of neonates (Roy & Basu, 1992). In comparison with regimens for labor analgesia that depend on the systemic absorption of drugs (e.g., parenterally administered opioids and inhalational analgesia), epidural and intrathecal analgesia have become established as the most effective and consistently reliable methods of providing pain relief in labor with minimal side effects for the neonate (Brownridge,

1991). However, in parturient women, even these methods may cause significant side effects such as pruritus, urinary retention, and headache (Herpolsheimer & Schretenthaler, 1994). It should be recognized that most women prefer to keep drug use during labor to a minimum, even though they expect labor to be very painful. Women who prefer to avoid drugs are more likely to do so and are often more satisfied with the overall birthing experience than women who use drugs (Green, 1993). Inadequate analgesia is also reported less frequently by women using nonpharmacologic methods such as breathing and relaxation exercises alone (Paech, 1991). The mechanisms of labor pain, the effect of pregnancy on pain, and the clinical implications of these have been reviewed by Faure (1991).

Sustained opioid treatment during pregnancy is rarely necessary because serious illness associated with chronic, intractable pain is, fortunately, an infrequent occurrence in pregnant women. In the United States the overall incidence of cancer during pregnancy is estimated at 1 in 1000. Invasive malignancies occur less commonly, and metastatic cancer even less so (Gusberg & Runowicz, 1991). However, other conditions associated with chronic pain syndromes such as sickle cell disease and AIDS may be encountered with greater frequency (Feinberg & Soper, 1992). The successful use of long-term, intravenous, patient-controlled meperidine analgesia in pregnancy has been reported (Aaen, Cowan, Sakala, & Small, 1993). McGrady, Malinow, Paly, and Mokriski (1993) have reported successful shorter-duration use of patient-controlled epidural sufentanil in a patient at 28 weeks gestation with severe pain due to metastatic gastric carcinoma.

Chronic opioid use in pregnancy causes physiologic dependence in fetuses and newborns, leading to symptoms of the neonatal withdrawal syndrome (NWS) after birth. Manifestations of NWS include irritability, hyperactivity, abnormal sleep pattern, high-pitched cry, tremor, vomiting, diarrhea, weight loss, and failure to gain weight (Levy & Spino, 1993). Neonatal withdrawal syndrome should be anticipated as an expected outcome in any pregnancy associated with chronic opioid exposure, whether due to planned therapy or to addiction. Neonatal withdrawal syndrome may also occur in infants born to alcoholic mothers as well as those chronically treated with or addicted to barbiturates and benzodiazepines. The onset, duration, and severity of the disorder differ based on such factors as the drug used, time and amount of the mother's last dose, and the rate of elimination of the drug from the newborn. Pharmacologic intervention with drugs such as phenobarbital, paregoric, chlorpromazine, and diazepam may be required to control severe signs and symptoms (Levy & Spino, 1993).

Additional deleterious effects of intrauterine opioid exposure on fetal and childhood development have been reported in the offspring of drug-addicted mothers. These include prematurity, low birth weight and length, smaller head circumference, and a twofold to threefold increase in perinatal mortality (Lam, To, Duthie, & Ma, 1992; Noia et al., 1994). Allowing for the contribution of socioeconomic conditions, prenatal opioid exposure has been associated with an increased risk of opioid addiction in later life, even when that exposure was confined to administration of opiates, barbiturates, and nitrous oxide to mothers during labor (Nyberg, Allebeck, Eklund, & Jacobson, 1992). School-age children exposed to maternal drug addiction, even those raised in foster homes, have shown high rates of behavioral and psychiatric morbidity, especially with respect to disruptive behavior disorders (Havens, Whitaker, Feldman, & Ehrhardt, 1994). Even controlled methadone exposure during pregnancy, although not associated with obvious cognitive impairments or IQ deficits in pre-school-age children—and although having a clearly preferable risk-to-benefit ratio than continued street-drug exposure—may sometimes increase the risk of fine motor coordination and attention deficit disorders that are likely to lead to poor school performance (Hutchings, Zmitrovich, Church, & Malowany, 1993). Ongoing studies should lead to greater understanding of the potential for developmental toxicity as a consequence of prenatal opioid exposure.

For pain management during labor and postpartum, the following findings are significant. Topical perineal application of 2% lidocaine gel during the second stage of labor can significantly ameliorate immediate postpartum pain (Collins et al., 1994). For relief of uterine cramps and episiotomy pain, both acetaminophen and naproxen appear equally effective (Skovlund, Fyllingen, Landre, & Nesheim, 1991). Although small amounts of codeine and morphine have been detected in breast milk, moderate codeine use in nursing mothers, not to exceed four 60-mg doses, is probably safe (Meny, Naumberg, Alger, Brill-Miller, & Brown, 1993). Furthermore, neither acetaminophen, meperidine, nor propoxyphene has been reported to cause problems in nursing babies (USP DI, 1993).

For situations in which pregnancy is prematurely terminated, there has been recent emphasis on the long-term effects of abortion on women but less emphasis on the painful and distressing aspects of the procedure itself. Findings indicate that abortion is both an anxiety-producing and painful, distressing medical procedure (Wells, 1991). During prostaglandin-induced abortions in the second trimester, intramuscular nalbuphine effectively relieved uterine pain during the myometrial contractility period, prevented the occurrence of prostaglandin-related gastrointestinal side effects, and provided good anesthesia during instrumental removal of the already detached but retained placenta (Kovacs, Herczeg, & Szabo, 1993). Concurrent use of intravenous metoclopramide promotes significantly earlier fetal and placental passage, reduces the requirement for opioid analgesics, and allows earlier discharge from the hospital (Rosenblatt, Cioffi, Sinatra, & Silverman, 1992).

NEUROPATHIC PAIN

Neuropathic pain, as described in Chapter 1, is defined as pain associated with injury to either the peripheral or central nervous system. Unlike nociceptive pain, which is generally localized to a defined site of tissue injury, neuropathic pain is commonly perceived in an anatomic distribution remote from the site of nerve injury and may "spread" to involve areas of the body whose innervation appears unconnected to the original injured nervous tissue. In order to understand neuropathic pain, it is important to remember that the nervous system cannot be thought of as a "hard-wired" electrical network in which a circuit can be broken by cutting a wire and then restored by splicing or soldering the cut ends together. Rather, it is more accurate to think of the nervous system in terms of "plasticity," or alteration in neuronal function and relationships in response to stimulation (the basis of memory) and injury (the basis of neuropathic pain). Nervous system plasticity involves a complex array of neuroactive substances and transmitters released by both inflammatory cells and neurons themselves. These alter intraneuronal neurochemistry and the network of interneuronal cell-cell interactions at varying levels of the nervous system, resulting in the following: hypersensitivity to mechanical and α-adrenergic stimulation; spontaneous electrical activity; abnormal "cross-talk" between neighboring neurons; wind-up phenomena in dorsal root neurons; and reengineering of the pain-inhibitory descending modulating system from the cortex, diencepahlon, and brainstem. These create a new central nervous system steady state that is spontaneously active and hyperexcitable (Twycross, 1993; Cross, 1994). Much of the evidence for these complex interactions has developed from the observation and study of two clinical neuropathic pain syndromes: reflex sympathetic dystrophy and phantom pain.

Reflex Sympathetic Dystrophy

Reflex sympathetic dystrophy (RSD) is a progressive, multisystem, disabling disease that can involve peripheral nerve, muscle, bone, blood vessel, and skin changes (Jackson, 1993). Other names for this disease include causalgia, Sudeck's atrophy, algodystrophy, and peripheral trophoneurosis (Veldman, Reynen, Arntz, & Goris, 1993). Reflex sympathetic dystrophy is most often initiated by surgery or even minor traumatic injury to a nerve, plexus, or soft tissue. It may follow stroke, head injury, tumor, or spinal cord injury

(Schwartzman, 1993; Veldman & Jacobs, 1994). It has been found with moderate frequency after Colles' fracture and less commonly after myocardial infarction (shoulder-hand syndrome), local cold injury (trench foot), revascularization of an ischemic extremity (Veldman et al.), mastectomy (Saddison & Vanek, 1993), and bone marrow transplantation (Stamatoullas, Ferrant, & Manicourt, 1993). Prednisone-responsive RSD has been reported in a patient with systemic lupus erythematosus (Ostrov, Eichenfield, Goldsmith, & Schumacher, 1993), has been associated with the use of antiepileptic drugs, and has been related to other fibrosing disorders associated with anticonvulsant therapy, including Dupuytren's contractures, frozen shoulder, and Peyronie's disease (Falasca, Toly, Reginato, Schraeder, & O'Conner, 1994). Reflex sympathetic dystrophy occurs in all age groups, including children and adolescents (Schwartzman; Stanton, Malcolm, Wesdock, & Singsen, 1993).

Reflex sympathetic dystrophy is invariably associated with pain and can cause major, progressive, and permanent disability. Nevertheless, because the manifestations of RSD are often disproportionate to the suspected inciting injury or trauma, patients suffering from this condition are commonly accused of malingering. Thus in the litigious climate currently prevailing in the United States, the diagnosis and verification of RSD takes on additional significance in the realm of liability and disability claims and employee compensation. Reflex sympathetic dystrophy has also been attributed to preexistent psychologic or psychiatric illness, depression, emotional instability, or anxiety, with the result that patient complaints are sometimes not taken seriously (Veldman et al., 1993). However, even though patients with RSD often demonstrate emotional distress and behavioral disturbance, there is no evidence that, relative to other chronic pain patients, RSD patients are uniquely disturbed in psychosocial functioning (DeGood, Cundiff, Adams, & Shutty, 1993; Schwartzman, 1993).

The major components of RSD are pain, edema, autonomic dysfunction, movement disorder, and trophic changes.

However, there is wide variation in the spectrum of clinical presentations, and there are no universally applied criteria for diagnosing RSD (Schwartzman, 1993). Veldman and colleagues (1993) propose that the following may support an RSD diagnosis:

1. The presence of four or five of these symptoms:
   - Unexplained diffuse pain
   - Difference in skin color relative to the other limb
   - Diffuse edema
   - Difference in skin temperature relative to the other limb
   - Limited active range of motion
2. Occurrence or increase of the preceding signs and symptoms after use
3. Presentation of the preceding signs and symptoms in an area larger than that of the of primary injury or operation and including the area distal to the primary injury

Diagnostic studies such as bone scans and radiographs often demonstrate evidence of osteopenia, but these abnormalities may not be found in the majority of patients with early disease (Veldman et al.). Improvement after phentolamine, an α-adrenergic receptor inhibitor, may be a useful diagnostic test in patients with early disease (Kozin, 1994) but may be useless in the later stages when the disorder may no longer be sympathetically driven.

The illness evolves insidiously over time at an unpredictable rate. The earliest, or acute, phase is often characterized by the classic signs and symptoms of inflammation in an area larger than the primary site of injury (Veldman et al., 1993). Increased vascular permeability for macromolecules, an important characteristic of inflammation, seems to be a hallmark of the early, acute phase but is rarely detected during the later stages (Oyen et al., 1993). The frequency of inflammatory pathophysiology, together with evidence for coexistent oxidative stress and decreased oxygen consumption in early-stage RSD, has prompted some investigators to question the centrality of the sympathetic nervous system in the pathogenesis of this disorder (Veldman et al.).

Pain is usually disproportionate to the degree of injury and is often described as deep, diffuse, and burning and as exacerbated by movement, exercise, emotional distress, and dependent posture. Hyperalgesia (increased sensitivity to a painful stimulus) and allodynia (a painful sensation caused by a stimulus not usually associated with pain, such as light touch) are common complaints. Half of the patients complain of one or more painful trigger points (Veldman et al., 1993). Most patients try to protect the affected part from exposure to all stimuli. Some patients obtain relief either by tightly wrapping the affected extremity with elastic bandages or by applying cold compresses (Schwartzman, 1993).

Additional manifestations of early-stage disease include edema, hyperhidrosis, discoloration, brown-gray scaly pigmentation, spontaneous hematomas, and increased hair and nail growth. Either hyperthermia or hypothermia may be present. The division into primarily warm (more prevalent) and primarily cold RSD may have prognostic significance, since more patients with cold RSD present with later-stage disease (Veldman et al., 1993). Muscular paresis and rapid fatigability are frequently present. Muscle atrophy, usually a sign of later disease, may be masked by the presence of edema. Bone changes may occasionally occur early but are typically found in later stages of RSD. However, decreases in bone mineral density and bone mineral content, as measured by x-ray bone densitometry, can be detected in many patients even in early-stage RSD (Arriagada & Arinoviche, 1994). Movement disorders are usually found in late-stage disease, but tremor akin to physiologic tremor may occur in the early phase and then disappear following sympatholytic intervention (Deuschl, Blumberg, & Lucking, 1991).

The later stages of RSD are associated with an increase in pain, hyperalgesia, and allodynia, often accompanied by other characteristic components of the chronic pain syndrome such as sleep disruption, anxiety, and depression. In general, the pain no longer responds to sympathetic blockade. Chronic, brawny edema may be accompanied by recurrent local tissue infections often resistant to treatment. Skin manifestations often include dusky cyanosis, mottling, livedo reticularis, and nodular fascitis of the palmar or plantar skin. In this phase hair loss is common and the nails become clubbed, ridged, dull, and brittle, a condition sometimes known as "hourglass nails" (Schwartzman, 1993). A movement disorder often occurs consisting of weakness, difficulty in initiating movement, tremor, spasms, dystonia, and increased reflex activity (Schwartzman), although electromyograms are usually normal (Veldman et al., 1993). Eventually, severe cartilage, muscle, and soft tissue atrophy and dystrophy occur, often associated with contractures, pseudoparalysis, and functional disability.

Reflex sympathetic dystrophy in one part of the body seems to sensitize patients so that a succeeding injury may initiate the process in the newly traumatized area (Schwartzman, 1993). However, multiple sites may be involved in the absence of an inciting cause for each affected location, and relapse without evident cause may occur in some patients after a period of few or no complaints (Veldman et al., 1993). This unpredictability, along with the insidious nature and variable progression of this disorder, often leads to patients being diagnosed as hysterical or as suffering from other psychiatric disorders; patients themselves often manifest psychophysiologic and behavioral aspects of helplessness (Van Houdenhove & Vasquez, 1993). Desperate patients with intractable pain and incapacity resulting from refractory RSD have attempted or committed suicide (Veldman et al.); this highlights the need for heightened understanding of the clinical features of this disorder and for early intervention and attempted treatment before irreversible disability occurs. Once RSD is diagnosed, prompt treatment is beneficial (Dzwierzynski & Sanger, 1994).

Success in treating RSD is never ensured, but it is enhanced by use of a multitherapy approach incorporating pharmacotherapy, sympathetic blockade or ablation, physical therapy and rehabilitation, distraction devices, relaxation therapy, biofeedback, counseling, stress management training, and psychotherapy. Medications reported to have been helpful in some patients include corticosteroids, NSAIDs, tricyclic antidepressants, anticonvulsants, systemic local anesthetics, and vasoactive drugs (Rogers & Valley, 1994). In children, analgesic and antiinflammatory medications, local injections, and regional blockades are reported to be unhelpful (Stanton et al., 1993). Phentolamine, an α-adrenergic receptor inhibitor, may temporarily alleviate pain, suggesting the likelihood of a positive response to longer-lasting sympathetic blockade techniques (Kozin, 1994). Transdermal clonidine may produce analgesia in the area around the application site, and sustained analgesia (sometimes complicated by sedation and hypotension) has been experimentally achieved by intraspinal and epidural clonidine infusion (Rauck, Eisenach, Jackson, Young, & Southern, 1993). Electromotive administration of guanethidine into affected areas of skin achieved short-term resolution of superficial symptoms of hyperalgesia, pain, pallor, coolness, and sweating in six out of eight patients (Bonezzi, Miotti, Bettaglio, & Stephen, 1994). Intravenous regional guanethidine (Geertzen, de Bruijn, de Bruijn-Kofman, & Arendzen, 1994) and bretyllium blocks (Dzwierzynski & Sanger, 1994) have been effective in patients who fail to respond to sympathetic ganglion blockade, as have dimethyl sulfoxide (Geertzen et al.) and calcitonin (Arriagada & Arinoviche, 1994).

Local anesthetic sympathetic blockade at the stellate ganglion or lumbar sympathetic chain (see Chapter 14) is often used as a therapeutic trial before attempting chemical neurolytic blockade. Long-acting ganglion blocks with a continuous catheter infusion (Dzwierzynski & Sanger, 1994), neurolytic blockade, and surgical sympathectomy are commonly offered to patients who show a limited, short-term response to local anesthetic blockade. Doppler ultrasound is useful for documenting the technical success of sympathetic blockade and for detecting failed sympathetic blockade in patients with RSD who have clinical relapse (Tu, Mailis, &

Simons, 1994). Unfortunately, sympathetic blockade or sympathectomy is not a panacea in RSD, because central nervous system plasticity prevents significant numbers of patients from achieving permanent or long-lasting relief (Veldman et al., 1993). Therefore it seems evident that consistently successful treatment of RSD will be achieved only with a comprehensive plan of care that addresses the central component of sympathetically maintained pain and the effects of sympathetic activity and mediators of inflammation on nociceptors, as well as with the provision of maximal rehabilitative and psychologic support.

Phantom Pain

Phantom pain can be thought of as a subset in the broad category of neuropathic pain. Phantom pain is defined as a painful sensation perceived in a missing body part, such as after an amputation, or in the paralyzed part of spinal cord injury or nerve root avulsion (Davis, 1993a). Phantom pain is different from stump pain, which arises in the residual body part and can be caused by multiple potential etiologies including improper prosthesis fitting, neuroma formation, arthritis, and ischemia. Phantom pain should also be distinguished from phantom sensations, which are ubiquitous after loss of a body part and which are defined as persisting sensory experiences in the absence of apparent afferent input (Stannard, 1993). Phantom sensation may assume many forms other than pain, including touch, pressure, cold, wetness, itching, tickling, fatigue, or a graphic feeling that the missing body part is still present. Other than the extremities, body parts with rich innervation, such as the teeth, tongue, breast, rectum, bladder, and genitalia, may be experienced as functionally active phantoms after surgical removal, sometimes leading in the case of the last three to attempts to defecate, urinate, or ejaculate (Davis). Phantom phenomena are often unreported to medical caregivers, which leads to the conclusion that they are generally benign (Stannard). Patients' reluctance to report unpleasant phantom phenomena as well as overt phantom pain may stem from fear that they will be either disbelieved or regarded as mentally ill (Davis, 1993a). Because pain is properly defined as any unpleasant sensory experience associated with real or potential tissue injury, a broader definition of phantom pain would include all phantom sensations that are perceived by the patient as troublesome. It should be emphasized that there is no etiologic psychologic basis for phantom pain nor any evidence that patients experiencing chronic phantom pain are psychologically abnormal or have abnormal personalities (Davis).

The incidence of phantom pain has often been underestimated. Recent studies suggest that the true incidence after extremity amputation ranges from 60% to 85% and that chronic, persistent pain is observed in 5% to 10% of amputees more than 2 years after amputation (Davis, 1993a; Stannard, 1993). Phantom pain is equally present in both traumatic and vascular amputees and appears to be related to the amount of preoperative pain (Houghton, Nicholls, Houghton, Saadeh, & McColl, 1994). Phantom pain occurs in adolescents and even in young children (Weinstein, 1994), but little research has been done regarding the incidence, prevalence, and nature of phantom pain and sensation in the pediatric population (McGrath & Hiller, 1992).

Phantom pain usually presents within the first week after amputation but may have its first appearance months or even years after amputation. Pain persisting longer than 6 months often becomes intractable. Pain may gradually decrease over time in some patients, but in others pain intensity may actually increase as time goes by. Even in the same patient, the pain often fluctuates in intensity, duration, and character. Pain may be variably described as aching, burning, dull, knifelike, sticking, squeezing, constricting, or electric. Pain is often exacerbated by emotional stress, exposure to cold, or local irritants. On the other hand, pain may sometimes be ameliorated by using a prosthesis, stroking the stump, applying heat, or employing a distraction

(Davis, 1993a). Unusual features of phantom pain are particularly challenging and require even more thorough evaluation. For example, pain perceived in a missing part may sometimes be referred pain and indicate the presence of significant coexistent disease such as angina pectoris (Martin, Margherita, & Amsterdam, 1994).

Phantom limb pain is notoriously difficult to treat. Prior to 1980, at least 68 different treatment methods had been reported, none of which was even moderately successful (Sherman, Sherman, & Gall, 1980). However, there have been some significant advances (Davis, 1993a) within the last decade. Treatment approaches have included medications, neurostimulation, ablation of peripheral and central nervous system structures, physical therapy, and psychologic and behavioral methods (Weinstein, 1994).

The provision of adequate analgesia and the establishment of a pain-free interval prior to amputation have been shown to reduce the incidence of phantom limb pain (Stannard, 1993). Additionally, through preoperative teaching, nurses can help prospective amputees through the grieving process associated with a change in body image and lay the groundwork for successful rehabilitation (Rounseville, 1992). Postoperatively, a holistic, multidisciplinary approach to rehabilitation incorporating the combined and coordinated use of medical, social, educational, and vocational measures results in higher functional levels, better management of pain, and more personal satisfaction in living for the individual who has undergone an amputation (Davis, 1993a).

A wide variety of pharmacologic interventions have been tried over the years with varying and unpredictable degrees of success. Oral and parenteral opioids and NSAIDs are minimally effective in the treatment of phantom limb pain. Opioid resistance may be related to nerve injury–induced loss of spinal opioid receptors and elaboration of dynorphins with antagonistic effects (Stannard, 1993). Intrathecal fentanyl was reported to reduce phantom limb pain in a few patients (Weinstein, 1994). Tricyclic antidepressants appear to decrease phantom pain in some patients. Amitriptyline may be effective in pediatric patients (Weinstein, 1994). A complete recovery from phantom limb pain of 5 years duration was observed in a 71-year-old man treated with the serotonin reuptake inhibitor fluoxetine (Power-Smith & Turkington, 1993). In a series of 31 patients with phantom pain, 18 patients had a good to excellent response to mexilitine alone, and 11 other patients responded to a combination of mexilitine and clonidine. Some patients could not tolerate mexilitine because of persistent nausea (Davis, 1993b). Salmon calcitonin also appears to be a valuable agent for the treatment of phantom pain in the early postoperative period, with approximately half the patients also having good to excellent long-term relief (Jaeger & Maier, 1992). Three patients with phantom limb pain were successfully treated with the NMDA receptor antagonist ketamine, an analgesic and anesthetic agent commonly used for surgical anesthesia (Stannard & Porter, 1993). Unfortunately, ketamine, which is chemically related to LSD, may cause significant psychomimetic side effects. Other medications with reported efficacy include carbamazepine, sodium valproate, and topical application of capsaicin (Weinstein).

Multiple surgical ablative approaches to the treatment of phantom pain including sympathectomy, cordotomy, gyrotomy, frontal leukotomy, stereotactic thalamotomy, and peripheral surgery for excision of neuromas have generally offered little relief. Dorsal root entry-zone lesions have been only marginally more successful (Davis, 1993a). Postoperative regional anesthesia by nerve sheath block prevented development of phantom pain in one series of 11 patients (Weinstein, 1994).

Physical stimulation of the stump by thermal, mechanical, or electrical means provides relief to some patients. The simplest and most frequently used of these techniques is transcutaneous electrical nerve stimulation (TENS), which is beneficial for some patients, whereas others experience no better than a placebo effect (Stannard, 1993). Auricular TENS has been associated with a modest decrease in phantom pain and unpleasant phantom sensations (Katz & Melzack,

1991). More complex techniques such as dorsal column stimulation and deep brain stimulation may be of value in selected patients (Stannard). Other physical modalities such as acupuncture and ultrasound may sometimes offer temporary relief.

Psychologic interventions including hypnosis, biofeedback, cognitive therapies, behavioral therapies, and support groups are often helpful adjunctive measures that facilitate adaptation to a change in body image and promote positive adaptive mechanisms for dealing with the anger and grief associated with loss of a body part (Davis, 1993a). It seems clear that, in the absence of a single, universally effective therapeutic technique, a multimodal and multidisciplinary approach to the patient with phantom pain is the most likely to accomplish effective pain relief and to promote successful functional rehabilitation and emotional, social, and spiritual well-being.

SUMMARY

The topics covered in this chapter are minimally related except in the difficult clinical challenges they present to the health care team committed to management of pain as reported, perceived, and experienced by each individual patient. The following clinical practice guidelines (Jacox et al., 1994) are applicable to all of the clinical problems discussed in this chapter:

1. Promise patients attentive care directed at achieving patient and family satisfaction with pain management and its impact on their quality of life.
2. Incorporate interdisciplinary collaboration and recognition of the diverse and complementary skills and contributions of each health care professional into the formal plan of care. Designate one person to be responsible for pain management and assign responsibilities to clinicians who are knowledgeable, experienced, interested, and able to respond to patients' needs in a timely fashion.

3. Define the roles of physicians, nurses, pharmacists, and psychosocial specialists and provide for professional accountability.
4. Document the assessment of pain and its relief.
5. Monitor the efficacy of pain treatment. Define pain and relief levels to trigger a review and modification of the current regimen.
6. Use oral analgesics (opioids and nonopioid adjuvant medications) and other noninvasive routes of administration whenever possible and administer them in accordance with the principles expressed in the WHO analgesic ladder.
7. Titrate analgesics to maximally effective doses or the appearance of dose-limiting side effects before using specialized invasive analgesic approaches (intraspinal opioids, systemic or intraspinal PCA, continuous opioid infusion, local anesthetic infusion, conscious or deep sedation).
8. Monitor use of specialized analgesic technologies.
9. Offer nonpharmacologic interventions (physical modalities and cognitive- and behavior-based interventions) as supplements to pharmacologic interventions.

Patients should be informed that effective pain management is an important part of their treatment, that their complaints of pain will be believed, and that health care professionals involved in their care will utilize all the resources available to manage their pain effectively.

References

Aaen, V., Cowan, L., Sakala, E. P., & Small, M. L. (1993). Prolonged parenteral meperidine analgesia during pregnancy for pain from an abdominal wall mesh graft. *Obstetrics and Gynecology, 82,* 721-722.

American Psychiatric Association. (1994). *Diagnostics and statistical manual of mental disorders* (4th ed.). Washington, DC: American Psychiatric Association.

Anand, A., Carmosino, L., & Glatt, A. E. (1994). Evaluation of recalcitrant pain in HIV-infected hospitalized patients. *Journal of Acquired Immune Deficiency Syndromes, 7,* 52-56.

Arriagada, M., & Arinoviche, R. (1994). X-ray bone densitometry in the diagnosis and followup of reflex sympathetic dystrophy syndrome. *Journal of Rheumatology, 21,* 498-500.

Blum, R. H., Kleinman Simpson, P., & Blum, D. S. (1990). Factors limiting the use of indicated opioid analgesics for cancer pain. *American Journal of Hospice and Palliative Care, 7,* 31-35.

Bonezzi, C., Miotti, D., Bettaglio, R., & Stephen, R. (1994). Electromotive administration of guanethidine for treatment of reflex sympathetic dystrophy: A pilot study in eight patients. *Journal of Pain Symptom Management, 9,* 39-43.

Brookoff, D., & Polomano, R. (1992). Treating sickle cell pain like cancer pain. *Annals of Internal Medicine, 116,* 364-368.

Brownridge, P. (1991). Treatment options for the relief of pain during childbirth. *Drugs, 41,* 69-80.

Bruera, E., MacEachern, T., Ripamonti, C., & Hanson, J. (1993). Subcutaneous morphine for dyspnea in cancer patients. *Annals of Internal Medicine, 119,* 906-907.

Cleeland, C. S., Gonin, R., Hatfield, A. K., Edmonson, J. H., Blum, R. H., Stewart, J. A., & Pandya, K. J. (1994). Pain and its treatment in outpatients with metastatic cancer. *New England Journal of Medicine, 330,* 592-596.

Collins, M. K., Porter, K. B., Brook, E., Johnson, L., Williams, M., & Jevitt, C. M., (1994). Vulvar application of lidocaine for pain relief in spontaneous vaginal delivery. *Obstetrics and Gynecology, 84,* 335-337.

Cross, S. A. (1994). Pathophysiology of pain. *Mayo Clinic Proceedings, 69,* 375-383.

Daly, J. M., Frame, P. S., & Rapoza, P. A. (1991). Sacroiliac subluxation: A common, treatable cause of low-back pain in pregnancy. *Family Practice Research Journal, 11,* 149-159.

Danziger, L. H., Martin, S. J., & Blum, R. A. (1994). Central nervous system toxicity associated with meperidine use in hepatic disease. *Pharmacotherapy, 14,* 235-238.

Davis, R. W. (1993a). Phantom sensation, phantom pain, and stump pain. *Archives of Physical Medicine and Rehabilitation, 74,* 79-91.

Davis, R. W. (1993b). Successful treatment for phantom pain. *Orthopedics, 16,* 691-695.

DeGood, D. E., Cundiff, G. W., Adams, L. E., & Shutty, M. S., Jr. (1993). A psychosocial and behavioral comparison of reflex sympathetic dystrophy, low back pain, and headache patients. *Pain, 54,* 317-322.

Deuschl, G., Blumberg, H., & Lucking, C. H. (1991). Tremor in reflex sympathetic dystrophy. *Archives of Neurology, 48,* 1247-1252.

Dildy, G. A., Moise, K. J., Jr., Smith, L. G., Kirshon, B., & Carpenter, R. J. (1992). Indomethacin for the treatment of symptomatic leiomyoma uteri during pregnancy. *American Journal of Perinatology, 9,* 185-189.

Drossman, D. A. (1994). Physical and sexual abuse and gastrointestinal illness: What is the link? *American Journal of Medicine, 97,* 105-107.

Dzwierzynski, W. W., & Sanger, J. R. (1994). Reflex sympathetic dystrophy. *Hand Clinics, 10,* 29-44.

Enck, R. E. (1991). Understanding tolerance, physical dependence and addiction in the use of opioid analgesics. *American Journal of Hospice and Palliative Care, 8,* 9-11.

Enck, R. E. (1994). *The medical care of terminally ill patients.* Baltimore: Johns Hopkins University Press.

Epstein, F. B. (1994). Acute abdominal pain in pregnancy. *Emergency Medicine Clinics of North America, 12,* 151-165.

Falasca, G. F., Toly, T. M., Reginato, A. J., Schraeder, P. L., & O'Connor, C. R. (1994). Reflex sympathetic dystrophy associated with antiepileptic drugs. *Epilepsia, 35,* 394-399.

Faure, E. A. M. (1991). The pain of parturition. *Seminars in Perinatology, 15,* 342-347.

Feinberg, B. B., & Soper, D. E. (1992). Miliary tuberculosis: Unusual cause of abdominal pain in pregnancy. *Southern Medical Journal, 85,* 184-186.

Friedman, D. P. (1990). Perspectives on the medical use of drugs of abuse. *Journal of Pain and Symptom Management, 5,* S2-S5.

Geertzen, J. H., de Bruijn, H., de Bruijn-Kofman, A. T., & Arendzen, J. H. (1994). Reflex sympathetic dystrophy: Early treatment and psychological aspects. *Archives of Physical Medicine and Rehabilitation, 75,* 442-446.

Glare, P. A., & Walsh, T. D. (1991). Clinical pharmacokinetics of morphine. *Therapeutic Drug Monitoring, 13,* 1-23.

Gonzalez, G. R., & Coyle, N. (1992). Treatment of cancer pain in a former opioid abuser: Fears of the patient and staff and their influence on care. *Journal of Pain and Symptom Management, 7,* 246-249.

Gran, J. T., & Husby, G. (1992). Ankylosing spondylitis: Current drug treatment. *Drugs, 44,* 585-603.

Green, J. M. (1993). Expectations and experiences of pain in labor: Findings from a large prospective study. *Birth, 20,* 65-72.

Gusberg, S. B., & Runowicz, C. D. (1991). Gynecologic cancers. In A. I. Holleb, D. J. Fink, & G. P. Murphy (Eds.), *American Cancer Society textbook of clinical oncology* (pp. 481-497). Atlanta: American Cancer Society.

Hammack, J. E., & Loprinzi, C. L. (1994). Use of orally administered opioids for cancer-related pain. *Mayo Clinic Proceedings, 69,* 384-390.

Hapidou, E. G., & DeCatanzaro, D. (1992). Responsiveness to laboratory pain in women as a function of age and childbirth pain experience. *Pain, 48,* 177-181.

Harrison, L. M., Zadina, J. E., Banks, W. A., & Kastin, A. J. (1993). Effects of neonatal treatment with Tyr-MIF-1, morphiceptin, and morphine on development, tail flick, and blood-brain barrier transport. *Brain Research: Developmental Brain Research, 75,* 207-212.

Havens, J. F., Whitaker, A. H., Feldman, J. F., & Ehrhardt, A. A. (1994). Psychiatric morbidity in school-age children with congenital human immunodeficiency virus infection: A pilot study. *Journal of Developmental and Behavioral Pediatrics, 15,* S18-S25.

Herpolsheimer, A., & Schretenthaler, J. (1994). The use of intrapartum intrathecal narcotic analgesia in a community-based hospital. *Obstetrics and Gynecology, 84,* 931-936.

Houghton, A. D., Nicholls, G., Houghton, A. L., Saadeh, E., & McColl, L. (1994). Phantom pain: Natural history and association with rehabilitation. *Annals of the Royal College of Surgeons of England, 76,* 22-25.

Hutchings, D. E., Zmitrovich, A., Church, S., & Malowany, D. (1993). Methadone during pregnancy: The search for a valid animal model. *Annali dell Istituto Superiore de Sanita, 29,* 439-444.

Inturrisi, C. E., & Hanks, G. (1993). Opioid analgesic therapy. In D. Derek, G. W. C. Hanks, & N. Macdonald (Eds.), *Oxford textbook of palliative medicine* (pp. 166-182). New York: Oxford University Press.

Jackson, D. A. (1993). Reflex sympathetic dystrophy syndrome: Two case studies. *Journal of Post Anesthesia Nursing, 8,* 327-331.

Jacox, A., Carr, D. B., Payne, R., Berde, C. B., Breitbart, W., Cain, J. M., Chapman, C. R., Cleeland, C. S., Ferrell, B. R., Finley, R. S., Hester, N. O., Hill, C. S., Leak, W. D., Lipman, A. G., Logan, C. L., McGarvey, C. L., Miaskowski, C. A., Mulder, D. S., Paice, J. A., Shapiro, B. S., Silberstein, E. B., Smith, R. S., Stover, J., Tsou, C. V., Vecchiarelli, L., & Weissman, D. E. (1994). *Management of cancer pain. Clinical practice guideline.* AHCPR Pub. No. 94-0592. Rockville, MD: Agency for Health Care Policy and Research, PHS, USDHHS.

Jaeger, H., & Maier, C. (1992). Calcitonin in phantom limb pain: A double-blind study. *Pain, 48,* 21-27.

Johansen, G. A. (1990). Should opioids or sedatives be used for dyspnea in end-stage disease? *American Journal of Hospice and Palliative Care, 7,* 12-13.

Kanner, R. M., & Foley, K. M. (1981). Patterns of narcotic drug use in a cancer pain clinic. *Annals of the New York Academy of Science, 362,* 161-172.

Katz, J., & Melzack, R. (1991). Auricular transcutaneous nerve stimulations (TENS) reduces phantom limb pain. *Journal of Pain and Symptom Management, 6,* 73-83.

Kovacs, L., Herczeg, J., & Szabo, L. (1993). Premedication and pain relief with Nubain during second trimester therapeutic pregnancy terminations. *International Journal of Gynaecology and Obstetrics, 40,* 51-58.

Kozin, F. (1994). Reflex sympathetic dystrophy syndrome. *Current Opinions in Rheumatology, 6,* 210-216.

Lam, S. K., To, W. K., Duthie, S. J., & Ma, H. K. (1992). Narcotic addiction in pregnancy with adverse maternal and perinatal outcome. *Australia and New Zealand Journal of Obstetrics and Gynecology, 32,* 216-221.

Lander, J. (1990). Fallacies and phobias about addiction and pain. *British Journal of Addiction, 85,* 803-809.

Levy, M., & Spino, M. (1993). Neonatal withdrawal syndrome: Associated drugs and pharmacologic management. *Pharmacotherapy, 13,* 202-211.

Martin, W. R., Margherita, A., & Amsterdam, E. (1994). Phantom angina. *Chest, 105,* 1271-1272.

McGrady, E. M., Malinow, A. M., Paly, D. A., & Mokriski, B. K. (1993). Metastatic pain in the parturient: Treatment with patient-controlled epidural sufentanil. *Acta Anaesthesiologica Scandinavica, 37,* 594-596.

McGrath, P. A., Hiller, L. M. (1992). Phantom limb sensations in adolescents: A case study to illustrate the utility of sensation and pain logs in pediatric clinical practice. *Journal of Pain and Symptom Management, 7*, 46-53.

Mehta, M. (Ed.). (1995). *PDR guide to drug interactions, side effects, indications.* Montvale, NJ: Medical Economics Data Production Company.

Meny, R. G., Naumberg, E. G., Alger, L. S., Brill-Miller, J. L., & Brown, S. (1993). Codeine and the breast-fed neonate. *Journal of Human Lactation, 9*, 237-240.

Morgan, J. P. (1986). *American opiophobia: Customary underutilization of opioid analgesia.* New York: Hawthorne, pp. 163-173.

Noia, G., de Santis, M., Fundaro, C., Mastromarino, C., Trivellini, C., Rosati, P., Caruso, A., Segni, G,. & Mancuso, S. (1994). Drug addiction in pregnancy: 13 years of experience. *Fetal Diagnosis and Therapy, 9*, 116-124.

Nyberg, K., Allebeck, P., Eklund, G., & Jacobson, B. (1992). Socioeconomic versus obstetric risk factors for drug addiction in offspring. *British Journal of Addiction, 87*, 1669-1676.

Orvieto, R., Achiron, A., Ben-Rafael, Z., Gelernter, I., & Achiron, R. (1994). Low-back pain of pregnancy. *Acta Obstetricia et Gynecologica Scandinavica, 73*, 209-214.

Ostgaard, H. C., Andersson, G. B., & Wennergren, M. (1991). The impact of low back and pelvic pain in pregnancy on the pregnancy outcome. *Acta Obstetricia Gynecologica Scandinavica, 70*, 21-24.

Ostgaard, H. C., Zetherstrom, G., Roos-Hansson, E., & Svanberg, B. (1994). Reduction of back and posterior pelvic pain in pregnancy. *Spine, 19*, 894-900.

Ostrov, B. E., Eichenfield, A. H., Goldsmith, D. P., & Schumacher, H. R. (1993). Recurrent reflex sympathetic dystrophy as a manifestation of systemic lupus erythematosus. *Journal of Rheumatology, 20*, 1774-1776.

Oyen, W. J., Arntz, I. E., Claessens, R. M., Van der Meer, J. W., Corstens, F. H. M., & Goris, R. J. A. (1993). Reflex sympathetic dystrophy of the hand: An excessive inflammatory response? *Pain, 55*, 151-157.

Paech, M. J. (1991). The King Edward Memorial Hospital 1,000 mother survey of methods of pain relief in labour. *Anaesthesiology and Intensive Care, 19*, 393-399.

Payne, R., & Gonzales, G. (1993). Pathophysiology of pain in cancer and other terminal diseases. In D. Derek, G. W. C. Hanks, & N. Macdonald (Eds.), *Oxford textbook of palliative medicine* (pp. 140-148). New York: Oxford University Press.

Portenoy, R. K. (1990). Chronic opioid therapy in nonmalignant pain. *Journal of Pain and Symptom Management, 5,* S46-S62.

Portenoy, R. K. (1993). Pathophysiology of cancer pain. *Advances in Oncology, 9,* 15-19.

Porter, J., & Jick, H. (1980). Addiction rare in inpatients treated with narcotics. *New England Journal of Medicine, 302,* 123.

Power-Smith, P., & Turkington, D. (1993). Fluoxetine in phantom limb pain. *British Journal of Psychiatry, 163,* 105-106.

Quill, T. E. (1993). Doctor, I want to die. Will you help me? *Journal of the American Medical Association, 270,* 874-875.

Rajan, L. (1993). Perceptions of pain and pain relief in labour: The gulf between experience and observation, *Midwifery, 9,* 136-145.

Rauck, R. L., Eisenach, J. C., Jackson, K., Young, L. D., & Southern, J. (1993). Epidural clonidine treatment for refractory reflex sympathetic dystrophy. *Anesthesiology, 79,* 1163-1169.

Rawlins, M. D. (1993). Non-opioid analgesics. In D. Derek, G. W. C. Hanks, & N. Macdonald (Eds.), *Oxford textbook of palliative medicine* (pp. 182-187). New York: Oxford University Press.

Rogers, J. N., Valley, M. A. (1994). Reflex sympathetic dystrophy. *Clinics of Podiatric Medicine and Surgery, 11,* 73-83.

Rosenblatt, W. H., Cioffi, A. M., Sinatra, R., & Silverman, D. C. (1992). Metoclopramide-enhanced analgesia for prostaglandin-induced termination of pregnancy. *Anesthesia and Analgesia, 75,* 760-763.

Rounseville, C. (1992). Phantom limb pain: The ghost that haunts the amputee. *Orthopedic Nursing, 11,* 67-71.

Roy, S., & Basu, R. K. (1992). Role of sublingual administration of tablet buprenorphine hydrochloride on relief of labour pain. *Journal of the Indian Medical Association, 90,* 151-153.

Saddison, D. K., & Vanek, V. W. (1993). Reflex sympathetic dystrophy after modified radical mastectomy: A case report. *Surgery, 114,* 116-120.

Savage, S. R. (1993). Addiction in the treatment of pain: Significance, recognition, and management. *Journal of Pain and Symptom Management, 8,* 265-278.

Schwartzman, R. J. (1993). Reflex sympathetic dystrophy. *Current Opinions in Neurology and Neurosurgery, 5,* 531-536.

Sees, K. L., & Clark, H. W. (1993). Opioid use in the treatment of chronic pain: Assessment of addiction. *Journal of Pain and Symptom Management, 8,* 257-264.

Sherman, R. A., Sherman, C. J., & Gall, N. G. (1980). A survey of current phantom limb pain treatment in the United States. *Pain, 8,* 85-99.

Simmons, W. D., & Johnson, C. A. (1991). Dialysis of drugs. *Pharmacy Practice News, 18,* 15-17.

Skovlund, E., Fyllingen, G., Landre, H., & Nesheim, B. I. (1991). Comparison of postpartum pain treatments using a sequential trial design: II. Naproxen versus paracetamol. *European Journal of Clinical Pharmacology, 40,* 539-542.

Stamatoullas, A., Ferrant, A., & Manicourt, D. (1993). Reflex sympathetic dystrophy after bone marrow transplantation. *Annals of Hematology, 67,* 245-247.

Stannard, C. F. (1993). Phantom limb pain. *British Journal of Hospital Medicine, 50,* 583-587.

Stannard, C. F., & Porter, G. E. (1993). Ketamine hydrochloride in the treatment of phantom limb pain. *Pain, 54,* 227-230.

Stanton, R. P., Malcolm, J. R., Wesdock, K. A., & Singsen, B. H. (1993). Reflex sympathetic dystrophy in children: An orthopedic perspective. *Orthopedics, 16,* 773-779.

Tu, E. S., Mailis, A., & Simons, M. E. (1994). Effect of surgical sympathectomy on arterial blood flow in reflex sympathetic dystrophy: Doppler US assessment. *Radiology, 191,* 833-834.

Twycross, R. G. (1993). Advances in cancer pain management. *Journal of Pharmacologic Care and Pain and Symptom Control, 1,* 5-29.

USP DI (1993). *Drug information for the health care professional: Vol. II. Advice for the patient* (13th ed.). Rockville, MD: United States Pharmacopeial Convention.

Van Houdenhove, B., & Vasquez, G. (1993). Is there a relationship between reflex sympathetic dystrophy and helplessness? Case reports and a hypothesis. *General Hospital Psychiatry, 15,* 325-329.

Veldman, P. H., Reynen, H. M., Arntz, I. E., & Goris, J. A. (1993). Signs and symptoms of reflex sympathetic dystrophy: Prospective study of 829 patients. *Lancet, 342,* 1012-1016.

Veldman, P. H., & Jacobs, P. B. (1994). Reflex sympathetic dystrophy of the head: Case report and discussion of diagnostic criteria. *Journal of Trauma, 36,* 119-121.

Ventafridda, V., Ripamonti, C., DeConno, F., Tamburini, M., & Cassileth, B. R. (1990). Symptom prevalence and control during cancer patients' last days of life. *Journal of Palliative Care, 6,* 7-11.

Viegas, O. A., Khaw, B., & Ratnam, S. S. (1993). Tramadol in labour pain in primiparous patients: A prospective comparative clinical trial. *European Journal of Obstetrics, Gynecology, and Reproductive Biology, 49,* 131-135.

Von Roenn, J. H., Cleeland, C. S., Gonin, R., Hatfield, A. K., & Pandya, K. J. (1993). Physician attitudes and practice in cancer pain management: A survey from the Eastern Cooperative Oncology Group. *Annals of Internal Medicine, 119,* 121-126.

Walker, J. J., Johnston, J., Fairlie, F. M., Lloyd, J., & Bullingham, R. (1992). A comparative study of intramuscular ketorolac and pethidine in labour pain. *European Journal of Obstetrics, Gynecology, and Reproductive Biology, 46,* 87-94.

Weinstein, S. M. (1994). Phantom pain. *Oncology, 8,* 65-70.

Weissman, D. E., & Haddox, J. D. (1989). Opioid pseudoaddiction—An iatrogenic syndrome. *Pain, 36,* 363-366.

Wells, N. (1991). Pain and distress during abortion. *Health Care Women International, 12,* 292-302.

Wesson, D. R., Ling, W., & Smith, D. E. (1993). Prescription of opioids for treatment of pain in patients with addictive disease. *Journal of Pain and Symptom Management, 8,* 289-296.

Whitcomb, D. C., & Block, G. D. (1994). Association of acetaminophen hepatotoxicity with fasting and ethanol use. *Journal of the American Medical Association, 272,* 1866-1867.

Woodcock, A. A., Gross, E. R., Gellert, A., Shah, S., Johnson, M., & Geddes, D. M. (1981). Effects of dihydrocodeine, alcohol, and caffeine on breathlessness and exercise tolerance in patients with chronic obstructive lung disease and normal blood gases. *New England Journal of Medicine, 305,* 1611-1616.

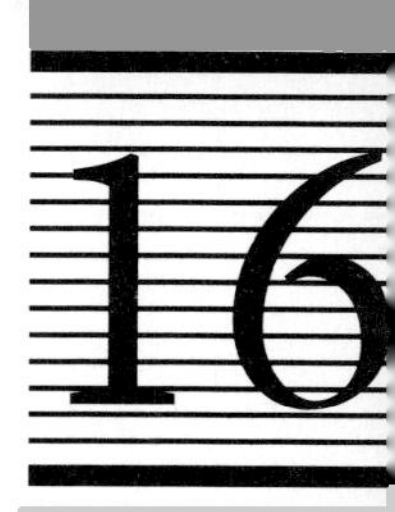

Symptom Management

Patricia M. Collins

Avery Spunt

Marianne B. Huml

Key Points

- Many of the side effects attributed to opioids are due to other drugs and treatments or to undiagnosed pathology within the patient.
- The nurse should collaborate with the physician, pharmacist, social worker, dietitian, and other health care team members, when appropriate, to provide the best possible care to patients experiencing the side effects of analgesics.
- Constipation should be treated prophylactically at the start of opioid therapy.
- The nurse often provides nursing care to patients over an extended period of time and is thus in a position to assess the side effects of pain management.
- The nurse prevents, monitors, and treats side effects due to analgesics but has an equally important role as patient and family educator and advocate. Nurses must encourage patients and families to report these side effects and to request relief for them.

This chapter is a review of the major side effects and adverse effects associated with the pharmacologic agents used for managing pain. Strategies for anticipating and treating these unwanted outcomes of therapy are outlined, with special attention given to patient and family education. If not managed, these symptoms can become a barrier to achieving adequate pain control because patients may choose to suffer pain rather than experience the side effects from the pain medication. The nurse must reassure patients and families that the side effects from analgesics can be relieved and often prevented.

Whether caring for the patient in the hospital, clinic, or home setting, the nurse is in an ideal position to prevent, diagnose, and treat the symptoms patients experience when taking analgesics. The nurse cares for patients over an extended period of time and is thus in a position to assess the side effects of pain management (Coyle, 1989). For the nurse to help patients manage these symptoms, a collaborative, interdisciplinary team approach, with the patient and family as key members of the team, is necessary. (See Chapter 6 for an in-depth discussion of the team concept.) To perform a thorough and accurate assessment, the nurse must possess excellent communication skills so that both verbal and nonverbal messages are interpreted correctly. Thorough knowledge of the pharmacokinetics and pharmacodynamics of analgesics and related drugs assists the nurse in knowing what to expect at any point in the treatment. The intended effects and the expected side effects can then be explained to the patient and family to facilitate symptom management. Many recommendations for symptom management are derived from anecdotal reports and the clinical consensus of pain management experts rather than from well-defined guidelines based on research.

MAJOR SIDE EFFECTS OF OPIOID ANALGESICS

Most side effects and adverse effects of opioid analgesics occur as an extension of their pharmacologic action on the opioid receptors located in the gastrointestinal (GI) tract and the central nervous system (CNS).

The degree to which these symptoms affect an individual depend on the following factors: age, concurrent medical conditions, acuity of present illness, previous exposure to analgesics, and drug-related factors. For example, a normal, healthy, older adult may experience a longer duration of pain relief from opioids and may accordingly be more sensitive to sedation and respiratory depression than a younger person because of the altered distribution, metabolism, and excretion rate of drugs that are associatied with aging (Ferrell &

Ferrell, 1992; Thomas, 1991). Older patients are more likely to have concurrent medical conditions—such as prostatic hypertrophy or renal, cardiac, hepatic, or pulmonary disease—that increase their risk for side effects. The accumulation of biologically active metabolites such as norproxyphene from propoxyphene or normeperidine from meperidine can cause neurologic changes such as confusion, agitation, and seizures in patients with impaired renal function (Portenoy, Thaler, Inturrisi, Klar, & Foley, 1992; USP DI, 1995). Opioids must be used with caution in patients with bronchial asthma and increased intracranial pressure (American Pain Society, 1993).

An example of an individual with previous drug exposure is a patient with cancer-related pain who has been taking oxycodone or acetaminophen tablets for months and now requires morphine. This individual would be at a lower risk for sedation and respiratory depression than the opioid-naive individual.

Drug-related factors that influence the occurrence and severity of side effects and adverse effects include the selected analgesic, dose, route and rate of administration, and dosing interval. Drugs vary greatly in the symptoms they induce, which have been well documented. For example, codeine causes more nausea than other drugs in its class (Schechter & Weisman, 1993). Intravenous fentanyl causes less pruritus than morphine (Schechter & Weisman). Methadone and levorphanol have a longer plasma half-life than hydromorphone; therefore drug accumulation with subsequent toxicity is more likely to occur with methadone or levorphanol than with hydromorphone (Hill, 1993).

The following situation is an example of how drug dose could affect the severity of a drug response: A patient with spinal cord compression due to metastatic cancer is receiving steroids, morphine, and radiation therapy. Within a week, the steroids and radiation therapy have significantly reduced the source of the pain. Because the patient is still on the same dose of morphine, he may experience increased sedation and respiratory depression. The sedative effects of the opioid are no longer opposed by the stimulating effects of the pain (Twycross, 1988). Thus, without proper adjustment of the dose, patients are more likely to encounter unpleasant and adverse effects associated with the very drugs that initially relieved their pain.

Similarly, route of administration can alter a drug's potential side effects. For instance, patients have more urinary retention and pruritus with the intraspinal administration of some opioids than with the other routes of administration (Waldman, Leak, Kennedy, & Patt, 1993). Yet compared with oral administration of opioids, intraspinal administration usually results in less sedation and constipation (American Pain Society, 1993).

Another factor affecting the patient's degree of sedation is the interval of drug administration. For example, reducing the dose of an opioid and administering it more frequently may decrease sedation (Ellison, 1993).

Many side effects attributed to opioids are actually due to other drugs and treatments or to undiagnosed pathology within the patient (McCaffery & Beebe, 1989). The nurse can play an important role in determining the etiology of a symptom that persists or is not consistent with the usual characteristics of opioid-induced side effects.

The nurse should collaborate with the physician, pharmacist, social worker, dietitian, and other health care team members, when appropriate, to provide the best possible care to patients experiencing the side effects of analgesics. The side effects to be discussed are sedation, respiratory depression, nausea and vomiting, constipation, and other potential adverse effects. Following the review of each side effect is a discussion on methods of assessment and interventions.

Sedation

Sedation is a "state of being calmed" (Thomas, 1993), and although many patients try to reach this state, others prefer to be more alert. Sedation and its lesser form, drowsiness, are common when opioids are initiated or when the dose is increased. These effects are usually resolved within a few days

(Ellison, 1993). During this period, previously sleep-deprived patients may sleep soundly for long periods because they are finally comfortable (Hill, 1993).

Assessment

Besides receiving subjective reports from their patients, nurses must be able to accurately assess the patient's respiratory rate, rhythm, and depth. The normal respiratory rate for an alert individual is 12 to 20 regular, unlabored breaths per minute, decreasing to 8 to 12 during sleep. Other signs the nurse must look for include level of consciousness, behavior, and cognitive functioning. It is important to ascertain patients' responsiveness to external stimuli and their degree of orientation. The presence of drowsiness is cause for concern, and the depth of sedation needs to be determined, reported, and evaluated as a possible signal that respiratory depression may follow. The box below shows suggested behaviors for different classifications of sedation that should be used consistently by all nurses to communicate patients' mental status.

The nurse should also have information about the patient's general medical condition and medication history. For example, is this a nontolerant patient receiving the first dose of an opioid? Is this a patient with pulmonary or renal

DEGREES OF SEDATION

Normal sleep	Easily aroused
0	Awake and alert
1	Occasionally drowsy, catnaps, easily aroused
2	Frequently drowsy, falls asleep during conversations, easily aroused
3	Sleeping most of the time, arousable
4	Somnolent, minimal or no response to stimuli

Modified from Pasero, C. L., & McCaffery, M. (1994): Avoiding opioid-induced respiratory depression. *American Journal of Nursing, 94* (4),25–30.

problems? Such vital information enables the nurse to make an accurate assessment of the patient's condition.

Interventions

When sedation and drowsiness are threatening to the patient's condition, intravenous naloxone should be titrated to an accepted level of consciousness and analgesia. For patients who merely find sedation a disturbing side effect, clinicians offer the following suggestions: decrease the dose; halve the unit dose and administer it twice as often; decrease the dose and add a nonopioid analgesic; change to a different analgesic; try caffeinated beverages or caffeine tablets; add an amphetamine (which also may enhance pain relief and improve mood); and encourage stimulating activities such as board games, outings, or exercises (Collins, 1994; Ellison, 1993; Hill, 1993; Jacox et al., 1994; McCaffery & Beebe, 1989).

Patient and Family Education

Patients and families should be informed that the patient may experience sedation when starting on an opioid. The box on p. 533 lists information to review when educating patients and families about the sedative effects of opioids.

Respiratory Depression

Opioids cause respiratory depression by depressing the respiratory center in the brainstem (Paice, 1992). Respiratory depression is characterized by a decrease in the rate and depth of respirations and a decrease in arterial oxygen saturation. A Cheyne-Stokes pattern may be established, which is identified by a continued succession of periods of rapid, deep breathing; periods of shallow, slow breathing; and periods of apnea (Bates, 1991). Persons at greatest risk for respiratory depression are those who are opioid naive, those whose cause of pain is gone but who are still receiving the same dose of opioids (pain is an antagonist to respiratory depression), those who have compromised pulmonary status, and those

PATIENT AND FAMILY HOME TEACHING TIPS: SEDATION

- Advise patient and family that sedation, drowsiness, and difficulty concentrating may occur at the beginning of opioid therapy but will usually disappear after a few days.
- Ascertain patient's recent sleep history. Advise patient and family that if sleeplessness has been a problem, whether due to unrelieved pain or another problem, the patient may sleep a great deal for the first few days after opioids are initiated.
- Educate the patient and family regarding the differences between being sedated (sleepy) but arousable and being sedated and unarousable. The latter demands immediate medical attention and possibly CPR.
- Instruct family members on emergency measures to be taken if sedation causes respiratory depression—for example, calling 911, trying to arouse patent by shaking, coaching patient to breathe, ensuring an open airway.
- Suggest that if drowsiness is unacceptable to the patient, stimulants such as caffeinated beverages, caffeine tablets, or amphetamines may be helpful. These suggestions are recommended for short-term use only because they carry their own side effects.
- Advise patient and family that driving a car or operating machinery is prohibited as long as sedation, drowsiness, or difficulty concentrating persist.
- If the patient has a terminal condition and death is imminent, sedation may be acceptable or desirable. Frequency and depth of respirations will decrease naturally until respiration finally ceases. Provide information for the family on how to manage this situation before death occurs, and suggest hospice care if appropriate.

who receive an overdose of an opioid (Cherny & Portenoy, 1993; Lindley, Dalton, & Fields, 1990).

An example of a patient who is at risk for respiratory depression is an opioid-naive patient in severe pain requiring high doses of hydromorphone administered intravenously. After several doses, the patient finally achieves pain relief and falls asleep. The patient is now at the greatest risk for respiratory depression. Conversely, risk for respiratory depression is low in those chronic-pain patients who have been taking opioids for an extended period (Hill, 1993).

Assessment

When assessing a patient's potential for experiencing respiratory depression, the nurse must be informed about the patient's medical condition and past history. Patients with neuromuscular disorders or chronic obstructive pulmonary disease or who are extremely young (neonates; see Chapter 11) or old (geriatrics; see Chapter 12) should be considered high-risk and be given close monitoring. The respiratory rate and depth, the ease of respirations, and the level of sedation (see the box on p. 531) should be carefully monitored. Knowing the onset and peak times of the opioid in use is important and serves as a guide for when to assess the patient and for how long. Table 16-1 shows onset and peak times for several opioids. High-risk patients should have arterial oxygen saturation levels checked frequently. Pulse oximeters should be readily available on all nursing units for measuring arterial oxygen saturation levels when necessary.

Interventions

If a patient exhibits the characteristics of respiratory depression, the nurse should use verbal and physical stimulation to arouse breathing. If these actions are not effective, the nurse should administer naloxone according to institutional protocol. Hospitals and clinics should have standard protocols for administering naloxone on units where opioids are given routinely. The cancer pain clinical guidelines (Jacox et al., 1994) suggest diluting 0.4 mg of naloxone

Table 16-1 Peak and Onset of Selected Opioids

Drug	Onset (minutes)*	Peak (minutes)
Oral Administration		
Morphine (immediate-release)	30-60	60-120
Hydromorphone (Dilaudid)	30	90-120
Levorphanol (Levo-Dromoran)	10-60	90-120
Intramuscular Administration		
Morphine	15-30	30-60
Hydromorphone (Dilaudid)	15	30-60
Levorphanol (Levo-Dromoran)	N/A	60
Meperidine (Demerol)	10-15	30-50
Intravenous Administration		
Morphine		20
Hydromorphone (Dilaudid)	10-15	15-30
Levorphanol (Levo-Dromoran)	N/A	Within 20
Meperidine (Demerol)	1	5-7
Fentanyl	1-2	3-5

From USP DI (1995). *Drug information for the health care professional* (Vol. 1, 15th ed.). Rockville, MD: 1995, U.S. Pharmacopeial Convention.
**N/A*, Not available.

in 10 ml of saline and then administering 0.5-ml boluses every minute, titrated to the individual's respiratory response. (See Chapter 4 for additional naloxone information.) Individuals skilled in airway management and the use of resuscitation equipment and drugs should be available (Carr et al., 1992).

When death from a terminal disease is imminent, periods of respiratory depression may occur until respirations finally cease. In this instance, resuscitation is inappropriate.

Patient and Family Education

Nurses should educate patients at risk and their families about respiratory depression. Although respiratory depression is rare, when it does occur it is a frightening experience for patients and their loved ones. For those patients and families who have experienced this adverse effect, the nurse should provide support and reassurance.

Nausea and Vomiting

Nausea is an unpleasant sensation that usually precedes vomiting, although nausea may occur without vomiting. Vomiting is the ejection through the mouth of gastric contents and can occur without the sensation of nausea. Opioids can cause nausea and vomiting in any of the following ways: stimulation of the chemoreceptor trigger zone (CTZ) in the brain, inhibition of gastric motility and decreased gastric emptying time, and stimulation of the vestibular nerve (Hammack & Loprinzi, 1994). As with sedation and respiratory depression, tolerance to nausea and vomiting usually develops early in the treatment of pain with opioids (Paice, 1992). If nausea and vomiting continue, look for other causes such as disease pathology or other medications. Some complications from severe vomiting are dehydration, electrolyte imbalance, aspiration, esophageal tears with hemorrhage (Mallory-Weiss syndrome), and weight loss.

Assessment

The character, frequency, and amount of emesis should be noted. Does movement aggravate the symptom? Does the patient feel bloated? Does the vomiting prevent the patient from eating, drinking, and taking medications? Rule out other causes such as constipation, hypercalcemia (check serum calcium level), presence of infection, liver metastasis (check blood chemistries), increased intracranial pressure (perform a neurological examination), and other medications and treatments such as chemotherapy and radiation therapy (Ajemian, 1993). Perform a hydration assessment.

Interventions

Prophylactic treatment of nausea is usually not routinely recommended because of the sedative effects of antiemetics and because many people do not experience this side effect when taking opioids. If the patient reports a past problem with nausea or vomiting, or if nausea or vomiting

Table 16-2 Selected Antiemetics, Proposed Site of Action, and Administration Forms

Antiemetic	Administration Forms*
CTZ inhibitors	
Prochlorperazine (Compazine)	PO (tablets, sustained-release capsules, liquid), IV, IM, rectal
Thiethylperazine (Torecan)	PO, IM, rectal
Droperidol (Inapsine)	IV, IM
Haloperidol (Haldol)	PO, IM
CTZ inhibitor and promotes gastric emptying	
Metoclopramide (Reglan)	PO, IV
Histamine blocker	
Dimenhydrinate (Dramamine)	PO, IM
Scopolamine (Transderm Scop)	Transdermal patch
Hydroxyzine (Atarax, Vistaril)	PO, IM

**CTZ,* Chemoreceptor trigger zone; *IM,* intramuscular; *IV,* intravenous; *PO,* per os.

occurs following opioid administration, then an antiemetic should be administered prophylactically. Table 16-2 shows the administration forms for several antiemetics. Monitor the patient closely for side effects or adverse effects. For example, if ambulation or sudden movement causes nausea or vomiting, request an antihistamine or anticholinergic drug and, unless this is contraindicated, suggest that the patient avoid ambulating for a time. Metoclopramide is recommended for patients who have delayed gastric emptying secondary to opioid-induced gastroparesis. These patients report feeling full or bloated (Ajemian, 1993).

When nausea and vomiting are severe, antiemetics should be administered parenterally and at regular intervals around the clock. Intravenous fluids should be prescribed to meet the patient's fluid requirements. Generally, unless the nausea and vomiting are due to other causes, these symptoms resolve in a few days. If the nausea and vomiting continue, the analgesic may need to be changed. For example, the postoperative patient taking meperidine who suffers from severe nausea and vomiting may benefit from being switched to another analgesic such as morphine or oxycodone (Twycross, 1994).

Other interventions to enhance the comfort of patients with nausea and vomiting are:

1. Reduce environmental stimuli that may contribute to nausea
2. Provide for privacy when the patient has a vomiting episode
3. Provide oral care after vomiting episodes
4. Involve the patient in decisions about food and fluids
5. Consult a dietitian if appropriate
6. Provide resources for distraction, such as music or relaxation tapes

Patient and Family Education

Reassure patients and families that nausea and vomiting are usually temporary and that there are several methods of treating these symptoms. Provide information when appropriate on managing nausea and vomiting at home. Consult the box on p. 539 for guidance.

Constipation

Constipation is "the passage of hard, dry stools, associated with an undue amount of straining, that may be decreased in frequency from normal and leave the patient with a sensation of incomplete evacuation" (Gross, 1994, p. 518). Constipation is a common, chronic problem for patients who take opioids for persistent pain. Unlike the side effects of opioids discussed earlier, constipation does not resolve with time. When opioid receptors in the GI tract are bound with opioids, the result is a decrease in peristalsis and a reduction in intestinal secretions (Canty, 1994; Paice, 1992). The stool moves slowly through the colon and is more compact or dry when it reaches the rectum. The sensory receptors in the rectum may fail to stimulate defecation, causing the stool to remain in the rectum and become more dehydrated and hard (Gross). Constipation is one of the most serious and unpleasant symptoms patients can experience. Unrelieved constipation can lead to abdominal pain and distension, decreased appetite, nausea,

PATIENT AND FAMILY HOME TEACHING TIPS: NAUSEA AND VOMITING

- Instruct patient that if nausea and vomiting occurs, it usually happens during the initial phase of taking the analgesic and usually resolves in a few days.
- Instruct patient to take the prescribed antiemetic if experiencing nausea and vomiting and to call the physician if nausea and vomiting persists.
- If ambulation aggravates nausea and vomiting, suggest that patient lie quietly in the recumbent position. If nausea and vomiting persists, instruct patient to call the physician for further evaluation. The physician may change the analgesic or add scopolamine, dimenhydrate, or hydroxyzine.
- Advise patient and family that antiemetics may cause increased sedation; therefore the patient should be closely monitored.
- Advise family members to seek immediate medical attention if patient is so sedated that arousal is not possible (see Patient and Family Home Teaching Tips for Sedation).
- If patient is interested, give instruction on various behavioral techniques such as relaxation and distraction.
- Advise patient to remove dentures during vomiting and to sit up to avoid aspiration.
- Suggest that patient perform oral hygiene after vomiting.
- Advise patient and family to note amount and frequency of vomiting to assist the physician or nurse evaluation for dehydration.
- Suggest ways to reduce environmental stimuli such as odors, food preparation, and sights that may contribute to nausea.
- Suggest nausea-reducing foods and fluids based on patient preferences and encourage small, frequent feedings. Peppermint-flavored water or chewing gum may be helpful.
- Review signs and symptoms to report to the physician or nurse.

increased anxiety, intestinal obstruction or pseudoobstruction, intestinal perforation, or the dreaded disimpaction procedure (Ajemian, 1993).

Examples of conditions that can aggravate constipation are intestinal obstruction, ileus, tumors, weakness, poor nutritional intake, dehydration, hemorrhoids, prolapsed rectum, and lack of exercise. Conversely, a number of medical conditions can cause diarrhea; therefore persons who suffer from unrelenting diarrhea and require opioids for an unrelated pain problem may benefit from the constipating effects of the analgesic (Hill, 1993).

Assessment

Obtaining information about the following will enable the nurse to better help the patient with this problem:

1. Normal bowel habits (frequency, consistency, amount, time of day, use of bowel aids)
2. Current bowel habits
3. Diet history, including fluid intake
4. Presence of symptoms related to constipation
5. Presence of medical conditions that contribute to constipation
6. Presence or absence of stool in the rectum
7. Character of bowel sounds
8. Condition of abdomen (soft, hard, distended, painful)
9. Patient's knowledge about managing constipation
10. Patient preference for a bowel program

A child with constipation may be reluctant to report this symptom because of fear of the treatment. In this case, assess for possible objective signs of constipation such as guarding, tenderness on palpation, bowel sounds, anorexia, nausea, or presence of hard stool in diaper or toilet.

Assessment may also be difficult with patients who are confused or very ill. The nurse must rely on the objective signs as previously noted and must perform a rectal examination if indicated. A flat plate x-ray of the abdomen can be another diagnostic tool.

Interventions

Constipation should be treated prophylactically at the start of opioid therapy. Bowel regimen usually includes the following actions:

1. Maintaining a daily fluid intake of at least 2 to 3 liters
2. Adding fiber and bulk-forming agents to diet
3. Avoiding caffeinated beverages
4. Increasing exercise regimen
5. Maintaining a daily schedule for bowel movements
6. Taking a stool softener daily if needed
7. Taking a mild laxative (senna, cascara, bisacodyl, or milk of magnesia) for mild constipation. For severe constipation, a strong laxative (lactulose, citrate of magnesia) is required. Enemas are suggested when stool is lodged in the rectum and the patient is unable to evacuate; however, enemas are contraindicated in patients with thrombocytopenia or neutropenia.

Many patients are not able to follow all of the guidelines listed. For example, concurrent conditions such as anorexia preclude patients from maintaining an optimal intake of fiber and fluids. Patients who cannot increase fluids should not take bulk laxatives (Metamucil, Citrucil) because these carry the risks of obstruction and bolus formation (Ajemian, 1993).

Choosing interventions for children involves careful consideration because most children fear and dislike invasive interventions such as enemas and suppositories. Debilitated older adults often have problems evacuating stool from the rectum because of decreased rectal sensory stimulation and decreased tone of the muscles required for evacuation (Gross, 1994).

Patient and Family Education

Although it is common knowledge among health care professionals that the chronic use of opioids causes constipation, too many patients are uninformed about this symptom (Ajemian, 1993). The nurse is responsible for educating the patient about the risk for this problem and counseling

PATIENT AND FAMILY HOME TEACHING TIPS: CONSTIPATION

- Advise patient and family that, without prevention, constipation will almost certainly occur if the patient takes opioid analgesics for more than a few days.
- Advise patient and family that the best approach to this problem is prevention.
- Ascertain patient's normal bowel pattern and previous experiences with constipation and its management.
- Make a list of foods that facilitate the patient's regular bowel movements.
- Provide a definition of constipation and related symptoms.
- Instruct patient to eat foods high in fiber if possible. Examples are wheat germ, cereals, kidney beans, cooked spinach, sweet potatoes, broccoli, brussels sprouts, and peanuts.
- Instruct patients who take bulk-forming laxatives such as Metamucil that a large amount of water must be taken with the material to prevent fecal impaction or small bowel obstruction.
- Instruct patient to increase fluid intake to 8 glasses of liquid a day.
- Explain to patient that caffeine is dehydrating and will decrease the amount of fluid available in the colon for softening stool. If the patient usually drinks coffee or tea in the morning to promote a bowel movement, suggest that they try decaffeinated coffee or tea.
- Suggest that the patient adhere to a regular routine for bowel movements. For the majority of individuals, bowel movements are most productive after breakfast.
- Encourage patient not to suppress the urge to move the bowels, as this can lead to decreased sensation in the rectum leading to retention and subsequent drying of the stool.
- Suggest using a bedside commode rather than a bedpan if patient is not able to get to a bathroom.

PATIENT AND FAMILY HOME TEACHING TIPS: CONSTIPATION—cont'd

- Encourage provisions for time for and privacy during bowel movements.
- Provide a bowel protocol that includes a stepwise approach to using softeners and laxatives.
- Advise patient that laxatives vary in their effects on individuals and that the patient may have to try several bowel aids before determining which is best.
- Advise against the use of castor oil (bad tasting and too strong) and mineral oil (interferes with absorption of fat-soluble vitamins, calcium, and phosphate, and if aspirated can lead to lipoid pneumonia), unless recommended by physician.
- Advise against the chronic use of enemas unless prescribed by the physician.
- Advise patient that regualr exercise, such as walking, stimulates the gastrointestinal system.
- Advise patient to notify physician or nurse if more than 2 or 3 days pass without a bowel movement.

the patient about the many ways to prevent and treat it. The box on pp. 542 and 543 contains guidelines for patient and family education about constipation.

Mental Changes

Patients undergoing opioid treatment may experience confusion, difficulty concentrating, mental clouding, mood changes (euphoria or dysphoria), or hallucinations. These effects usually occur only in the acute phase of treatment (Paice, 1992). Nonetheless, any of these symptoms—especially hallucinations—can be very disturbing to patients.

Assessment

The nurse should determine the patient's mental status by the patient's subjective reports and by observations of the patient's behavior. The nurse should perform a neurologic assessment and check records for the patient's level of functioning prior to taking opioids.

Interventions and Patient and Family Education

Educate the patient and family about the possibility of these side effects. If mental changes occur, provide for the patient's safety and offer reassurance and reorientation. Depending on the severity and persistence of symptoms, the drug or dose may need to be changed.

Seizures

Opioids can cause seizures, but this usually occurs when the drug dose is higher than that required for analgesia (Ellison, 1993). However, the accumulation of the metabolite normeperidine can cause seizures in patients taking analgesic doses of meperidine for chronic pain (American Pain Society, 1993; McCaffery & Beebe, 1989; Hill, 1993). Meperidine is contraindicated in patients who are currently receiving monoamine oxidase inhibitors or who have recently received them because of the risk of sudden death (American Pain Society; PDR, 1995).

Assessment

The nurse should identify patients at risk for seizures and monitor for signs of CNS hyperactivity such as tremors, twitching, and restlessness.

Interventions and Patient and Family Education

The nurse should consult with the patient's physician if the patient is at risk for seizures. For patients taking meperidine, the nurse should suggest an alternative analgesic. For a patient receiving an opioid other than meperidine, the nurse should monitor the patient closely, and if the patient begins to develop signs of neurologic toxicity (tremors, myoclonus), the nurse should suggest that the physician lower the dose and add a benzodiazepine to help reduce symptoms (Ellison, 1993).

If a patient has an opioid-induced seizure, the nurse should follow the usual procedures in responding to seizure. The patient experiencing normeperidine-induced seizures should not be given naloxone because such seizures result from CNS hyperactivity, which can be aggravated by naloxone. Experts recommend an anticonvulsant or a benzodiazepine, either of which should be continued for several days until the metabolite is excreted (McCaffery & Beebe, 1989).

Myoclonus

Myoclonus (involuntary jerking movements) is a form of central nervous system hyperactivity and may be seen in patients receiving high doses of any opioid, patients with renal or liver failure, and patients receiving meperidine (Baird, McCorkle, & Grant, 1991; Cherny & Portenoy, 1993; Hammack & Loprinzi, 1994). Benzodiazepines, especially clonazepam (Klonopin), will usually reduce this hyperactivity (Ellison, 1993).

Pruritus

Pruritus and flushing are caused by histamine release. Pruritus is seen on the face, palate, and torso, and although it may occur with any of the routes of administration, it is seen mainly in patients receiving intraspinal opioids. The effects of pruritus may be reduced by the administration of an antihistamine. For severe cases of pruritus, small doses of naloxone may relieve the symptom (Ellison, 1993).

Urinary Retention

Urinary retention and urgency may develop due to an opioid's effect on the muscle tone of the bladder. This effect may be seen in older men or in individuals with preexisting urinary problems who are opioid naive. Intermittent catheterization may be necessary for a day or two until tolerance to the opioid develops (Paice, 1992). If the pain is not severe, the physician may stop the opioid and prescribe another type of analgesic.

Allergic Reactions

Patients will frequently report that they are "allergic" to an opioid after having experienced a side effect such as vomiting. True allergies are rare, but when they do happen, urticaria, hives, bronchospasms, or anaphylaxis is seen (Ellison, 1993; Hill, 1993).

MAJOR SIDE EFFECTS OF NONOPIOID ANALGESICS

Nonsteroidal Antiinflammatory Drugs (NSAIDs)

Gastrointestinal and Hematologic Effects

When tissues are injured, the enzyme cyclooxygenase breaks down arachidonic acid, releasing several chemicals including prostaglandins, which cause inflammation and pain. Nonsteroidal antiinflammatory drugs (NSAIDs) inhibit cyclooxygenase, thus blocking the formation of prostaglandins and decreasing pain. Prostaglandins also play a role in maintaining the mucus lining of the stomach. Unfortunately, rather than limiting their action to the pain-producing prostaglandins, NSAIDs reduce the production of the helpful gastric prostaglandins as well (Stambaugh, 1993). Consequently, there is an increase in gastric acid secretion and a reduction in the protective gastric mucin production, potentially resulting in gastrointestinal distress. Prostaglandins are also important in the production of thromboxane, the chemical that helps platelets clump together to stop bleeding. Gastrointestinal bleeding may occur through a combination of these effects. Choline magnesium trisalicylate (Trilisate) and nabumetone (Relafen) reportedly have little effect on platelet aggregation compared with other NSAIDs (Stambaugh; Hilleman, Mohiuddin, & Lucas, 1993). Efforts to reduce the GI effects by administering H_2-receptor antagonists, antacids, and misoprostol (Cytotec) have met with varying success (Stambaugh).

Other System Effects

Central nervous system effects associated with some NSAIDs are headache, depression, and subtle cognitive impairment (Stambaugh, 1993). Other reported side effects are tinnitus, fluid retention, decreased growth of new bone, bone marrow suppression, allergic reactions, and renal and hepatic toxicity (McCaffery & Beebe, 1989; McEvoy, 1994; Paice, 1992).

Drug Interactions

Multiple drug interactions have been associated with NSAIDs, either causing serious drug reactions or rendering the NSAID a less effective analgesic. (See Chapter 4 for additional information.)

Assessment

Nursing assessment of patients taking NSAIDs should include subjective and objective data on all body systems. It is vital to evaluate concurrent medical problems and identify all medications the patient is taking. Inform patients that ingestion of alcohol with NSAIDs is contraindicated due to the risk of increased GI toxicity (Price & Fletcher, 1990). Misoprostol is contraindicated in pregnancy due to risk of miscarriage (PDR, 1995).

Interventions

Notify the patient's physician if new or potential problems are identified during the assessment. If cost is an issue for the patient, suggest that the physician prescribe a less expensive yet potentially equally effective NSAID such as ibuprofen. NSAIDs are available in a variety of dose forms; therefore if the patient is having problems with one route, suggest that the physician evaluate the patient and recommend another route of administration (McCaffery & Beebe, 1989).

Patient and Family Education

Provide patients with information about their prescribed NSAIDs and instruct them to report any side effects to their nurses or physicians. To prevent drug interactions, instruct patients to inform their primary physicians when other physicians prescribe new drugs.

Aspirin

Common side effects of aspirin are gastrointestinal disturbances and decreased platelet aggregation. One of aspirin's important applications is related to this platelet side effect, as evidenced by the number of people taking aspirin in hopes of preventing heart attack and stroke. A normal dose of aspirin will cause an irreversible effect on the platelets and double the mean bleeding time of normal persons for 4 to 7 days (McCaffery & Beebe, 1989). Other adverse effects are tinnitus, hypersensitivity, and Reye's syndrome (primarily in pediatric patients) (American Pain Society, 1993).

Assessment

People taking aspirin as a normal part of their daily routine may fail to inform their physicians or nurses of this fact when surgery or invasive procedures are planned. Consequently, nurses must specifically ask patients whether they are currently taking aspirin or have taken aspirin in the last week. Failure to discover this information could lead to bleeding complications during or after a procedure. Additional subjective data the nurse should collect include the existence of side effects to aspirin and the patient's method of treating them.

Interventions and Patient and Family Education

Advise patients to inform their physicians before invasive procedures that they are taking aspirin. Generally, aspirin should be stopped at least 10 days before an invasive procedure (Paice, 1992). For symptoms of mild gastric distress, suggest that the patient take the drug with food or switch to enteric-coated aspirin (Paice).

Acetaminophen

Acetaminophen is the best tolerated of the nonopioid analgesics and is therefore contained in many over-the-counter medications. Patients may not be aware that they could be taking potentially toxic doses of this drug. Experts recommend that the total daily dose of acetaminophen not exceed 4000 mg (McCaffery & Beebe, 1989; USP DI, 1995). The major toxic effect is on the liver; therefore this drug is contraindicated in patients with liver disease because even therapeutic doses are known to cause liver failure (American Pain Society, 1993).

Assessment

In addition to the basic components of a nursing assessment, the nurse should question patients about all medications they are taking, including over-the-counter medications. Monitor blood chemistry and check for jaundice.

Interventions and Patient and Family Education

Provide information about the prevalence of acetaminophen in over-the-counter drugs and instruct the patient and family not to exceed the total recommended daily dose.

SIDE EFFECTS OF ADJUVANT MEDICATIONS

Tricyclic Antidepressants

Amitriptyline (Elavil) is the most frequently prescribed adjuvant drug of the tricyclic antidepressants, yet it is associated with more anticholinergic effects and sedation than several other tricyclics, including doxepin, desipramine, and nortriptyline (American Pain Society, 1993; Richlin, 1991; Twycross, 1988). Amitriptyline may be toxic for older and debilitated patients (Twycross). The common use of amitriptyline as an adjuvant for neuropathic pain is probably attributable to its frequent citation in the literature. Moreover, many physicians are more familiar with amitriptyline than with the other tricyclics.

Assessment

The nurse should assess the patient for dry mouth, sedation, orthostatic hypotension, blurred vision, urinary retention, and the cardiac effects of palpations, extrasystole, and dysrhythmia. A sleep assessment is essential.

Interventions and Patient and Family Education

Educate patients and families about the side effects of the drug. Encourage patients to report intolerable side effects. For dry mouth, suggest that the patient keep a small bottle of water readily available, suck on sugarless candy, chew sugarless gum, or try artificial saliva. For patients taking amitriptyline who report excessive daytime drowsiness, question the time of drug administration. Clinicians recommend that amitriptyline be taken at bedtime to reduce daytime drowsiness. These patients should be cautioned about nocturnal orthostatic hypotension. If drowsiness persists, suggest a physician consultation. For patients taking desipramine or nortriptyline who develop insomnia, suggest that they take the medication during the day (American Pain Society, 1993).

Anticonvulsants

Carbamazepine (Tegretol), clonazepam (Klonopin), phenytoin (Dilantin), and sodium valproate (Depakene) are anticonvulsants. Baclofen (Lioresal), a muscle relaxant, may relieve lancinating pain arising from peripheral nerve syndromes or nerve injury (American Pain Society, 1993). Because carbamazepine is the most effective and is prescribed most frequently, the discussion will be limited to the side effects of this drug only (Payne, 1989). Common side effects of carbamazepine are bone marrow depression, dizziness, epigastric pain, diplopia, nausea, and drowsiness (Bruera & Ripamonti, 1993; Payne).

Assessment

The nurse should question the patient about the presence of side effects and observe for obvious effects. Monitor complete blood cell and platelet counts.

Interventions and Patient and Family Education

Educate the patient and family about the side effects of the drug. Encourage the patient to report intolerable side effects. A patient who develops a rash must stop the drug immediately and notify the physician. Exfoliative dermatitis and the Stevens-Johnson syndrome have been reported in patients taking carbamazepine and phenytoin (Payne, 1989).

Corticosteroids

For many patients experiencing pain, two side effects of corticosteroids that are pleasant are elevated mood and increased appetite. Some unpleasant effects are immunosuppression, affective disorders (ranging from mild mood changes to severe psychosis), Cushing's syndrome, GI bleeding, myopathy, osteoporosis, cataracts, moon face, headache, and facial flushing (Bruera & Ripamonti, 1993). Some clinicians have reported that administering intravenous dexamethasone too rapidly can cause severe perineal burning and itching.

Assessment

The nurse should question the patient about side effects and perform cephalocaudal assessment, carefully checking for any signs of infection. Pay special attention to the oral and vaginal areas, venous access sites, wounds, and incisions. Monitor for signs of GI bleeding. Assess the patient's mood.

Intervention and Patient and Family Education

Educate the patient and family about the side effects of the drug. Encourage the patient to report intolerable side effects.

SUMMARY

The nurse prevents, monitors, and treats the side effects of analgesics. The nurse's additional role as patient and family educator and advocate is equally important. Nurses must encourage patients and families to report side effects and request relief for them. The effective nurse will know the patient's health situation and the relevant psychosocial issues influencing the patient's symptoms. Also, the nurse must use problem-solving techniques to treat symptoms effectively and, most importantly, must collaborate with colleagues from other disciplines as the patient's needs demand.

References

Ajemian, I. C. (1993). Treatment of related symptoms. In R. B. Patt (Ed.), *Cancer pain* (pp. 197-208) Philadelphia: Lippincott.

American Pain Society (1993). *Principles of analgesic use in the treatment of acute pain and cancer pain.* Skokie, IL: American Pain Society.

Baird, S. B., McCorkle, R., & Grant, M. (1991). *Cancer nursing.* Philadelphia: Saunders.

Bates, B. (1991). *Physical examination and history taking.* Philadelphia: Lippincott.

Bruera, E., & Ripamonti, C. (1993). Adjuvants to opioid analgesics. In R. B. Patt (Ed.), *Cancer pain* (pp. 143-159). Philadelphia: Lippincott.

Canty, S. L. (1994). Constipation as a side effect of opioids. *Oncology Nursing Forum, 21*(4), 739-745.

Carr, D. B., Jacox, A., Chapman, C. R., Ferrell, B., Fields, H. L., Heidrich, G., Hester, N. K., Hill, C. S., Lipman A. G., McGarvey, C. L., Miaskowski, C., Mulder, D., Payne, R., Schechter, N., Shapiro, B. S., Smith, R. S., Tsou, C. V., Vecchiarelli, L. (1992). *Acute pain management: Operative or medical procedures and trauma. Clinical practice guideline.* AHCPR Pub. No. 92-0032. Rockville, MD: Agency for Health Care Policy and Research, PHS, USDHHS.

Cherny, N. I., & Portenoy, R. K. (1993). Cancer pain management. *Cancer, 72*, 3393-3415.

Collins, P. M. (1994). Comfort-pain. In J. Gross & B. L. Johnson (Eds.), *Handbook of oncology nursing* (pp. 285-309). Boston: Jones and Bartlett.

Coyle, N. (1989). Role of the nurse in pain management. In K. M. Foley & R. M. Payne (Eds.), *Current therapy of pain* (pp. 63-69). Toronto: Decker.

Ellison, N. M. (1993). Opioid analgesics for cancer pain: Toxicities and their treatments. In R. B. Patt (Ed.), *Cancer pain* (pp. 185-194). Philadelphia: Lippincott.

Ferrell, B. R., & Ferrell, B. (1992). Pain in the elderly. In J. H. Watt-Watson & M. I. Donovan (Eds.), *Pain management—Nursing perspective* (pp. 349-369). St. Louis: Mosby.

Gross, J. (1994). Functional alterations: Bowel. In J. Gross & B. L. Johnson (Eds.), *Handbook of oncology nursing* (pp. 517-528). Boston: Jones and Bartlett.

Hammack, J. E. & Loprinzi C. L. (1994). Use of orally administered opioids for cancer-related pain. *Mayo Clinic Proceedings, 69,* 384-390.

Hill, C. S. (1993). Oral opioid analgesics. In R. B. Patt (Ed.), *Cancer pain* (pp. 129-142). Philadelphia: Lippincott.

Hilleman, D. E., Mohiuddin, S. M., & Lucas, B. D. (1993). Nonsteroidal anti-inflammatory drug use in patients receiving warfarin: Emphasis on nabmetone. *American Journal of Medicine, 95*(suppl. 2A), 30-34.

Jacox, A., Carr, D. B., Payne, R., Berde, C. B., Breitbart, W., Cain, J. M., Chapman, C. R., Cleeland, C. S., Ferrell, B. R., Finley, R. S., Hester, N. O., Hill, C. S., Leak, W. D., Lipman, A. G., Logan, C. L., McGarvey, C. L., Miaskowski, C. A., Mulder, D. S., Paice, J. A., Shapiro, B. S., Silberstein, E. B., Smith, R. S., Stover, J., Tsou, C. V., Vecchiarelli, L., & Weissman, D. E. (1994). *Management of cancer pain: Clinical practice guideline.* AHCPR Pub. No. 94-0592. Rockville, MD: Agency for Health Care Policy and Research, PHS, USDHHS.

Lindley, C. M., Dalton, J. A., & Fields, S. M. (1990). Narcotic analgesics. *Cancer Nursing, 13,* 28-38.

McCaffery, M., & Beebe, A. (1989). *Pain: Clinical manual for nursing practice.* St. Louis: Mosby.

McEvoy, G. K. (Ed.). (1994). *AHFS drug information.* Bethesda, MD: American Society of Hospital Pharmacists.

Paice, J. A. (1992). Pharmacological management. In J. H. Watt-Watson & M. I. Donovan (Eds.), *Pain management—Nursing perspective* (pp. 124-161). St. Louis: Mosby.

Pasero, C. L., & McCaffery, M. (1994). Avoiding opioid-induced respiratory depression. *American Journal of Nursing, 94*(4), 25-30.

Payne, R. M. (1989). Pain in peripheral neuropathy. In K. M. Foley & R. M. Payne (Eds.), *Current therapy of pain* (pp. 235-244). Toronto: Decker.

PDR (1995). *Physicians' desk reference* (49th ed.). Montvale, NJ: Medical Economics.

Portenoy, R. K., Thaler, H. T., Inturrisi, C. E., Klar, H. F., & Foley, K. M. (1992). The metabolite morphine-6-glucuronide contributes to the analgesia produced by morphine infusion in patients with pain and normal renal function. *Clinical Pharmacology and Therapeutics, 51*(4), 422–431.

Price, A. H., & Fletcher, M. (1990). Mechanisms of NSAID-induced gastroenteropathy. *Drugs, 40*(suppl. 5), 1–11.

Richlin, D. M. (1991). Nonnarcotic analgesics and tricyclic antidepressants for the treatment of chronic nonmalignant pain. *Mount Sinai Journal of Medicine, 53*(3), 221-228.

Schechter, N. L., & Weisman, S. J. (1993). The management of pain in childhood cancer. In R. B. Patt (Ed.), *Cancer pain* (pp. 509-526). Philadelphia: Lippincott.

Stambaugh, J. E. (1993). Role of nonsteroidal anti-inflammatory drugs in the management of cancer pain. In R. B. Patt (Ed.), *Cancer pain* (pp. 105-117). Philadelphia: Lippincott.

Thomas, B. L. (1991). Pain management for the elderly: Alternative interventions (part II). *Journal of the Association of Operating Room Nurses, 53*(1), 126–132.

Thomas, C. L. (Ed.). (1993). *Taber's cyclopedic medical dictionary.* Philadelphia: Davis.

Twycross, R. G. (1988). The management of pain in cancer: A guide to drugs and dosages. *Oncology, 2*(4), 35-42.

Twycross, R. (1994). *Pain relief in advanced cancer.* Edinburgh: Churchill Livingstone.

USP DI (1995). *Drug information for the health care professional.* (Vol. 1, 15th ed.). Rockville, MD: U.S. Pharmacopeial Convention.

Waldman, S. D., Leak, D. W., Kennedy, L. D., & Patt, R. B. (1993). Intraspinal opioid therapy. In R. B. Patt (Ed.), *Cancer pain* (pp. 285-328). Philadelphia: Lippincott.

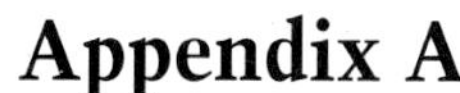

Appendix A

Trade Name List

Trade Name	Generic Name
Acephen	Acetaminophen
Aceta	Acetaminophen
Acetaminophen Elixir	Acetaminophen
Acetaminophen Uniserts	Acetaminophen
Advil	Ibuprofen
Alka-Seltzer	Aspirin with buffers
Aleve	Naproxen sodium
Amoxapine	Amoxapine
Anacin	Aspirin with caffeine
Anacin-3	Acetaminophen
Anaprox	Naproxen sodium
Anexsia	Hydrocodone bitartrate and acetaminophen
Anodynos-DHC	Hydrocodone bitartrate and acetaminophen
Antrocol	Atropine sulfate and phenobarbital
Argesic	Salsalate
Arthra-G	Salsalate
Arthropan	Choline salicylate
Ascriptin	Aspirin with buffers
Ascriptin A/D	Aspirin with buffers
Asendin	Amoxapine
Aspergum	Aspirin
Aspirin Uniserts	Aspirin
Astramorph	Morphine sulfate (preservative free)

Continued.

Trade Name	Generic Name
Atarax	Hydroxyzine HCl
Ativan	Lorazepam
Aventyl	Nortriptyline HCl
Azdone	Hydrocodone bitartrate and aspirin
Azolid	Phenylbutazone
Azotal	Aspirin with butalbital
Bayer's Children's Aspirin	Aspirin
Buffaprin	Aspirin with buffers
Buffered Aspirin	Aspirin with buffers
Bufferin	Aspirin with buffers
Buffex	Aspirin with buffers
Buffinol	Aspirin with buffers
Buprenex	Buprenorphine HCl
Butazolidin	Phenylbutazone
Capital and Codeine	Codeine phosphate and acetaminophen
Carbamazepine	Carbamazepine
Catapres	Clonidine HCl
Catapres TTS	Clonidine HCl—transdermal therapeutic system
Children's Aspirin	Aspirin
Clinoril	Sulindac
Cocaine	Cocaine HCl
Codeine Phosphate	Codeine phosphate
Codeine Sulfate	Codeine sulfate
Codoxy	Oxycodone HCl and aspirin
Co-Gesic	Hydrocodone bitartrate and acetaminophen
Colace	Docusate sodium
Colace Liquid	Docusate sodium
Compazine	Prochlorperazine
Correctol	Docusate sodium and phenolphthalein
Cortan	Prednisone
Cytotec	Misoprostol
Dalalone Decaject	Dexamethasone sodium phosphate
Dalalone D.P.	Dexamethasone acetate
Dalalone L.A.	Dexamethasone acetate
Damason-P	Hydrocodone bitartrate and aspirin
Dapa	Acetaminophen
Darvon	Aspirin with propoxyphene napsylate
Darvon Compound	Propoxyphene HCl, aspirin, and caffeine
Darvon-N	Propoxyphene napsylate
DC 240	Docusate calcium

Trade Name	Generic Name
Decadrol	Dexamethasone sodium phosphate
Decadron	Dexamethasone
Decadron-L.A.	Dexamethasone acetate
Decadron Phosphate	Dexamethasone sodium phosphate
Decadron Phosphate with Xylocaine	Dexamethasone sodium phosphate and lidocaine HCl
Dekasol	Dexamethasone sodium phosphate
Dekasol-L.A.	Dexamethasone acetate
Deltasone	Prednisone
Demerol	Meperidine HCl
Dexacene-4	Dexamethasone sodium phosphate
Dexamethasone	Dexamethasone
Dexamethasone Sodium Phosphate	Dexamethasone sodium phosphate
Dexamethasone Intensol	Dexamethasone
Dexasone	Dexamethasone sodium phosphate
Dexone	Dexamethasone
Dexone L.A.	Dexamethasone acetate
Dialose	Docusate potassium
Dialose Plus	Docusate potassium and casanthranol
Diazepam Solution	Diazepam
Dilantin	Phenytoin sodium
Dilantin Kapseals	Phenytoin sodium extended
Dilaudid	Hydromorphone HCl
Dilaudid HP	Hydromorphone HCl (high potency)
Dilocaine	Lidocaine HCl
Dioctocal	Docusate calcium
Diocto-K	Docusate potassium
Diocto-K Plus	Docusate potassium and casanthranol
Diocto Liquid	Docusate sodium
Dioctolose Plus	Docusate potassium and casanthranol
Dioeze	Docusate sodium
Dionex	Docusate sodium
Diosuccin	Docusate sodium
Diphenylan Sodium	Phenytoin sodium prompt
Disalcid	Salsalate
Disanthrol	Docusate sodium and casanthranol
Disolan	Docusate sodium and phenolphthalein
Disolan Forte	Docusate sodium and carboxymethylcellulose sodium and casanthranol
Disonate	Docusate sodium
Disonate Liquid	Docusate sodium

Continued.

Trade Name	Generic Name
Disoplex	Docusate sodium and carboxymethylcellulose
Di-Sosul	Docusate sodium
Docusate Potassium	Docusate potassium
Docusate Potassium with Casanthranol	Docusate potassium and casanthranol docusate sodium
Dolacet	Hydrocodone bitartrate and acetaminophen
Dolobid	Diflunisal
Dolophine	Methadone HCl
DOS	Docusate sodium
Doxidan Liquigel	Docusate calcium and phenolphthalein
Doxinate	Docusate sodium
Doxinate Solution	Docusate sodium
D-S-Duosol	Docusate sodium
DSMC	Docusate potassium
DSMC Plus	Docusate potassium and casanthranol
D-S-S Plus	Docusate sodium and casanthranol
DuoCet	Hydrocodone bitartrate and acetaminophen
Duradyne DHC	Hydrocodone bitartrate and acetaminophen
Duragesic	Fentanyl citrate (topical transdermal system)
Duramorph	Morphine sulfate (preservative free)
E-Lor	Propoxyphene HCl and acetaminophen
Elavil	Amitriptyline HCl
EMLA	Lidocaine and prilocaine
Endep	Amitriptyline HCl
Enovil	Amitriptyline HCl
Epitol	Carbamazepine
Etrafon	Amitriptyline HCl and perphenazine
Etrafon-A	Amitriptyline HCl and perphenazine
Etrafon-Forte	Amitriptyline HCl and perphenazine
Excedrin P.M.	Acetaminophen and diphenhydramine citrate
Ex-Lax Extra Gentle	Docusate sodium and phenolphthalein
Feen-A-Mint	Docusate sodium and phenolphthalein
Feldene	Piroxicam
Gemnisyn	Acetaminophen with aspirin
Genagesic	Acetaminophen and propoxyphene HCl
Genapap	Acetaminophen
Genapap Children's	Acetaminophen
Genebs	Acetaminophen
Genpril	Ibuprofen
Gentlax S	Docusate sodium and senna concentrate
Haldol	Haloperidol lactate

Trade Name	Generic Name
Haldol Decanoate	Haloperidol decanoate
Halenol	Acetaminophen
Haloperidol	Haloperidol lactate
Hexadrol	Dexamethasone
Hexadrol Phosphate	Dexamethasone sodium phosphate
Hydrocet	Hydrocodone bitartrate and acetaminophen
Hy-Pam	Hydroxyzine pamoate
Hy-Phen	Hydrocodone bitartrate and acetaminophen
Hyzine	Hydroxyzine HCl
Ibuprin	Ibuprofen
Indocin	Indomethacin
Indocin SR	Indomethacin (slow release)
Infumorph	Morphine sulfate (preservative free)
Janimine	Imipramine HCl
Kasof	Docusate potassium
Levo-Dromoran	Levorphanol
Lidocaine	Lidocaine HCl
Lidoject	Lidocaine HCl
Limbitrol	Amitriptyline HCl and chlordiazepoxide
Lioresal	Baclofen
Lodine	Etodolac
Lorazepam Intensol	Lorazepam
Lorcet	Hydrocodone bitartrate and acetaminophen
Lortab	Hydrocodone bitartrate and acetaminophen
Lortab ASA	Hydrocodone bitartrate and aspirin
Magnaprin	Aspirin with buffers
Marcaine	Bupivacaine HCl
Meclomen	Meclofenamate sodium
Medipren	Ibuprofen
Menadol	Ibuprofen
Mepergan	Promethazine HCl and meperidine HCl
Mepro-Analgesic	Aspirin with meprobamate
Meticorten	Prednisone
Mexitil	Mexiletine HCl
Modane Plus	Docusate sodium and phenolphthalein
Modane Soft	Docusate sodium
Morphine Sulfate	Morphine sulfate
Motrin	Ibuprofen
MS Contin	Morphine sulfate (slow release)
MSIR	Morphine sulfate
Nalfon	Fenoprofen
Naprosyn	Naproxen
Neopap Supprettes	Acetaminophen

Continued.

Trade Name	Generic Name
Nervocaine	Lidocaine HCl
Nesacaine	Chloroprocaine HCl
Nesacaine-MPF	Chloroprocaine HCl
Neucalm	Hydroxyzine HCl
Norcet	Hydrocodone bitartrate and acetaminophen
Novocain	Procaine HCl
Nubain	Nalbuphine HCl
Numorphan	Oxymorphone HCl
Nuprin	Ibuprofen
Oramorph SR	Morphine sulfate (slow release)
Orasone	Prednisone
Orudis	Ketoprofen
Oruvail	Ketoprofen
Oxycet	Oxycodone HCl and acetaminophen
Pamelor	Nortriptyline HCl
Panadol	Acetaminophen
Panadol Children's	Acetaminophen
Panasol	Prednisone
Paxil	Paroxetine HCl
Pepcid	Famotidine
Percocet	Oxycodone HCl and acetaminophen
Percodan	Oxycodone HCl and aspirin
Percodan-Demi	Oxycodone HCl and aspirin
Perestan	Docusate potassium and casanthranol
Peri-Colace	Docusate sodium and casanthranol
Peri-DOS	Docusate sodium and casanthranol
Permitil	Fluphenazine HCl
Pertofrane	Desipramine HCl
Phenaphen	Acetaminophen
Phenaphen with Codeine	Codeine phosphate and acetaminophen
Phenazine 25	Promethazine HCl
Phencen	Promethazine HCl
Phenergan	Promethazine HCl
Phenergan VC	Promethazine HCl and phenylephrine HCl
Phenoject	Promethazine HCl
Phenytoin Sodium	Phenytoin sodium
Pherazine	Promethazine HCl
Phillips LaxCaps	Docusate sodium and phenolphthalein sodium
Polocaine	Mepivacaine HCl
Ponstel	Mefenamic acid
Pontocaine	Tetracaine HCl

Trade Name	Generic Name
Prednicen-M	Prednisone
Prednisone	Prednisone
Primatene Mist	Epinephrine
Pro-Cal-Sof	Docusate calcium
Prolixin	Fluphenazine HCl
Prolixin Decanoate	Fluphenazine decanoate
Prolixin Enanthate	Fluphenazine enanthate
Promethazine Hydrochloride	Promethazine HCl
Promethegan	Promethazine HCl
Prorex	Promethazine HCl
Prozac	Fluoxetine HCl
Quiess	Hydroxyzine HCl
Reglan	Metoclopramide HCl
Regutol	Docusate sodium
RMS	Morphine sulfate
Robaxin	Methocarbamol
Robaxisal	Methocarbamol and aspirin
Roxanol	Morphine sulfate
Roxanol SR	Morphine sulfate (slow release)
Roxicodone	Oxycodone HCl
Roxicet	Oxycodone HCl and acetaminophen
Roxilox	Oxycodone HCl and acetaminophen
Roxiprin	Oxycodone HCl and aspirin
Senokot S	Docusate sodium and senna concentrate
Sensorcaine	Bupivacaine HCl
Sereen	Chlordiazepoxide HCl
Sinequan	Doxepin HCl
Solurex L.A.	Dexamethasone acetate
Stadol	Butorphanol
Sublimaze	Fentanyl citrate
Sufenta	Sufentanil citrate
Suppap	Acetaminophen
Surfak	Docusate calcium
Surmontil	Trimipramine HCl
Tagamet	Cimetidine HCl
Talacen Caplets	Pentazocine HCl with acetaminophen
Talwin Nx Caplets	Pentazocine HCl and naloxone HCl
Talwin	Pentazocine lactate
Talwin Compound Caplets	Pentazocine HCl with aspirin
Tegretol	Carbamazepine
Therevac Plus Enema	Docusate sodium and benzocaine
Therevac S.B. Enema	Docusate sodium

Continued.

Trade Name	Generic Name
Tofranil	Imipramine HCl
Tofranil-PM	Imipramine pamoate
Tolectin	Tolmetin sodium
Toradol	Ketorolac tromethamine
Trexan	Naltrexone HCl
Triavil	Perphenazine and amitriptyline HCl
Tri-buffered Bufferin	Aspirin with buffer
Trilafon	Perphenazine
Trilax	Docusate sodium and dehydrocholic acid and phenolphthalein
Trisilate	Choline salicylate with magnesium salicylate
Tylenol	Acetaminophen
Tylenol with Codeine	Acetaminophen and codeine phosphate
Tylenol Children's	Acetaminophen
Tylox	Acetaminophen and oxycodone HCl
Uni Ace	Acetaminophen
Valium	Diazepam
Valrelease	Diazepam
Versed	Midazolam hydrochloride
Vicodin	Hydrocodone bitartrate and acetaminophen
Vidocin ES	Hydrocodone bitartrate and acetaminophen
Vistacon	Hydroxyzine HCl
Vistaject	Hydroxyzine HCl
Vistaril	Hydroxyzine HCl
Vistaril	Hydroxyzine pamoate
Vistazine	Hydroxyzine HCl
Vivactil	Protriptyline HCl
V-Gan	Promethazine HCl
Voltaren	Diclofenac sodium
Wygesic	Propoxyphene HCl and acetaminophen
Xanax	Alprazolam
Xylocaine	Lidocaine HCl
Zantac	Ranitidine
Zetran	Diazepam
Zostrix	Capsaicin
Zostrix HP	Capsaicin
Zovirax	Acyclovir
Zydone	Hydrocodone bitartrate and acetaminophen

Modified from Omoigui, S. (1995). *The pain drugs handbook.* St. Louis: Mosby.

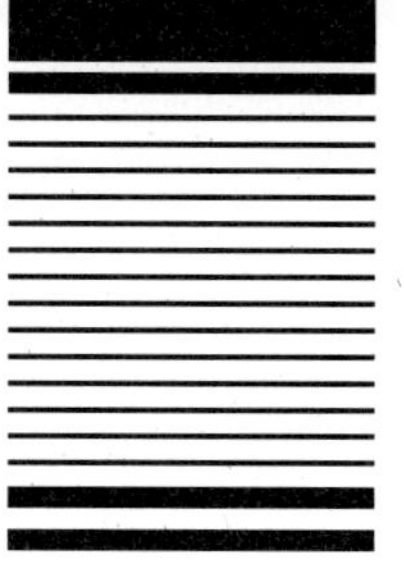

Appendix B

Glossary

Allodynia: Strange or abnormal sensation.

Analgesia: Loss of sensitivity to pain.

Dysethesias: Condition in which a disagreeable sensation is produced by ordinary stimuli.

Equianalgesic: The dose and route of administration of one drug that produces approximately the same degree of analgesia as the dosage and route of administration of another drug.

Hypalgesia: Diminished sensitivity to painful stimuli.

Hyperalgesia: Extreme sensitivity to mildly painful stimuli.

Hypesthesia: Diminished sensitivity to normal stimuli.

Neuropathic (deafferentation) pain: Pain that is the result of peripheral nerve injury and not stimulation.

Nociceptive pain: Pain that is the result of the stimulation of intact afferent nerve endings.

NSAIDs: Abbreviation for *nonsteroidal antiinflammatory drugs.* Such drugs have antiinflammatory and analgesic properties.

Opioid: A natural (opiate) or synthetic product that has morphinelike effects.

Opioid agonist-antagonist: A drug that acts as an agonist at one type of opioid receptor and as an antagonist at another receptor.

Psychotropic: Exerting an effect on the mind or modifying mental activity.

Selective tolerance: Tolerance to some of the effects of a drug with no interference with its analgesic effect.

Somatic pain: Pain that arises from the skeletal muscles, facies, ligaments, vessels, or joints.

Step system approach: A three-step approach to pain management using nonopioid analgesics initially and progressing to stronger analgesics in the second and third steps.

Visceral pain: Pain that has its origins in the smooth musculature or organ systems.

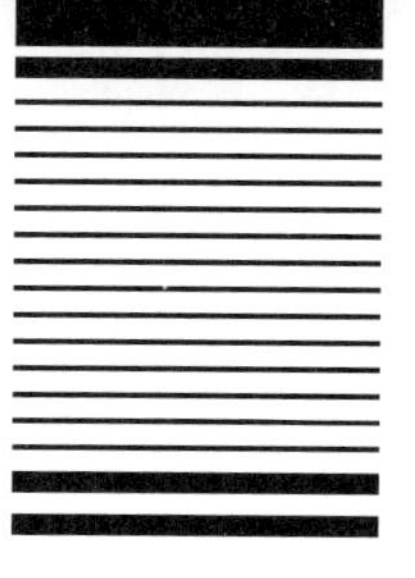

Appendix C

Adverse Central Nervous System Reaction to Drugs Used in Pain Control

Marguerite Geer-Pyron

Adverse Central Nervous System Reactions to Drugs Used in Pain Control

Adverse Reactions	Drugs
Euphoria or dysphoria, headache, agitation, tremor, disorientation, delirium, uncoordinated movements, transient hallucinations	Opioid analgesics
More common at high doses or prolonged use: headache, dizziness, confusion Severe intoxication may cause delirium and hallucination	Salicylates
More common with chronic use of high doses: CNS stimulation, psychologic changes Severe intoxication may cause excitement, delirium, toxic depression, toxic psychosis followed by CNS depression	Acetominophen
Headache, fatigue, drowsiness, depression, nervousness, anxiety, confusion, insomnia, muscle weakness, syncope, involuntary movements, psychic disturbances, convulsions, peripheral neuropathy, depersonalization	NSAIDs
Dizziness	Gold compounds
Overdose may cause muscle weakness, delirium, and convulsions	Antigout drugs
Sedation, anxiety, restlessness, agitation, irritability, insomnia, nightmares, disorientation, confusion, delusions, hallucinations	Tricyclic antidepressants
Confusion, slurred speech, dizziness, insomnia, nervousness, fatigue, irritability, headache, depression, behavioral disturbance	Anticonvulsants
Drowsiness, fatigue, dizziness, ataxia, headache, blurred vision, insomnia, confusion, irritability	Muscle relaxants
Vertigo, headache, syncope, personality changes, irritability, insomnia, convulsions, catatonia	Corticosteroids
Nervousness, insomnia, dizziness, drowsiness, headache, agitation, toxic psychoses	Stimulants
Headache, insomnia, drowsiness, dizziness, confusion or excitation in elderly patients, nervousness, weakness	Antispasmodics

From Malseed, R. T., Goldstein, F. J., & Balkon, N. (1995). *Pharmacology, drug therapy, and nursing considerations.* Philadelphia: Lippincott; *Nursing 94 drug handbook.* (1994). Springhouse, PA: Springhouse Corp.

* *CNS,* Central nervous system; *NSAIDs,* nonsteroidal antiinflammatory drugs.

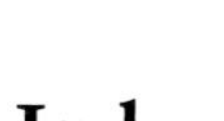

Index

Page numbers followed by n *indicate notes.*

Q

R

S